CT・MRI画像解剖ポケットアトラス 3

第4版

脊椎・四肢・関節

監訳 町田 徹 山王病院放射線科部長
　　　　　　　 国際医療福祉大学臨床医学研究センター教授
訳　 小林有香 東京共済病院放射線科部長

Torsten B. Moeller, M.D.
Department of Radiology
Marienhaus Klinikum
Saarlouis/Dillingen, Germany

Emil Reif, M.D.
Department of Teleradiology
reif & moeller diagnostic-network
Dillingen, Germany

Pocket Atlas of Sectional Anatomy
Computed Tomography and Magnetic Resonance Imaging
Volume 3: Spine, Extremities, Joints
2nd edition

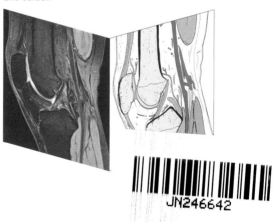

メディカル・サイエンス・インターナショナル

米国のわが親類たち Bernie & Arlene, Bryan & Nancy, Rick, Krista & Ella Rose, Bill, Kayla, Abby & Liviana, Shirley, Mike, Austin & Amanda, Michael & Kendall, Audrey, Mike & Kristen, Katelyn & Matt, Claudia & Larry, Bryan & Stacy, Jamie & Shawn, Meghan & Jason に捧げる.

Authorized translation of the original English edition,
"Pocket Atlas of Sectional Anatomy; Computed Tomography and
Magnetic Resonance Imaging, Volume 3: Spine, Extremities, Joints",
Second Edition
by Torsten B. Moeller and Emil Reif

Copyright © 2017 by Georg Thieme Verlag KG, Stuttgart, Germany
All rights reserved.

©Fourth Japanese Edition 2018 by Medical Sciences International, Ltd.,
Tokyo

Printed and Bound in Japan

監訳者序文

　本書は『CT・MRI 画像解剖ポケットアトラス』第 3 巻の改訂版である．内容は旧版と同じで，「脊椎・四肢・関節」である．旧版との違いは，著者らも述べているように，関節近傍の部位に焦点を当て，上腕・前腕・大腿・下腿全体の二方向画像とイラストを第 3 版の画像に新たに加えたことにある．そのため，さらにボリュームを増し，480 ページに及ぶアトラスとなり，小さいポケットに入りきらないくらい充実した内容になった．読影端末や机の上に置いて，適宜参照していただければと思う．

　本シリーズの特徴は何といっても，断層画像とそれに対比するイラストにある．イラストは臓器別に色分けされ，複雑な解剖をわかりやすく表示している．このため読者は複雑な解剖構造を容易にかつ正確に認識することができるであろう．各スライスには撮像レベルを示す小さなシェーマがついており，実際の画像との対比が容易となるように工夫されている．一枚のイラストには多数の引出線がついており，やや煩雑なきらいはあるが，それぞれ重要な構造物であるので，じっくりと画像と見比べていただきたい．

　本書には単純撮影と CT が掲載されていないので，骨病変の診断などに若干不便を感じるかもしれないが，適宜姉妹編『X 線画像解剖ポケットアトラス』や成書を参照すれば解剖学的知識の整理・習得に一層役立つであろう．

　本書の作成に尽力された東京共済病院放射線科部長 小林 有香先生，株式会社メディカル・サイエンス・インターナショナル代表取締役社長 金子浩平氏，出版部 藤堂 保行氏，菅野 明氏に深謝する．

　2018 年 2 月　見ごろを迎えた紅梅に来るべき桜の花を想いつつ

町田　徹

序　文

『CT・MRI 画像解剖ポケットアトラス』第3巻「筋骨格系のアトラス」は，幸い非常に好評を博し，諸外国で翻訳・出版されていることは大変光栄である．前著が好評であったので，再度本書を改訂しようという動機付けになった．そこで，初版の画像は尊重し，関節近傍の部位に焦点を当て，二方向画像とイラストを追加し，上腕・前腕・大腿・下腿全体画像を網羅した．このようにして，炎症や腫瘍などの骨幹の骨・軟部病変についての理解も十分になるように前回の不足部位を補った．一方，本書の元々の構成はそのまま踏襲した．すなわち，筋肉，血管，神経，その他の構造物を色分けし，高精細 MR 画像（3テスラ）とイラストを対照させた．こうすることで解剖学的構造の局在を正確にかつ容易に認識できると考えた．

　シリーズの他の巻と同様に，多くの助手達の熱意あふれる貴重な助力なしにこの本はできなかったであろう．本書の作成に携わった方々に深謝する．

　また，われわれの全MRIグループに最適な画像が撮像できるよう常に的確な助言を与えてくれた Carina Engler と3テスラの画像を撮像してくれた Nicole Bigga に深謝する．

　この本の読者の皆さんが，私たちが画像とイラストを楽しみながら作ったのと同様に，旧版同様，楽しんで本書を使っていただけることを確信する．

Torsten B. Moeller, MD
Emil Reif, MD

目　次

上　肢 1

上肢 軸位断	2
肩 冠状断	70
肩 矢状断	82
上腕 冠状断	96
上腕 矢状断	108
肘 冠状断	124
肘 矢状断	132
前腕 矢状断	142
前腕 冠状断	154
手 冠状断	164
手 矢状断	172

下　肢 185

下肢 軸位断	186
股関節 冠状断	254
股関節 矢状断	266
大腿 冠状断	280
大腿 矢状断	292
膝 冠状断	302
膝 矢状断	318
下腿 冠状断	338
下腿 矢状断	348
足 冠状断	358
足 矢状断	382

脊 椎 ……………………………………………………… 395

脊椎 矢状断 …………………………………………… 396
頸椎 矢状断 …………………………………………… 398
頸椎 冠状断 …………………………………………… 404
頸椎 軸位断 …………………………………………… 410
胸椎 矢状断 …………………………………………… 420
胸椎 軸位断 …………………………………………… 426
腰椎 矢状断 …………………………………………… 428
腰椎 冠状断 …………………………………………… 436
腰椎 軸位断 …………………………………………… 442
仙骨 …………………………………………………… 448

参考文献 ………………………………………………… 452

和文索引 ………………………………………………… 454

欧文索引 ………………………………………………… 466

注 意

　本書に記載した情報に関しては，正確を期し，一般臨床で広く受け入れられている方法を記載するよう注意を払った．しかしながら，著者，監訳者，訳者ならびに出版社は，本書の情報を用いた結果生じたいかなる不都合に対しても責任を負うものではない．本書の内容の特定な状況への適用に関しての責任は，医師各自のうちにある．

　著者，監訳者，訳者ならびに出版社は，本書に記載した薬物の選択，用量については，出版時の最新の推奨，および臨床状況に基づいていることを確認するよう努力を払っている．しかし，医学は日進月歩で進んでおり，政府の規制は変わり，薬物療法や薬物反応に関する情報は常に変化している．読者は，薬物の使用にあたっては個々の薬物の添付文書を参照し，適応，用量，付加された注意・警告に関する変化を常に確認することを怠ってはならない．これは，推奨された薬物が新しいものであったり，汎用されるものではない場合に，特に重要である．

凡 例

本書に使用した和名用語は原則として日本解剖学会により制定された用語に従った．また臨床で一般に使用されている用語も適宜使用した．

色分けコード：上肢　*1*

- 動脈
- 神経
- 静脈
- 骨
- 脂肪組織
- 軟骨
- 腱
- 関節円板, 関節唇など
- 液体

体幹の筋:
　前鋸筋
　肩甲舌骨筋
　僧帽筋
　鎖骨下筋
　肋間筋

肩の筋:
　三角筋
　棘下筋
　大胸筋
　小胸筋
　肩甲下筋
　烏口腕筋
　広背筋

前腕背側の筋:
　回外筋
　長母指伸筋
　短母指伸筋
　示指伸筋

手の筋:
　背側骨間筋
　掌側骨間筋
　虫様筋

上腕掌側の筋:
　上腕二頭筋
　上腕筋

上腕背側の筋:
　上腕三頭筋
　肘筋

前腕背側の筋(浅層):
　指伸筋
　小指伸筋
　尺側手根伸筋

前腕橈側の筋:
　腕橈骨筋
　長橈側手根伸筋
　短橈側手根伸筋

前腕掌側の筋(浅層):
　円回内筋
　浅指屈筋
　橈側手根屈筋
　尺側手根屈筋
　長掌筋
　短掌筋

前腕掌側の筋(深層):
　深指屈筋
　長母指屈筋
　方形回内筋

小指(第5指)の筋:
　小指外転筋
　短小指屈筋
　小指対立筋

母指の筋:
　長母指外転筋
　短母指外転筋
　母指対立筋
　短母指屈筋
　母指内転筋

2 上 肢

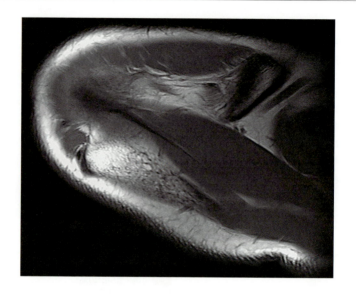

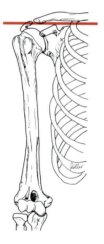

腹側

外側 内側

背側

上肢，軸位断 3

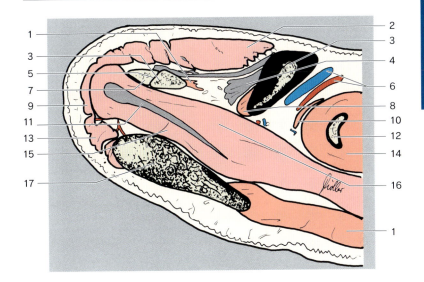

1 僧帽筋 Trapezius muscle
2 三角筋(鎖骨部) Deltoid muscle (clavicular part)
3 鎖骨 Clavicle
4 烏口鎖骨靱帯 Coracoclavicular ligament
5 肩鎖関節 Acromioclavicular joint
6 肩甲上動静脈 Suprascapular artery and vein
7 肩峰 Acromion
8 鎖骨下筋 Subclavius muscle
9 三角筋(肩峰部) Deltoid muscle (acromial part)
10 肩甲舌骨筋 Omohyoid muscle
11 棘上筋(中心腱) Supraspinatus muscle (central tendon)
12 肋骨 Rib
13 三角筋(肩甲棘部) Deltoid muscle (spinal part)
14 前鋸筋 Serratus anterior muscle
15 棘上筋(背側部) Supraspinatus muscle (dorsal part)
16 棘上筋(腹側部) Supraspinatus muscle (ventral part)
17 肩甲棘 Spine of scapula

4　上肢

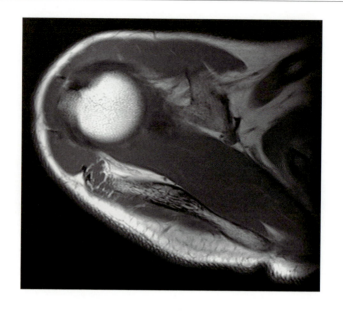

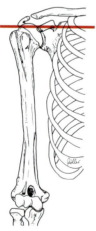

腹側

外側　□　内側

背側

上肢，軸位断　5

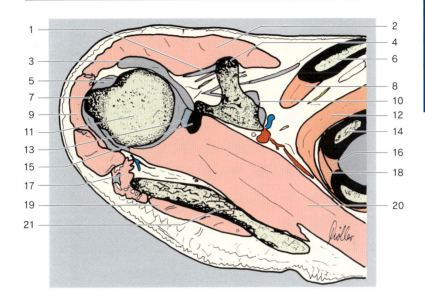

1 烏口上腕靱帯 Coracohumeral ligament
2 三角筋(鎖骨部) Deltoid muscle (clavicular part)
3 中関節上腕靱帯 Middle glenohumeral ligament
4 烏口突起 Coracoid process
5 棘上筋(腱) Supraspinatus muscle (tendon)
6 鎖骨 Clavicle
7 上腕骨(大結節) Humerus (greater tubercle)
8 鎖骨下筋 Subclavius muscle
9 三角筋(肩峰部) Deltoid muscle (acromial part)
10 烏口鎖骨靱帯 Coracoclavicular ligament
11 上腕骨(頭) Humerus (head)
12 前鋸筋 Serratus anterior muscle
13 上方関節唇 Superior glenoid labrum
14 肋骨 Rib
15 関節窩 Glenoid
16 内肋間筋 Internal intercostal muscle
17 三角筋(肩甲棘部) Deltoid muscle (spinal part)
18 外肋間筋 External intercostal muscle
19 棘下筋 Infraspinatus muscle
20 棘上筋 Supraspinatus muscle
21 肩甲棘 Spine of scapula

6　上　肢

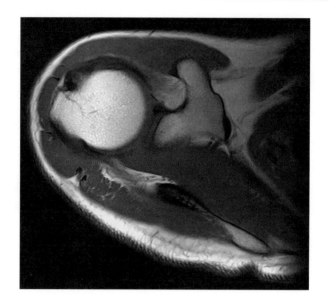

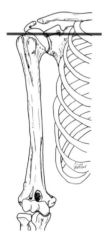

腹側

外側　□　内側

背側

上肢，軸位断

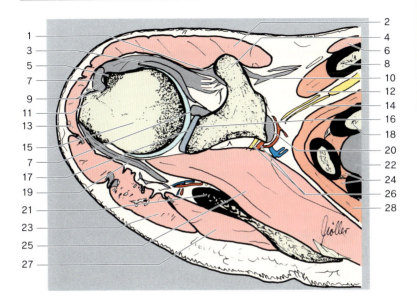

1 烏口上腕靱帯 Coracohumeral ligament
2 三角筋(鎖骨部) Deltoid muscle (clavicular part)
3 中関節上腕靱帯 Middle glenohumeral ligament
4 烏口突起 Coracoid process
5 上腕骨(小結節) Humerus (lesser tubercle)
6 大胸筋 Pectoralis major muscle
7 上腕二頭筋(長頭，腱) Biceps brachii muscle (long head, tendon)
8 鎖骨 Clavicle
9 結節間溝(上腕二頭筋溝) Intertubercular sulcus (bicipital groove)
10 小胸筋(腱) Pectoralis minor muscle (tendon)
11 上腕骨(大結節) Humerus (greater tubercle)
12 鎖骨下筋 Subclavius muscle
13 三角筋(肩峰部) Deltoid muscle (acromial part)
14 腕神経叢 Brachial plexus
15 上腕骨(頭) Humerus (head)
16 関節窩 Glenoid
17 上方関節唇 Superior glenoid labrum
18 肋骨 Rib
19 棘下筋(腱付着部) Infraspinatus muscle (tendon attachment)
20 烏口鎖骨靱帯 Coracoclavicular ligament
21 肩甲棘 Spine of scapula
22 肺 Lung
23 三角筋(肩甲棘部) Deltoid muscle (spinal part)
24 内肋間筋 Internal intercostal muscle, 外肋間筋 External intercostal muscle
25 棘上筋 Supraspinatus muscle
26 肩甲上動静脈 Suprascapular artery and vein
27 棘下筋 Infraspinatus muscle
28 前鋸筋 Serratus anterior muscle

8　上　肢

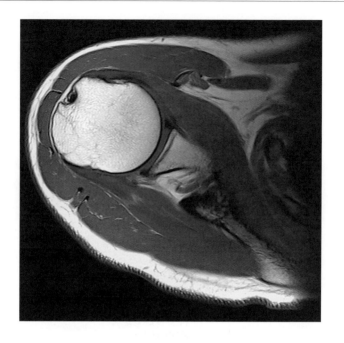

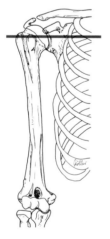

腹側

外側　□　内側

背側

上肢，軸位断

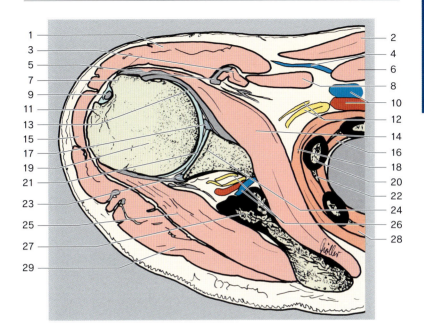

1 三角筋(鎖骨部) Deltoid muscle (clavicular part)
2 大胸筋 Pectoralis major muscle
3 烏口腕筋(+腱) Coracobrachialis muscle (+tendon)
4 橈側皮静脈 Cephalic vein
5 上腕二頭筋(短頭，腱) Biceps brachii muscle (short head, tendon)
6 鎖骨下筋 Subclavius muscle
7 上腕骨(小結節) Humerus (lesser tubercle)
8 小胸筋 Pectoralis minor muscle
9 上腕二頭筋(長頭，腱) Biceps brachii muscle (long head, tendon)
10 腋窩動静脈 Axillary artery and vein
11 上腕骨(大結節) Humerus (greater tubercle)
12 腕神経叢 Brachial plexus, 肩甲下神経 Subscapular nerve
13 中関節上腕靱帯 Middle glenohumeral ligament
14 肩甲下筋 Subscapularis muscle
15 三角筋(肩峰部) Deltoid muscle (acromial part)
16 内肋間筋 Internal intercostal muscle
17 前方関節唇 Anterior glenoid labrum
18 前鋸筋 Serratus anterior muscle
19 上腕骨(頭) Humerus (head)
20 肋骨 Rib
21 肩関節(関節窩上腕関節) Glenohumeral joint
22 肋間動静脈，神経 Intercostal artery, vein, and nerve
23 後方関節唇 Posterior glenoid labrum
24 関節窩 Glenoid
25 棘下筋 Infraspinatus muscle
26 肩甲上動静脈，神経 Suprascapular artery, vein, and nerve
27 肩甲骨 Scapula
28 外肋間筋 External intercostal muscle
29 三角筋(肩甲棘部) Deltoid muscle (spinal part)

10 上 肢

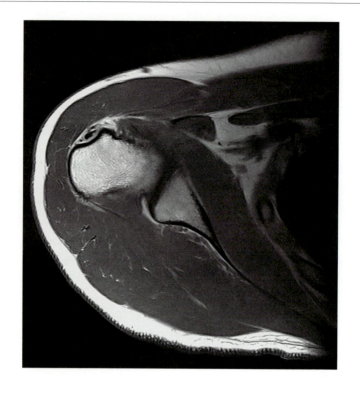

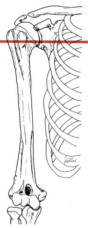

腹側
外側 ☐ 内側
背側

上肢，軸位断

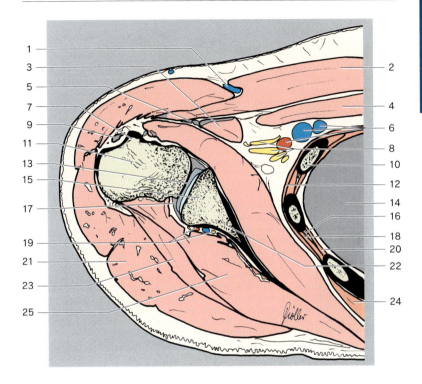

1 橈側皮静脈 Cephalic vein
2 大胸筋 Pectoralis major muscle
3 烏口腕筋(＋腱) Coracobrachialis muscle (＋tendon)
4 小胸筋 Pectoralis minor muscle
5 上腕二頭筋(短頭，腱) Biceps brachii muscle (short head, tendon)
6 腋窩動静脈 Axillary artery and vein
7 上腕骨(小結節) Humerus (lesser tubercle)
8 腕神経叢 Brachial plexus
9 上腕二頭筋(長頭，腱) Biceps brachii muscle (long head, tendon)
10 肋骨 Rib
11 上腕骨 Humerus
12 前鋸筋 Serratus anterior muscle
13 下方関節唇 Posterior glenoid labrum
14 肺 Lung
15 関節窩 Glenoid
16 肋間動静脈，神経 Intercostal artery, vein, and nerve
17 関節包 Joint capsule
18 外肋間筋 External intercostal muscle
19 肩甲上動静脈，神経 Suprascapular artery, vein, and nerve
20 内肋間筋 Internal intercostal muscle
21 三角筋 Deltoid muscle
22 肩甲骨 Scapula
23 小円筋 Teres minor muscle
24 後鋸筋 Serratus posterior muscle
25 棘下筋 Infraspinatus muscle

12 上　肢

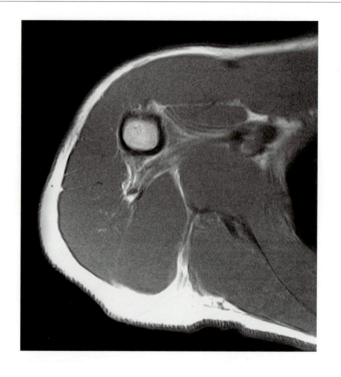

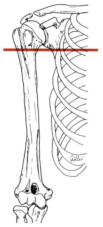

腹側

外側 □ 内側

背側

上肢，軸位断

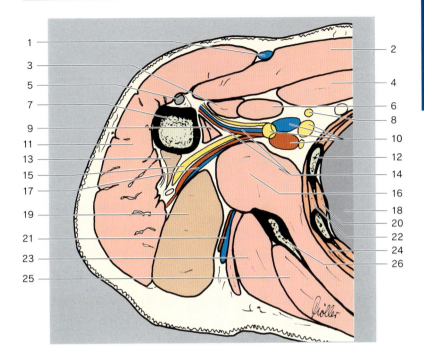

1 橈側皮静脈 Cephalic vein
2 大胸筋 Pectoralis major muscle
3 上腕二頭筋(短頭, 腱) Biceps brachii muscle (short head, tendon)
4 小胸筋 Pectoralis minor muscle
5 上腕二頭筋(長頭, 腱) Biceps brachii muscle (long head, tendon)
6 烏口腕筋 Coracobrachialis muscle
7 上腕骨 Humerus
8 長胸神経 Long thoracic nerve
9 広背筋 Latissimus dorsi muscle, 大円筋 Teres major muscle
10 腋窩動静脈 Axillary artery and vein, 腕神経叢 Brachial plexus
11 三角筋 Deltoid muscle
12 肋骨 Rib
13 上腕三頭筋(外側頭) Triceps brachii muscle (lateral head)
14 前上腕回旋動静脈 Anterior circumflex humeral artery and vein
15 腋窩神経 Axillary nerve
16 肩甲下筋 Subscapularis muscle
17 後上腕回旋動静脈 Posterior circumflex humeral artery and vein
18 肺 Lung
19 上腕三頭筋(長頭) Triceps brachii muscle (long head)
20 内肋間筋 Internal intercostal muscle, 最内肋間筋 Innermost intercostal muscle
21 肩甲回旋動静脈 Circumflex scapular artery and vein
22 外肋間筋 External intercostal muscle
23 小円筋 Teres minor muscle
24 前鋸筋 Serratus anterior muscle
25 棘下筋 Infraspinatus muscle
26 肩甲骨 Scapula

14 上 肢

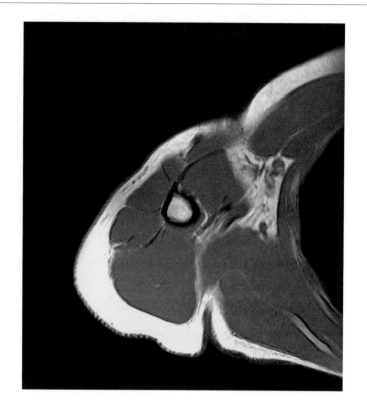

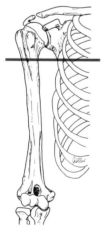

腹側
外側 □ 内側
背側

上肢, 軸位断 15

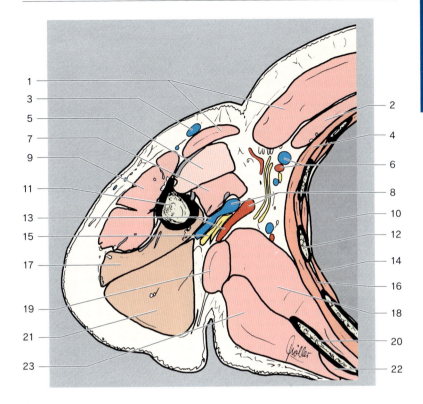

1 大胸筋 Pectoralis major muscle
2 小胸筋 Pectoralis minor muscle
3 橈側皮静脈 Cephalic vein
4 前鋸筋 Serratus anterior muscle
5 上腕二頭筋 Biceps brachii muscle
6 外側胸動静脈 Lateral thoracic artery and vein
7 烏口腕筋 Coracobrachialis muscle
8 腋窩動静脈 Axillary artery and vein
9 三角筋 Deltoid muscle
10 肺 Lung
11 上腕骨 Humerus
12 肋骨 Rib
13 上腕動静脈 Brachial artery and vein
14 内肋間筋 Internal intercostal muscle,
最内肋間筋 Innermost intercostal muscle
15 橈骨神経 Radial nerve
16 外肋間筋 External intercostal muscle
17 上腕三頭筋(外側頭) Triceps brachii muscle (lateral head)
18 肩甲下筋 Subscapularis muscle
19 大円筋 Teres major muscle
20 肩甲骨 Scapula
21 上腕三頭筋(長頭) Triceps brachii muscle (long head)
22 棘下筋 Infraspinatus muscle
23 大円筋 Teres major muscle,
広背筋 Latissimus dorsi muscle

16 上肢

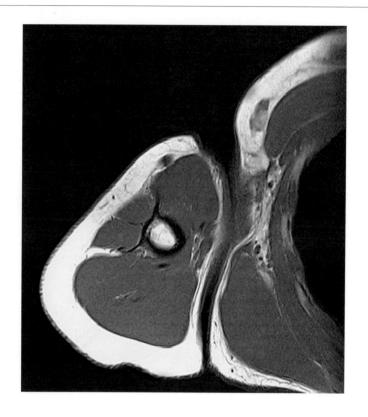

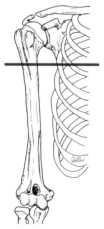

腹側
外側　内側
背側

上肢，軸位断

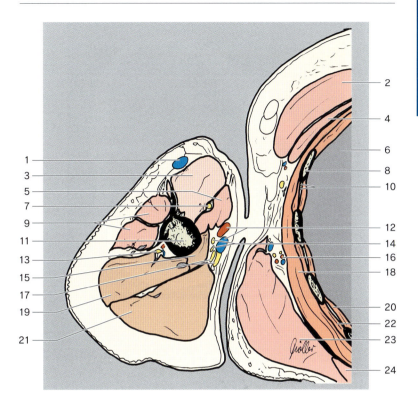

1 橈側皮静脈 Cephalic vein
2 大胸筋 Pectoralis major muscle
3 上腕二頭筋 Biceps brachii muscle
4 小胸筋 Pectoralis minor muscle
5 烏口腕筋 Coracobrachialis muscle
6 肺 Lung
7 筋皮神経 Musculocutaneous nerve
8 肋骨 Rib
9 三角筋 Deltoid muscle
10 肋間動静脈，神経 Intercostal artery, vein, and nerve
11 上腕骨（体）Humerus (shaft)
12 上腕動静脈 Brachial artery and vein
13 橈骨神経 Radial nerve
14 正中神経 Median nerve
15 上腕三頭筋（内側頭）Triceps brachii muscle (medial head)
16 胸背動脈，神経 Thoracodorsal artery and nerve
17 尺骨神経 Ulnar nerve
18 前鋸筋 Serratus anterior muscle
19 上腕三頭筋（外側頭）Triceps brachii muscle (lateral head)
20 内肋間筋 Internal intercostal muscle, 最内肋間筋 Innermost intercostal muscle
21 上腕三頭筋（長頭）Triceps brachii muscle (long head)
22 外肋間筋 External intercostal muscle
23 大円筋 Teres major muscle, 広背筋 Latissimus dorsi muscle
24 棘下筋 Infraspinatus muscle

18　上　肢

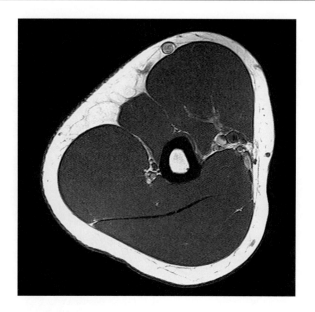

腹側

外側　内側

背側

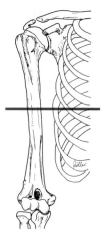

上肢，軸位断 **19**

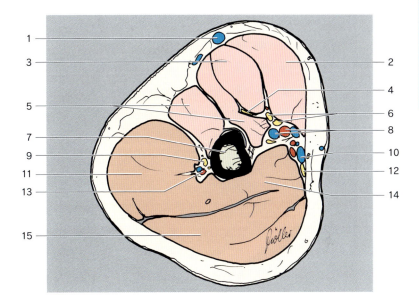

1 橈側皮静脈 Cephalic vein
2 上腕二頭筋(短頭) Biceps brachii muscle (short head)
3 上腕二頭筋(長頭) Biceps brachii muscle (long head)
4 筋皮神経 Musculocutaneous nerve
5 上腕筋 Brachialis muscle
6 正中神経 Median nerve
7 上腕骨(体) Humerus (shaft)
8 上腕動静脈 Brachial artery and vein
9 橈骨神経 Radial nerve
10 尺側皮静脈 Basilic vein
11 上腕三頭筋(外側頭) Triceps brachii muscle (lateral head)
12 尺骨神経 Ulnar nerve
13 上腕深動静脈 Deep brachial artery and vein
14 上腕三頭筋(内側頭) Triceps brachii muscle (medial head)
15 上腕三頭筋(長頭) Triceps brachii muscle (long head)

20　上肢

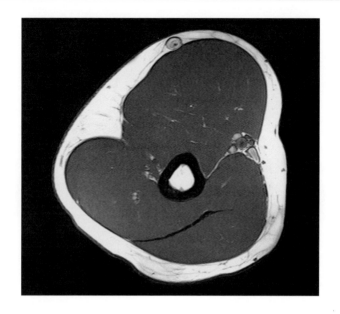

腹側

外側　☐　内側

背側

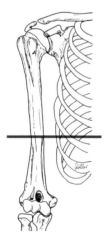

上肢，軸位断 **21**

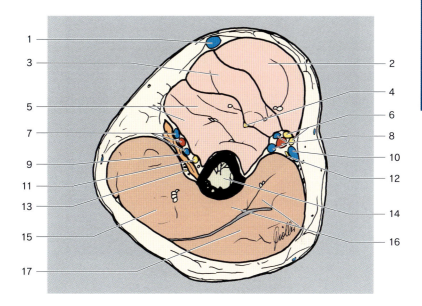

1 **橈側皮静脈** Cephalic vein
2 **上腕二頭筋(短頭)** Biceps brachii muscle (short head)
3 **上腕二頭筋(長頭)** Biceps brachii muscle (long head)
4 **筋皮神経** Musculocutaneous nerve
5 **上腕筋** Brachialis muscle
6 **正中神経** Median nerve
7 **上腕深動静脈** Deep brachial artery and vein
8 **上腕動静脈** Brachial artery and vein
9 **腕橈骨筋** Brachioradialis muscle
10 **尺側皮静脈** Basilic vein
11 **橈骨神経** Radial nerve
12 **尺骨神経** Ulnar nerve
13 **後前腕皮神経(枝)** Posterior cutaneous nerve of forearm (branch)
14 **上腕骨(体)** Humerus (shaft)
15 **上腕三頭筋(外側頭)** Triceps brachii muscle (lateral head)
16 **上腕三頭筋(内側頭)** Triceps brachii muscle (medial head)
17 **上腕三頭筋(長頭)** Triceps brachii muscle (long head)

上 肢

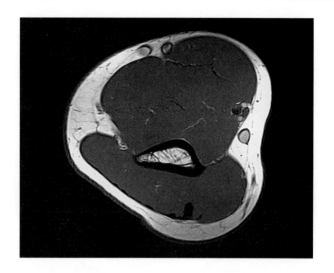

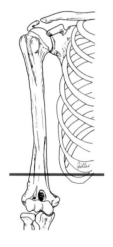

腹側

外側 □ 内側

背側

上肢，軸位断 **23**

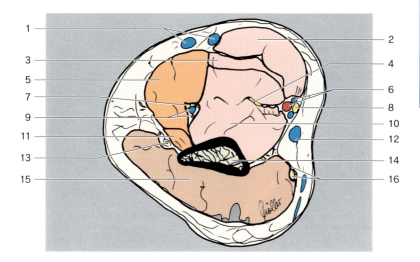

1 **橈側皮静脈** Cephalic vein
2 **上腕二頭筋（短頭）** Biceps brachii muscle (short head)
3 **上腕二頭筋（長頭）** Biceps brachii muscle (long head)
4 **筋皮神経** Musculocutaneous nerve
5 **腕橈骨筋** Brachioradialis muscle
6 **上腕動静脈** Brachial artery and vein
7 **橈骨神経** Radial nerve
8 **正中神経** Median nerve
9 **上腕深動静脈** Deep brachial artery and vein
10 **上腕筋** Brachialis muscle
11 **長橈側手根伸筋** Extensor carpi radialis longus muscle
12 **尺側皮静脈** Basilic vein
13 **後前腕皮神経** Posterior cutaneous nerve of forearm
14 **上腕骨（体）** Humerus (shaft)
15 **上腕三頭筋** Triceps brachii muscle
16 **尺骨神経，動静脈** Ulnar nerve, artery, and vein

24 上肢

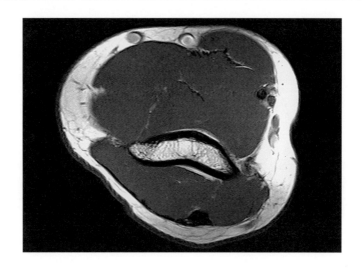

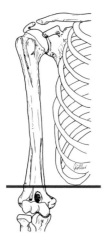

腹側

外側 　　 内側

背側

上肢，軸位断 25

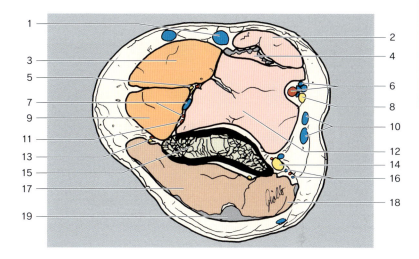

1 橈側皮静脈 Cephalic vein
2 上腕二頭筋(短頭) Biceps brachii muscle (short head)
3 腕橈骨筋 Brachioradialis muscle
4 上腕二頭筋(長頭＋腱) Biceps brachii muscle (long head+tendon)
5 橈骨神経 Radial nerve
6 上腕動静脈 Brachial artery and vein
7 上腕深動静脈 Deep brachial artery and vein
8 正中神経 Median nerve
9 長橈側手根伸筋 Extensor carpi radialis longus muscle
10 尺側皮静脈 Basilic vein
11 中側副動脈 Medial collateral artery
12 上腕筋 Brachialis muscle
13 後前腕皮神経 Posterior cutaneous nerve of forearm
14 尺骨神経 Ulnar nerve
15 上腕骨(体) Humerus(shaft)
16 尺骨動静脈 Ulnar artery and vein
17 上腕三頭筋(外側頭) Triceps brachii muscle(lateral head)
18 上腕三頭筋(内側頭) Triceps brachii muscle(medial head)
19 上腕三頭筋(腱) Triceps brachii muscle (tendon)

26 上肢

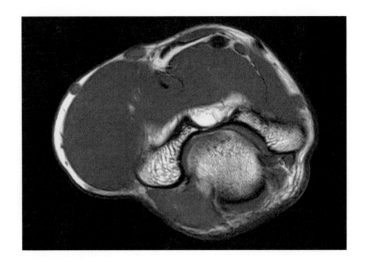

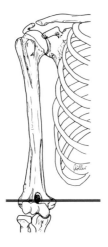

腹側
外側　　内側
背側

上肢，軸位断

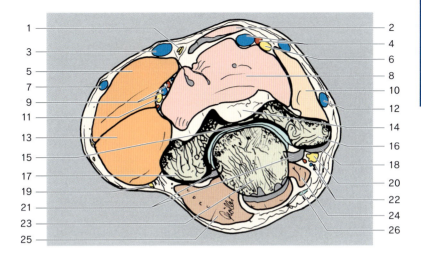

1 前腕の皮神経 Cutaneous nerve of forearm
2 上腕二頭筋（＋腱）Biceps brachii muscle (+tendon)
3 肘正中皮静脈 Median cubital vein
4 上腕動静脈 Brachial artery and vein
5 腕橈骨筋 Brachioradialis muscle
6 正中神経 Median nerve
7 橈側皮静脈 Cephalic vein
8 上腕筋 Brachialis muscle
9 橈側側副動静脈 Radial collateral artery and vein
10 円回内筋 Pronator teres muscle
11 橈骨神経 Radial nerve
12 尺側皮静脈 Basilic vein
13 長橈側手根伸筋 Extensor carpi radialis longus muscle
14 鈎突窩 Coronoid fossa
15 腕尺関節 Humeroulnar joint
16 上腕骨の内側上顆 Medial epicondyle of humerus
17 上腕骨の外側上顆 Lateral epicondyle of humerus
18 前腕腹側浅層筋群の腱付着部 Tendon attachment of ventral superficial muscles of forearm,
側副靱帯 Collateral ligaments
19 後前腕皮神経（橈骨神経）Posterior cutaneous nerve of forearm (radial nerve)
20 尺骨神経 Ulnar nerve
21 関節包 Joint capsule
22 上尺側側副動脈，神経 Superior collateral ulnar artery and nerve
23 肘頭 Olecranon
24 上腕三頭筋（＋腱）Triceps brachii muscle (+tendon)
25 肘筋 Anconeus muscle
26 肘頭皮下包 Subcutaneous olecranon bursa

28　上　肢

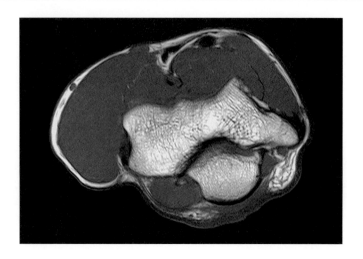

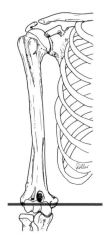

腹側

外側　　　内側

背側

上肢，軸位断

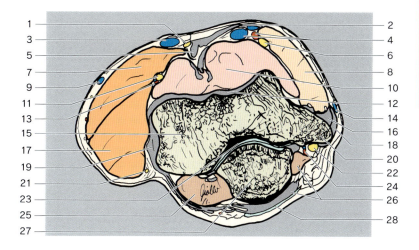

1 前腕の皮神経 Cutaneous nerve of forearm
2 上腕二頭筋腱膜 Bicipital aponeurosis
3 肘正中皮静脈 Median cubital vein
4 上腕動静脈 Brachial artery and vein
5 上腕二頭筋（腱）Biceps brachii muscle (tendon)
6 正中神経 Median nerve
7 腕橈骨筋 Brachioradialis muscle
8 円回内筋 Pronator teres muscle
9 橈側皮静脈 Cephalic vein
10 上腕筋（+腱）Brachialis muscle (+tendon)
11 橈骨神経 Radial nerve
12 肘関節の関節包 Articular capsule of elbow
13 橈側側副動静脈 Radial collateral artery and vein
14 尺側皮静脈 Basilic vein
15 上腕骨（小頭）Humerus (capitulum)
16 橈側手根屈筋（腱付着部）Flexor carpi radialis muscle (tendon attachment)
17 長橈側手根伸筋 Extensor carpi radialis longus muscle
18 長掌筋（腱付着部）Palmaris longus muscle (tendon attachment)
19 外側側副靱帯 Lateral collateral ligament
20 上腕骨の内側上顆 Medial epicondyle of humerus
21 後前腕皮神経（橈骨神経）Posterior cutaneous nerve of forearm (radial nerve)
22 尺骨神経 Ulnar nerve
23 腕尺関節 Humeroulnar joint
24 上尺側側副動静脈 Superior collateral ulnar artery and vein
25 肘筋 Anconeus muscle
26 上腕三頭筋（+腱）Triceps brachii muscle (+tendon)
27 肘頭 Olecranon
28 肘頭皮下包 Subcutaneous olecranon bursa

30　上　肢

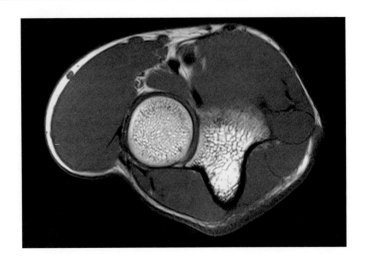

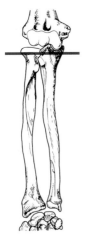

腹側

橈側 □ 尺側

背側

上肢，軸位断

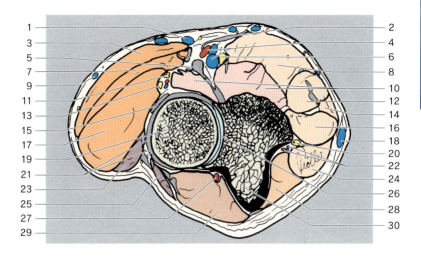

1 肘正中皮静脈 Median cubital vein
2 上腕二頭筋腱膜 Bicipital aponeurosis
3 腕橈骨筋 Brachioradialis muscle
4 上腕動静脈 Brachial artery and vein
5 上腕二頭筋(腱) Biceps brachii muscle (tendon)
6 正中神経 Median nerve
7 長橈側手根伸筋 Extensor carpi radialis longus muscle
8 円回内筋 Pronator teres muscle
9 橈側皮静脈 Cephalic vein
10 上腕筋(＋腱) Brachialis muscle (+tendon)
11 橈骨神経(浅枝) Radial nerve (superficial branch)
12 橈側手根屈筋 Flexor carpi radialis muscle
13 橈骨神経(深枝) Radial nerve (deep branch)
14 長掌筋 Palmaris longus muscle
15 回外筋(腱) Supinator muscle (tendon)
16 浅指屈筋 Flexor digitorum superficialis muscle
17 短橈側手根伸筋 Extensor carpi radialis brevis muscle
18 尺側皮静脈 Basilic vein
19 橈骨(頭) Radius (head)
20 尺骨神経 Ulnar nerve
21 橈骨輪状靱帯 Anular ligament
22 上尺側側副動静脈 Superior ulnar collateral artery and vein
23 指伸筋 Extensor digitorum muscle
24 尺側手根屈筋 Flexor carpi ulnaris muscle
25 尺側手根伸筋 Extensor carpi ulnaris muscle
26 上橈尺関節 Proximal radioulnar joint
27 反回骨間動脈 Recurrent interosseous artery
28 深指屈筋 Flexor digitorum profundus muscle
29 肘筋 Anconeus muscle
30 尺骨 Ulna

32 上肢

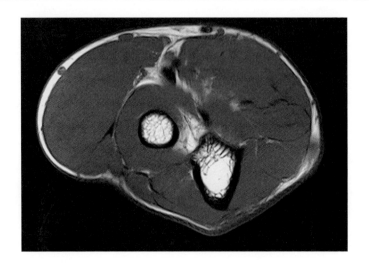

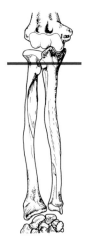

腹側
橈側 □ 尺側
背側

上肢，軸位断 33

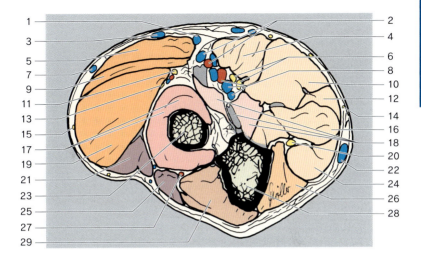

1 肘正中皮静脈 Median cubital vein
2 橈骨動静脈 Radial artery and vein
3 副橈側皮静脈 Accessory cephalic vein
4 円回内筋 Pronator teres muscle
5 腕橈骨筋 Brachioradialis muscle
6 正中神経 Median nerve
7 橈側皮静脈 Cephalic vein
8 尺骨動静脈 Ulnar artery and vein
9 長橈側手根伸筋 Extensor carpi radialis longus muscle
10 橈側手根屈筋 Flexor carpi radialis muscle
11 橈骨神経(浅枝) Radial nerve (superficial branch)
12 長掌筋 Palmaris longus muscle
13 橈骨神経(深枝) Radial nerve (deep branch)
14 内側前腕皮神経 Medial cutaneous nerve of forearm
15 後前腕皮神経 Posterior cutaneous nerve of forearm
16 浅指屈筋 Flexor digitorum superficialis muscle
17 回外筋 Supinator muscle
18 上腕筋(+腱付着部) Brachialis muscle (+tendon attachment)
19 短橈側手根伸筋 Extensor carpi radialis brevis muscle
20 尺骨神経 Ulnar nerve
21 指伸筋 Extensor digitorum muscle
22 尺側皮静脈 Basilic vein
23 橈骨 Radius
24 尺側手根屈筋 Flexor carpi ulnaris muscle
25 尺側手根伸筋 Extensor carpi ulnaris muscle
26 深指屈筋 Flexor digitorum profundus muscle
27 反回骨間動静脈 Recurrent interosseous artery and vein
28 尺骨 Ulna
29 肘筋 Anconeus muscle

34　上 肢

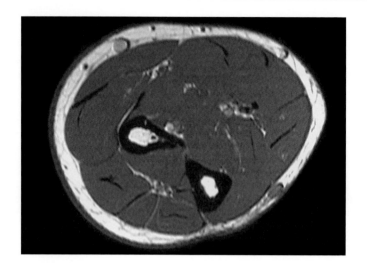

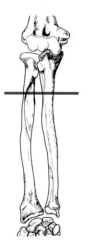

腹側

橈側 ☐ 尺側

背側

上肢，軸位断

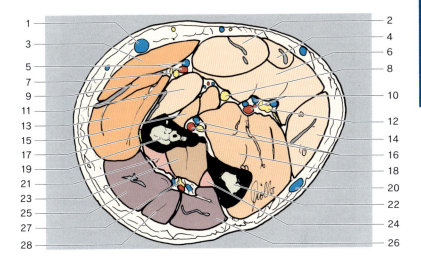

1 肘正中皮静脈 Median cubital vein
2 橈側手根屈筋 Flexor carpi radialis muscle
3 腕橈骨筋 Brachioradialis muscle
4 長掌筋 Palmaris longus muscle
5 橈骨動静脈 Radial artery and vein
6 浅指屈筋 Flexor digitorum superficialis muscle
7 橈骨神経(浅枝) Radial nerve (superficial branch)
8 正中神経 Median nerve
9 長橈側手根伸筋(＋腱) Extensor carpi radialis longus muscle (+tendon)
10 尺骨動静脈 Ulnar artery and vein
11 円回内筋 Pronator teres muscle
12 尺骨神経 Ulnar nerve
13 短橈側手根伸筋 Extensor carpi radialis brevis muscle
14 尺側手根屈筋 Flexor carpi ulnaris muscle
15 長母指屈筋 Flexor pollicis longus muscle
16 前骨間動静脈,神経 Anterior interosseous artery, vein and nerve
17 橈骨神経(深枝) Radial nerve (deep branch)
18 深指屈筋 Flexor digitorum profundus muscle
19 橈骨 Radius
20 尺側皮静脈 Basilic vein
21 回外筋 Supinator muscle
22 尺骨 ulna
23 長母指外転筋 Abductor pollicis longus muscle
24 長母指伸筋 Extensor pollicis longus muscle
25 指伸筋 Extensor digitorum muscle
26 尺側手根伸筋 Extensor carpi ulnaris muscle
27 後骨間動静脈,神経 Posterior interosseous artery, vein, and nerve
28 小指伸筋 Extensor digiti minimi muscle

36　上　肢

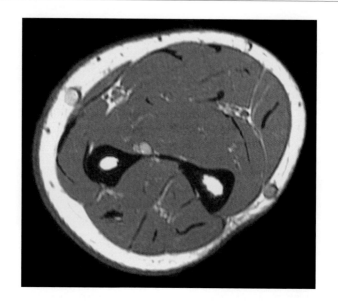

腹側
橈側 ☐ 尺側
背側

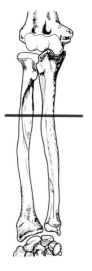

上肢，軸位断 **37**

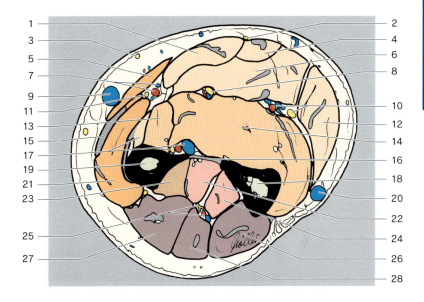

1 橈側手根屈筋 Flexor carpi radialis muscle
2 内側前腕皮神経（前枝）Medial cutaneous nerve of forearm (anterior branch)
3 外側前腕皮神経（筋皮神経）Lateral cutaneous nerve of forearm (musculocutaneous nerve)
4 長掌筋 Palmaris longus muscle
5 腕橈骨筋 Brachioradialis muscle
6 浅指屈筋 Flexor digitorum superficialis muscle
7 橈骨動静脈 Radial artery and vein
8 正中神経 Median nerve
9 橈側皮静脈 Cephalic vein
10 尺骨動静脈，神経 Ulnar artery, vein, and nerve
11 橈骨神経（浅枝）Radial nerve (superficial branch)
12 尺側手根屈筋 Flexor carpi ulnaris muscle
13 長母指屈筋 Flexor pollicis longus muscle
14 深指屈筋 Flexor digitorum profundus muscle
15 長橈側手根伸筋（＋腱）Extensor carpi radialis longus muscle (+tendon)
16 前腕骨間膜 Interosseous membrane of forearm
17 円回内筋 Pronator teres muscle, 前骨間動静脈，神経 Anterior interosseous artery, vein, and nerve
18 尺骨 Ulna
19 橈骨 Radius
20 尺側皮静脈 Basilic vein
21 短橈側手根伸筋 Extensor carpi radialis brevis muscle
22 短母指伸筋 Extensor pollicis brevis muscle
23 長母指外転筋 Abductor pollicis longus muscle
24 長母指伸筋 Extensor pollicis longus muscle
25 後骨間動静脈，神経 Posterior interosseous artery, vein, and nerve
26 尺側手根伸筋 Extensor carpi ulnaris muscle
27 指伸筋 Extensor digitorum muscle
28 小指伸筋 Extensor digiti minimi muscle

38 上 肢

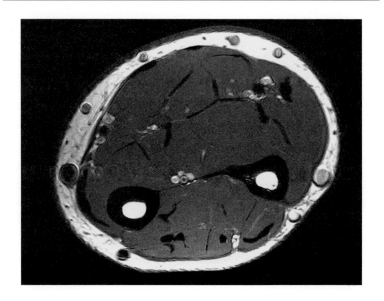

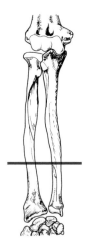

腹側

橈側 ☐ 尺側

背側

上肢，軸位断　**39**

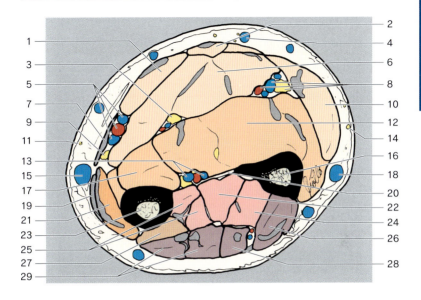

1 橈側手根屈筋 Flexor carpi radialis muscle
2 長掌筋 Palmaris longus muscle
3 正中神経 Median nerve
4 皮静脈 Cutaneous vein
5 橈骨動静脈 Radial artery and veins
6 浅指屈筋 Flexor digitorum superficialis muscle
7 腕橈骨筋(腱) Brachioradialis muscle(tendon)
8 尺骨動静脈，神経 Ulnar artery, vein, and nerve
9 橈骨神経(浅枝) Radial nerve(superficial branch)
10 尺側手根屈筋 Flexor carpi ulnaris muscle
11 後前腕皮神経 Posterior cutaneous nerve of forearm
12 深指屈筋 Flexor digitorum profundus muscle
13 前骨間動静脈，神経 Anterior interosseous artery, vein, and nerve
14 内側前腕皮神経 Medial cutaneous nerve of forearm
15 橈側皮静脈 Cephalic vein
16 尺骨 Ulna
17 長母指屈筋 Flexor pollicis longus muscle
18 尺側皮静脈 Basilic vein
19 長橈側手根伸筋(腱) Extensor carpi radialis longus muscle(tendon)
20 前骨間膜 Interosseous membrane of forearm
21 短橈側手根伸筋(＋腱) Extensor carpi radialis brevis muscle(+tendon)
22 長母指伸筋 Extensor pollicis longus muscle
23 橈骨 Radius
24 示指伸筋 Extensor indicis muscle
25 短母指伸筋 Extensor pollicis brevis muscle
26 尺側手根伸筋 Extensor carpi ulnaris muscle
27 長母指外転筋 Abductor pollicis longus muscle
28 小指伸筋 Extensor digiti minimi muscle
29 指伸筋 Extensor digitorum muscle

40 上 肢

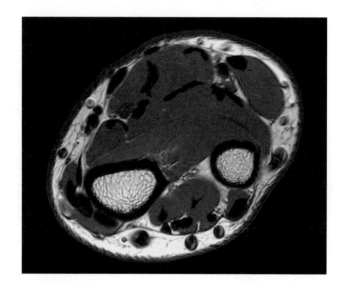

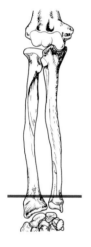

腹側

橈側 ☐ 尺側

背側

上肢，軸位断 **41**

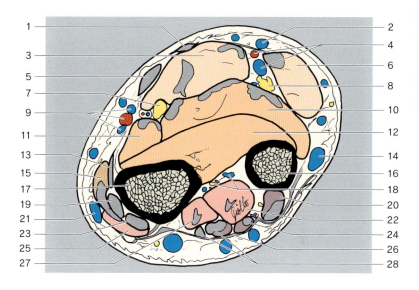

1 長掌筋(腱) Palmaris longus muscle(tendon)
2 皮静脈 Cutaneous vein
3 浅指屈筋 Flexor digitorum superficialis muscle
4 尺骨動静脈 Ulnar artery and vein
5 橈側手根屈筋(腱) Flexor carpi radialis muscle(tendon)
6 尺側手根屈筋 Flexor carpi ulnaris muscle
7 正中神経 Median nerve
8 尺骨神経 Ulnar nerve
9 橈骨動静脈 Radial artery and veins
10 深指屈筋 Flexor digitorum profundus muscle
11 長母指屈筋 Flexor pollicis longus muscle
12 方形回内筋 Pronator quadratus muscle
13 腕橈骨筋(腱) Brachioradialis muscle(tendon)
14 尺側皮静脈 Basilic vein
15 長母指外転筋(+腱) Abductor pollicis longus muscle(+tendon)
16 尺骨 Ulna
17 橈骨 Radius
18 前骨間動静脈, 神経 Anterior interosseous artery, vein, and nerve
19 長橈側手根伸筋(腱) Extensor carpi radialis longus muscle(tendon)
20 尺側手根伸筋 Extensor carpi ulnaris muscle
21 橈側皮静脈 Cephalic vein
22 示指伸筋 Extensor indicis muscle
23 短橈側手根伸筋(腱) Extensor carpi radialis brevis muscle(tendon)
24 小指伸筋 Extensor digiti minimi muscle
25 短母指伸筋 Extensor pollicis brevis muscle
26 伸筋支帯 Extensor retinaculum
27 長母指伸筋 Extensor pollicis longus muscle
28 指伸筋(+腱) Extensor digitorum muscle (+tendon)

42 上 肢

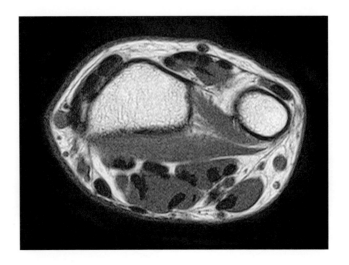

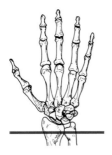

手背側

橈側 ☐ 尺側

手掌側

上肢，軸位断

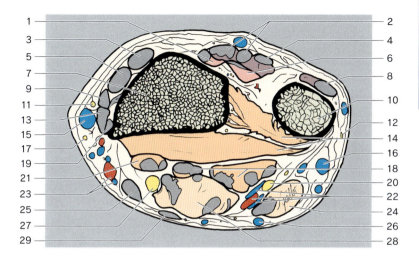

1 長母指伸筋 Extensor pollicis longus muscle
2 指伸筋 Extensor digitorum muscle
3 短橈側手根伸筋(腱) Extensor carpi radialis brevis muscle(tendon)
4 小指伸筋 Extensor digiti minimi muscle
5 長橈側手根伸筋(腱) Extensor carpi radialis longus muscle(tendon)
6 示指伸筋 Extensor indicis muscle
7 橈骨 Radius
8 尺側手根伸筋 Extensor carpi ulnaris muscle
9 短母指伸筋(腱) Extensor pollicis brevis muscle(tendon)
10 尺骨 Ulna
11 橈骨神経(浅枝) Radial nerve(superficial branch)
12 内側前腕皮神経 Medial cutaneous nerve of forearm
13 長母指外転筋(腱) Abductor pollicis longus muscle(tendon)
14 方形回内筋 Pronator quadratus muscle
15 橈側皮静脈 Cephalic vein
16 尺側皮静脈 Basilic vein
17 外側前腕皮神経 Lateral cutaneous nerve of forearm
18 深指屈筋(＋腱) Flexor digitorum profundus muscle(＋tendon)
19 腕橈骨筋(腱) Brachioradialis muscle (tendon)
20 尺骨神経 Ulnar nerve
21 長母指屈筋 Flexor pollicis longus muscle
22 尺骨動静脈 Ulnar artery and veins
23 橈骨動静脈 Radial artery and veins
24 尺側手根屈筋 Flexor carpi ulnaris muscle
25 橈側手根屈筋(腱) Flexor carpi radialis muscle(tendon)
26 皮静脈 Cutaneous vein
27 正中神経 Median nerve
28 浅指屈筋 Flexor digitorum superficialis muscle
29 長掌筋(＋腱) Palmaris longus muscle (＋tendon)

44　上肢

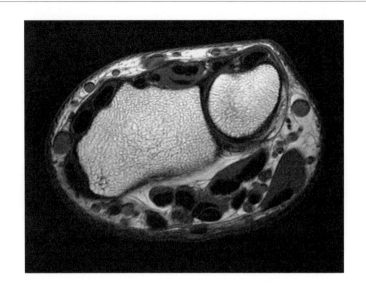

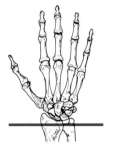

手背側

橈側　□　尺側

手掌側

上肢，軸位断

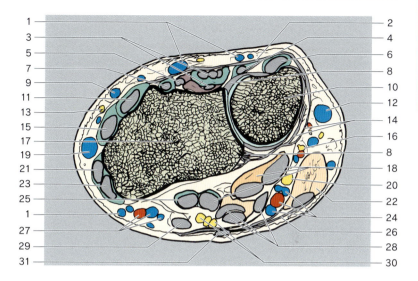

1 皮静脈 Cutaneous vein
2 伸筋支帯 Extensor retinaculum
3 指伸筋(＋腱) Extensor digitorum muscle (＋tendon)
4 小指伸筋(腱) Extensor digiti minimi muscle (tendon)
5 示指伸筋(腱) Extensor indicis muscle (tendon)
6 尺側手根伸筋(腱) Extensor carpi ulnaris muscle (tendon)
7 長母指伸筋(腱) Extensor pollicis longus muscle (tendon)
8 関節包 Joint capsule
9 副橈側皮静脈 Accessory cephalic vein
10 尺骨 Ulna
11 短橈側手根伸筋(腱) Extensor carpi radialis brevis muscle (tendon)
12 尺側皮静脈 Basilic vein
13 橈骨神経(浅枝) Radial nerve (superficial branch)
14 掌側尺骨手根靱帯 Palmar ulnocarpal ligament
15 長橈側手根伸筋(腱) Extensor carpi radialis longus muscle (tendon)
16 尺骨神経(手背枝) Ulnar nerve (dorsal branch)
17 橈骨 Radius
18 深指屈筋(＋腱) Flexor digitorum profundus muscle (＋tendon)
19 橈側皮静脈 Cephalic vein
20 尺骨神経 Ulnar nerve
21 短母指伸筋(腱) Extensor pollicis brevis muscle (tendon)
22 尺側手根屈筋 Flexor carpi ulnaris muscle
23 長母指外転筋(腱) Abductor pollicis longus muscle (tendon)
24 尺骨動静脈 Ulnar artery and veins
25 長母指屈筋(腱) Flexor pollicis longus muscle (tendon)
26 前腕筋膜 Antebrachial fascia
27 橈骨動静脈 Radial artery and veins
28 浅指屈筋(＋腱) Flexor digitorum superficialis muscle (＋tendon)
29 橈側手根屈筋(腱) Flexor carpi radialis muscle (tendon)
30 正中神経 Median nerve
31 長掌筋(腱) Palmaris longus muscle (tendon)

46　上　肢

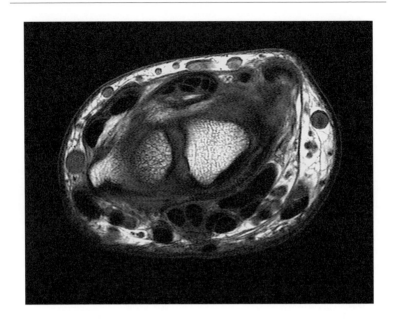

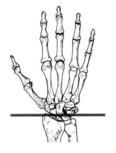

手背側

橈側　□　尺側

手掌側

上肢，軸位断

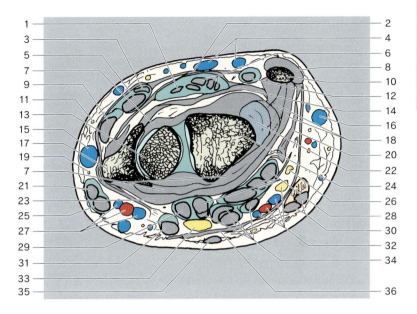

1. 示指伸筋(腱) Extensor indicis muscle (tendon)
2. 伸筋支帯 Extensor retinaculum
3. 長母指伸筋(腱) Extensor pollicis longus muscle(tendon)
4. 皮静脈 Cutaneous vein
5. 短橈側手根伸筋(腱) Extensor carpi radialis brevis muscle(tendon)
6. 指伸筋(腱) Extensor digitorum muscle(tendon)
7. 関節包 Joint capsule
8. 尺側手根伸筋(腱) Extensor carpi ulnaris muscle(tendon)
9. 長橈側手根伸筋(腱) Extensor carpi radialis longus muscle(tendon)
10. 尺骨茎状突起 Ulnar styloid process
11. 後前腕皮神経(橈骨神経) Posterior cutaneous nerve of forearm (radial nerve)
12. 小指伸筋(腱) Extensor digiti minimi muscle (tendon)
13. 舟状骨 Scaphoid
14. 背側橈骨手根靱帯 Dorsal radiocarpal ligament
15. 橈側皮静脈 Cephalic vein
16. 尺側皮静脈 Basilic vein
17. 橈骨 Radius
18. 掌側尺骨手根靱帯 Palmar ulnocarpal ligament
19. 橈骨神経(浅枝) Radial nerve(superficial branch)
20. 内側手根側副靱帯 Ulnar collateral ligament of wrist joint
21. 短母指伸筋(腱) Extensor pollicis brevis muscle(tendon)
22. 三角線維軟骨 Triangular fibrocartilage
23. 掌側橈骨手根靱帯 Palmar radiocarpal ligament
24. 月状骨 Lunate
25. 長母指外転筋(腱) Abductor pollicis longus muscle(tendon)
26. 尺骨神経(手背枝) Ulnar nerve(dorsal branch)
27. 橈骨動静脈 Radial artery and veins
28. 深指屈筋(腱) Flexor digitorum profundus muscle(tendons)
29. 長母指屈筋(腱) Flexor pollicis longus muscle(tendon)
30. 尺側手根屈筋(＋腱) Flexor carpi ulnaris muscle(+tendon)
31. 橈側手根屈筋(腱) Flexor carpi radialis muscle(tendon)
32. 尺骨神経，尺骨動静脈 Ulnar nerve, artery, and veins
33. 正中神経 Median nerve
34. 浅指屈筋(腱) Flexor digitorum superficialis muscle(tendons)
35. 長掌筋(腱) Palmaris longus muscle(tendon)
36. 屈筋支帯 Flexor retinaculum

48　上　肢

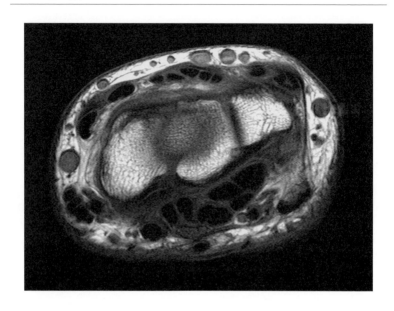

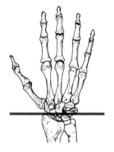

手背側

橈側　□　尺側

手掌側

上肢，軸位断 49

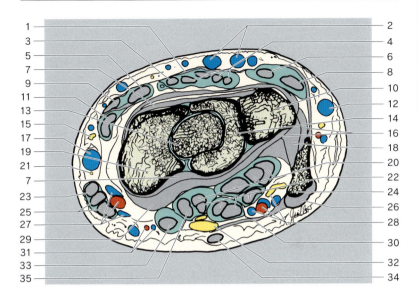

1 伸筋支帯 Extensor retinaculum
2 皮静脈 Cutaneous vein
3 示指伸筋(腱) Extensor indicis muscle(tendon)
4 指伸筋(腱) Extensor digitorum muscle (tendons)
5 短橈側手根伸筋(腱) Extensor carpi radialis brevis muscle(tendon)
6 小指伸筋(腱) Extensor digiti minimi muscle (tendon)
7 関節包 Joint capsule
8 尺側手根伸筋(腱) Extensor carpi ulnaris muscle(tendon)
9 長母指伸筋(腱) Extensor pollicis longus muscle(tendon)
10 三角骨 Triquetrum
11 長橈側手根伸筋(腱) Extensor carpi radialis longus muscle(tendon)
12 尺側皮静脈 Basilic vein
13 有頭骨 Capitate
14 月状骨 Lunate
15 後前腕皮神経(橈骨神経) Posterior cutaneous nerve of forearm(radial nerve)
16 掌側尺骨手根靱帯 Palmar ulnocarpal ligament
17 橈側皮静脈 Cephalic vein
18 掌側手根間靱帯 Palmar intercarpal ligament
19 舟状骨 Scaphoid
20 深指屈筋(腱) Flexor digitorum profundus muscle(tendons)
21 橈骨神経(浅枝) Radial nerve(superficial branch)
22 浅指屈筋(腱) Flexor digitorum superficialis muscle(tendons)
23 短母指伸筋(腱) Extensor pollicis brevis muscle(tendon)
24 豆状骨 Pisiform
25 長母指外転筋(腱) Abductor pollicis longus muscle(tendon)
26 尺側手根屈筋(腱付着部) Flexor carpi ulnaris muscle(tendon attachment)
27 橈骨動静脈 Radial artery and veins
28 尺骨神経，尺骨動静脈 Ulnar nerve, artery, and veins
29 掌側橈骨手根靱帯 Palmar radiocarpal ligament
30 屈筋支帯 Flexor retinaculum
31 橈骨動静脈(浅掌枝) Radial artery and vein (superficial palmar branch)
32 正中神経 Median nerve
33 橈側手根屈筋(腱) Flexor carpi radialis muscle(tendon)
34 長掌筋 Palmaris longus muscle
35 長母指屈筋 Flexor pollicis longus muscle

50 上 肢

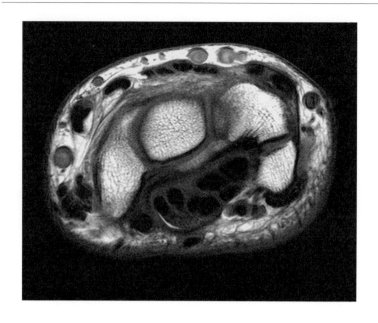

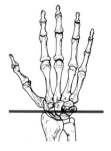

手背側

橈側 □ 尺側

手掌側

上肢，軸位断 **51**

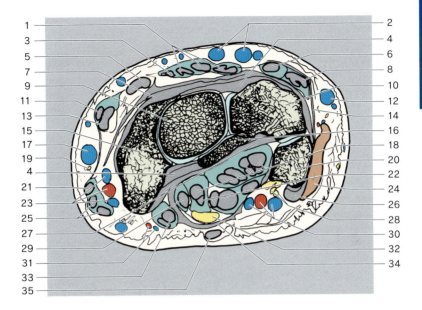

1 指伸筋(腱) Extensor digitorum muscle (tendons)
2 皮静脈 Cutaneous vein
3 示指伸筋(腱) Extensor indicis muscle (tendon)
4 関節包 Joint capsule
5 短橈側手根伸筋(腱) Extensor carpi radialis brevis muscle (tendon)
6 小指伸筋(腱) Extensor digiti minimi muscle (tendon)
7 背側手根間靱帯 Dorsal intercarpal ligament
8 尺側手根伸筋(腱) Extensor carpi ulnaris muscle (tendon)
9 有頭骨 Capitate
10 三角骨 Triquetrum
11 長母指伸筋(腱) Extensor pollicis longus muscle (tendon)
12 尺側皮静脈 Basilic vein
13 長橈側手根伸筋(腱) Extensor carpi radialis longus muscle (tendon)
14 掌側尺骨手根靱帯 Palmar ulnocarpal ligament
15 舟状骨 Scaphoid
16 月状骨 Lunate
17 橈側皮静脈 Cephalic vein
18 深指屈筋(腱) Flexor digitorum profundus muscle (tendons)
19 橈骨神経(浅枝) Radial nerve (superficial branch)
20 豆状骨 Pisiform
21 短母指伸筋(腱) Extensor pollicis brevis muscle (tendon)
22 浅指屈筋(腱) Flexor digitorum superficialis muscle (tendons)
23 橈骨動静脈 Radial artery and veins
24 小指外転筋 Abductor digiti minimi muscle
25 長母指外転筋(腱) Abductor pollicis longus muscle (tendon)
26 尺側手根屈筋 Flexor carpi ulnaris muscle
27 掌側橈骨手根靱帯 Palmar radiocarpal ligament
28 尺骨神経 Ulnar nerve
29 長母指屈筋(腱) Flexor pollicis longus muscle (tendon)
30 尺骨動静脈 Ulnar artery and veins
31 橈骨動静脈(浅掌枝) Radial artery and vein (superficial palmar branch)
32 正中神経 Median nerve
33 橈側手根屈筋(腱) Flexor carpi radialis muscle (tendon)
34 屈筋支帯 Flexor retinaculum
35 長掌筋(腱) Palmaris longus muscle (tendon)

52　上　肢

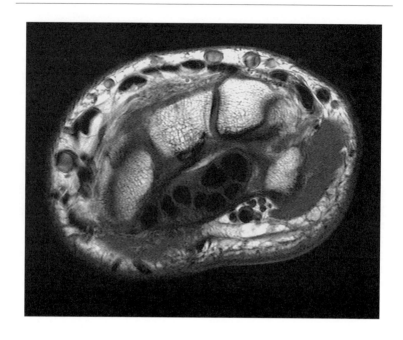

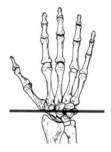

手背側

橈側　□　尺側

手掌側

上肢，軸位断

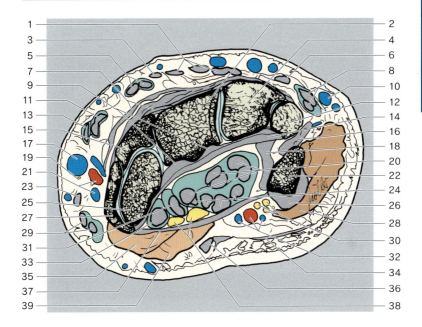

1 指伸筋（腱）Extensor digitorum muscle (tendons)
2 有頭骨 Capitate
3 示指伸筋（腱）Extensor indicis muscle (tendon)
4 有鈎骨 Hamate
5 短橈側手根伸筋（腱）Extensor carpi radialis brevis muscle (tendon)
6 小指伸筋（腱）Extensor digiti minimi muscle (tendon)
7 背側手根間靱帯 Dorsal intercarpal ligament
8 尺側手根伸筋（腱）Extensor carpi ulnaris muscle (tendon)
9 関節包 Joint capsule
10 尺側皮静脈 Basilic vein
11 長橈側手根伸筋（腱）Extensor carpi radialis longus muscle (tendon)
12 三角骨 Triquetrum
13 長母指伸筋（腱）Extensor pollicis longus muscle (tendon)
14 掌側手根間靱帯 Palmar intercarpal ligament
15 小菱形骨 Trapezoid
16 豆中手靱帯 Pisometacarpal ligament
17 橈側皮静脈 Cephalic vein
18 豆鈎靱帯 Pisohamate ligament
19 橈骨神経（浅枝）Radial nerve (superficial branch)
20 深指屈筋（腱）Flexor digitorum profundus muscle (tendons)
21 橈骨動静脈 Radial artery and veins
22 豆状骨 Pisiform
23 短母指伸筋（腱）Extensor pollicis brevis muscle (tendon)
24 浅指屈筋（腱）Flexor digitorum superficialis muscle (tendons)
25 舟状骨 Scaphoid
26 尺側手根屈筋（腱）Flexor carpi ulnaris muscle (tendon)
27 大菱形骨 Trapezium
28 小指外転筋 Abductor digiti minimi muscle
29 長母指外転筋（腱）Abductor pollicis longus muscle (tendon)
30 尺骨神経 Ulnar nerve
31 長母指屈筋（腱）Flexor pollicis longus muscle (tendon)
32 尺骨動静脈 Ulnar artery and veins
33 橈側手根屈筋（腱）Flexor carpi radialis muscle (tendon)
34 短掌筋（腱）Palmaris brevis muscle (tendon)
35 母指対立筋 Opponens pollicis muscle
36 長掌筋（腱）Palmaris longus muscle (tendon)
37 屈筋支帯 Flexor retinaculum
38 正中神経 Median nerve
39 短母指外転筋 Abductor pollicis brevis muscle

54 上 肢

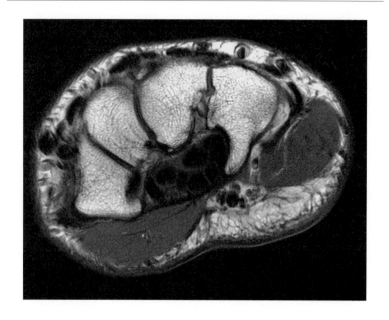

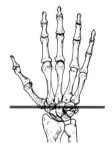

手背側

橈側 ☐ 尺側

手掌側

上肢，軸位断　55

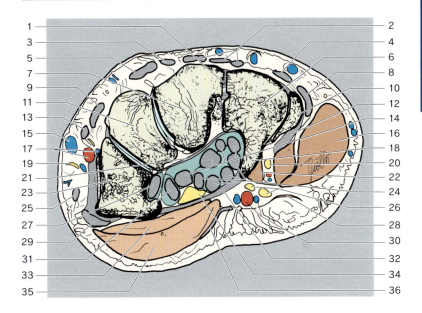

1 (有頭有鈎)手根間関節 Intercarpal (capitato-hamate) joint
2 指伸筋(腱) Extensor digitorum muscle (tendons)
3 示指伸筋(腱) Extensor indicis muscle (tendon)
4 小指伸筋(腱) Extensor digiti minimi muscle (tendon)
5 短橈側手根伸筋(腱) Extensor carpi radialis brevis muscle (tendon)
6 有鈎骨 Hamate
7 有頭骨 Capitate
8 尺側手根伸筋(腱) Extensor carpi ulnaris muscle (tendon)
9 長橈側手根伸筋(腱) Extensor carpi radialis longus muscle (tendon)
10 第5中手骨(底) Metacarpal V (base)
11 小菱形骨 Trapezoid
12 豆中手靱帯 Pisometacarpal ligament
13 長母指伸筋(腱) Extensor pollicis longus muscle (tendon)
14 深指屈筋(腱) Flexor digitorum profundus muscle (tendons)
15 橈側皮静脈 Cephalic vein
16 小指外転筋 Abductor digiti minimi muscle
17 橈骨動静脈 Radial artery and veins
18 有鈎骨(鈎) Hamate (hook)
19 橈骨神経(浅枝) Radial nerve (superficial branch)
20 尺骨神経(深枝) Ulnar nerve (deep branch)
21 掌側手根間靱帯 Palmar intercarpal ligament
22 短小指屈筋 Flexor digiti minimi brevis muscle
23 大菱形骨 Trapezium
24 浅指屈筋(腱) Flexor digitorum superficialis muscle (tendons)
25 短母指伸筋(腱) Extensor pollicis brevis muscle (tendon)
26 尺骨神経 Ulnar nerve
27 橈側手根屈筋(腱) Flexor carpi radialis muscle (tendon)
28 短掌筋 Palmaris brevis muscle
29 長母指外転筋(腱) Abductor pollicis longus muscle (tendon)
30 尺骨動静脈 Ulnar artery and veins
31 長母指屈筋(腱) Flexor pollicis longus muscle (tendon)
32 屈筋支帯 Flexor retinaculum
33 母指対立筋 Opponens pollicis muscle
34 正中神経 Median nerve
35 短母指外転筋 Abductor pollicis brevis muscle
36 手掌腱膜 Palmar aponeurosis

56　上 肢

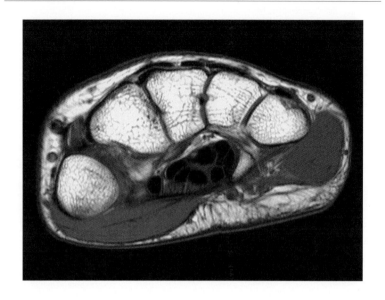

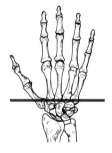

　　　　　手背側

橈側　☐　尺側

　　　　　手掌側

上肢, 軸位断

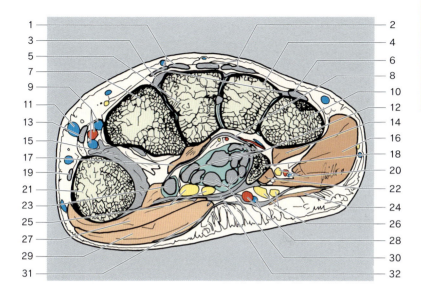

1 示指伸筋(腱) Extensor indicis muscle (tendon)
2 指伸筋(腱) Extensor digitorum muscle (tendons)
3 背側中手靭帯 Dorsal metacarpal ligament
4 第4中手骨(底) Metacarpal Ⅳ (base)
5 第3中手骨(底) Metacarpal Ⅲ (base)
6 小指伸筋(腱) Extensor digiti minimi muscle (tendon)
7 第2中手骨(底) Metacarpal Ⅱ (base)
8 掌側手根間靭帯 Palmar intercarpal ligament
9 橈骨動静脈 Radial artery and veins
10 第5中手骨(底) Metacarpal Ⅴ (base)
11 橈側皮静脈 Cephalic vein
12 深指屈筋(腱) Flexor digitorum profundus muscle (tendons)
13 長母指伸筋(腱) Extensor pollicis longus muscle (tendon)
14 小指対立筋 Opponens digiti minimi muscle
15 関節包 Joint capsule
16 小指外転筋 Abductor digiti minimi muscle
17 母指内転筋(斜頭) Adductor pollicis muscle (oblique head)
18 有鈎骨(鈎) Hamate (hook)
19 短母指伸筋(腱) Extensor pollicis brevis muscle (tendon)
20 尺骨神経, 尺骨動静脈(深枝) Ulnar nerve, artery, and vein (deep branch)
21 第1中手骨(底) Metacarpal Ⅰ (base)
22 短小指屈筋 Flexor digiti minimi brevis muscle
23 長母指屈筋(腱) Flexor pollicis longus muscle (tendon)
24 短掌筋 Palmaris brevis muscle
25 正中神経 Median nerve
26 尺骨神経 Ulnar nerve
27 母指対立筋 Opponens pollicis muscle
28 尺骨動静脈 Ulnar artery and vein
29 短母指外転筋 Abductor pollicis brevis muscle
30 浅指屈筋(腱) Flexor digitorum superficialis muscle (tendons)
31 手掌腱膜 Palmar aponeurosis
32 屈筋支帯 Flexor retinaculum

58 上　肢

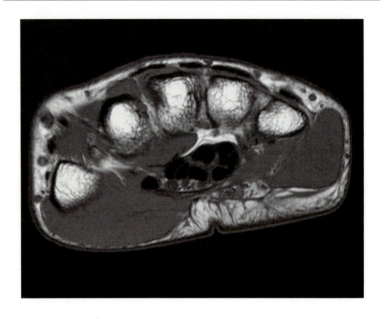

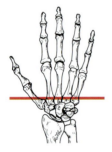

手背側
橈側　□　尺側
手掌側

上肢，軸位断

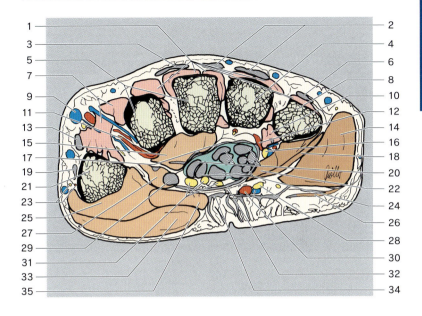

1 背側骨間筋 Dorsal interosseous muscles
2 指伸筋(腱) Extensor digitorum muscle (tendons)
3 示指伸筋(腱) Extensor indicis muscle (tendon)
4 第4中手骨(底) Metacarpal Ⅳ(base)
5 第2, 第3中手骨(底) Metacarpals Ⅱ and Ⅲ (bases)
6 小指伸筋(腱) Extensor digiti minimi muscle(tendon)
7 第1背側骨間筋 Dorsal interosseous muscle Ⅰ
8 第5中手骨 Metacarpal Ⅴ
9 橈側皮静脈 Cephalic vein
10 掌側骨間筋 Palmar interosseous muscles
11 深掌動脈弓 Deep palmar arch 橈骨動脈から
12 深掌動脈弓 Deep palmar arch 尺骨動脈から
13 長母指伸筋(腱) Extensor pollicis longus muscle(tendon)
14 小指外転筋 Abductor digiti minimi muscle
15 母指内転筋(斜頭) Adductor pollicis muscle (oblique head)
16 尺骨神経(深枝) Ulnar nerve(deep branch)
17 掌側手根間靱帯 Palmar intercarpal ligament
18 短小指屈筋 Flexor digiti minimi brevis muscle
19 短母指伸筋(腱) Extensor pollicis brevis muscle(tendon)
20 深指屈筋(腱) Flexor digitorum profundus muscle(tendons)
21 第1中手骨 Metacarpal Ⅰ
22 小指対立筋 Opponens digiti minimi muscle
23 母指の背側指神経, 動脈 Dorsal nerve and artery of thumb
24 浅指屈筋(腱) Flexor digitorum superficialis muscle(tendons)
25 母指対立筋 Opponens pollicis muscle
26 短掌筋 Palmaris brevis muscle
27 短母指屈筋(深頭) Flexor pollicis brevis muscle(deep head)
28 尺骨神経 Ulnar nerve
29 長母指屈筋(腱) Flexor pollicis longus muscle (tendon)
30 尺骨動静脈 Ulnar artery and veins
31 正中神経 Median nerve
32 屈筋支帯 Flexor retinaculum
33 短母指外転筋 Abductor pollicis brevis muscle
34 手掌腱膜 Palmar aponeurosis
35 短母指屈筋(浅頭) Flexor pollicis brevis muscle(superficial head)

60　上　肢

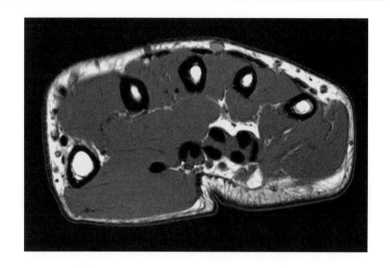

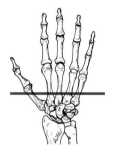

手背側

橈側　□　尺側

手掌側

上肢，軸位断

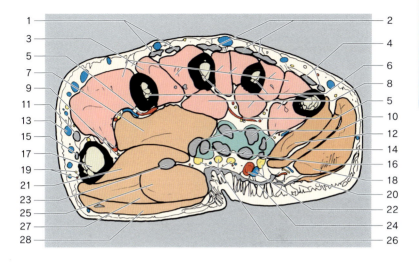

1 示指伸筋(腱) Extensor indicis muscle (tendon)
2 指伸筋(腱) Extensor digitorum muscle (tendons)
3 背側骨間筋 Dorsal interosseous muscles
4 小指伸筋(腱) Extensor digiti minimi muscle (tendon)
5 深掌動脈弓 Deep palmar arch
6 第2-第5中手骨(体) Metacarpals II - V (shafts)
7 母指内転筋(斜頭) Adductor pollicis muscle (oblique head)
8 掌側骨間筋 Palmar interosseous muscles
9 母指主動脈 Princeps pollicis artery，(母指の)掌側指神経 Palmar digital nerve(of thumb)
10 深指屈筋(腱) Flexor digitorum profundus muscle(tendons)
11 長母指伸筋(腱) Extensor pollicis longus muscle(tendon)
12 小指対立筋 Opponens digiti minimi muscle
13 (母指の)橈側皮静脈 Cephalic vein(of thumb)
14 短小指屈筋 Flexor digiti minimi brevis muscle
15 短母指伸筋(腱) Extensor pollicis brevis muscle(tendon)
16 浅指屈筋(腱) Flexor digitorum superficialis muscle(tendons)
17 第1中手骨(体) Metacarpal I (shaft)
18 小指外転筋 Abductor digiti minimi muscle
19 母指の背側指動脈，神経 Dorsal digital artery and nerve of thumb
20 短掌筋 Palmaris brevis muscle
21 短母指屈筋(深頭) Flexor pollicis brevis muscle(deep head)
22 尺骨神経,動静脈 Ulnar nerve, artery, and vein
23 長母指屈筋 Flexor pollicis longus muscle
24 手掌腱膜 Palmar aponeurosis
25 短母指屈筋(浅頭) Flexor pollicis brevis muscle(superficial head)
26 正中神経 Median nerve
27 母指対立筋 Opponens pollicis muscle
28 短母指外転筋 Abductor pollicis brevis muscle

62　上 肢

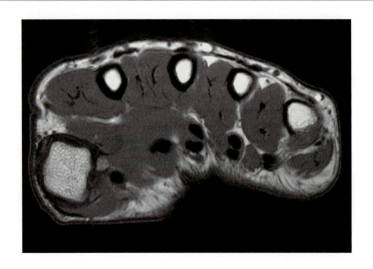

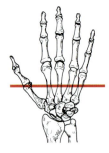

手背側

橈側 □ 尺側

手掌側

上肢，軸位断　63

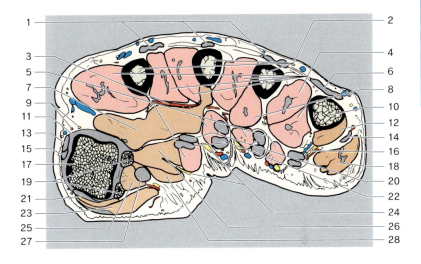

1 **指伸筋（腱）** Extensor digitorum muscle (tendons)
2 **第2-第4中手骨（体）** Metacarpals II-IV (shafts)
3 **深掌動脈弓** Deep palmar arch
4 **背側骨間筋** Dorsal interosseous muscles
5 **虫様筋** Lumbrical muscles
6 **小指伸筋（腱）** Extensor digiti minimi muscle (tendon)
7 **母指内転筋（横頭）** Adductor pollicis muscle (transverse head)
8 **掌側骨間筋** Palmar interosseous muscles
9 **母指の背側指神経, 動脈** Dorsal digital nerve and artery of thumb
10 **第5中手骨（頭）** Metacarpal V (head)
11 **側副靱帯** Collateral ligament
12 **小指対立筋（腱）** Opponens digiti minimi muscle (tendon)
13 **長母指伸筋（腱）** Extensor pollicis longus muscle (tendon)
14 **短小指屈筋（+腱）** Flexor digiti minimi brevis muscle (+tendon)
15 **短母指伸筋（腱）** Extensor pollicis brevis muscle (tendon)
16 **尺骨神経（浅枝）** Ulnar nerve (superficial branch)
17 **第1中手骨（頭）** Metacarpal I (head)
18 **小指外転筋** Abductor digiti minimi muscle
19 **種子骨** Sesamoid bones
20 **深指屈筋（腱）** Flexor digitorum profundus muscle (tendons)
21 **母指対立筋（+腱付着部）** Opponens pollicis muscle (+tendon attachment)
22 **浅指屈筋（腱）** Flexor digitorum superficialis muscle (tendons)
23 **短母指外転筋** Abductor pollicis brevis muscle
24 **総掌側指神経（正中神経）** Common palmar digital nerves (median nerve)
25 **短母指屈筋（浅頭）** Flexor pollicis brevis muscle (superficial head)
26 **母指内転筋（斜頭）** Adductor pollicis muscle (oblique head)
27 **長母指屈筋（腱）** Flexor pollicis longus muscle (tendon)
28 **短母指屈筋（深頭）** Flexor pollicis brevis muscle (deep head)

64　上 肢

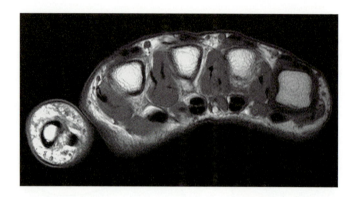

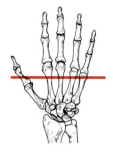

手背側

橈側　□　尺側

手掌側

上肢，軸位断

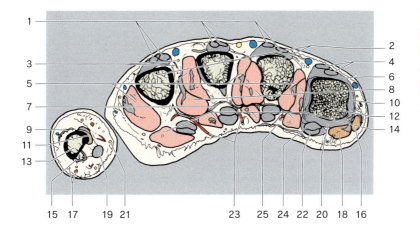

1 指伸筋(腱) Extensor digitorum muscle (tendons)
2 第2-第4中手骨(体) MetacarpalsⅡ-Ⅳ (shafts)
3 背側指動脈,神経 Dorsal digital artery and nerve
4 小指伸筋(腱) Extensor digiti minimi muscle(tendon)
5 背側骨間筋 Dorsal interosseous muscles
6 指背(伸筋)腱膜展開部 Dorsal(extensor) expansion
7 深横中手靱帯 Deep transverse metacarpal ligament
8 掌側骨間筋 Palmar interosseous muscles
9 母指伸筋(腱膜) Extensor pollicis muscle (aponeurosis)
10 側副靱帯 Collateral ligament
11 母指内転筋(腱付着部) Adductor pollicis muscle(tendon attachment)
12 第5中手骨(頭) Metacarpal Ⅴ(head)
13 第1基節骨 Proximal phalanx Ⅰ
14 虫様筋 Lumbrical muscles
15 短母指屈筋 Flexor pollicis brevis muscle, 短母指外転筋 Abductor pollicis brevis muscle (腱付着部 tendon attachment)
16 小指外転筋 Abductor digiti minimi muscle
17 母指の背側指神経,動脈 Dorsal digital nerve and artery of thumb
18 短小指屈筋 Flexor digiti minimi brevis muscle
19 長母指屈筋(腱) Flexor pollicis longus muscle (tendon)
20 掌側靱帯 Palmar ligament
21 母指の掌側指動脈,神経 Palmar digital artery and nerve of thumb
22 浅指屈筋(腱) Flexor digitorum superficialis muscle(tendons)
23 掌側指動脈,神経 Palmar digital arteries and nerves
24 深指屈筋(腱) Flexor digitorum profundus muscle(tendons)
25 手掌腱膜 Palmar aponeurosis, 縦束 Longitudinal fasciculi

66　上　肢

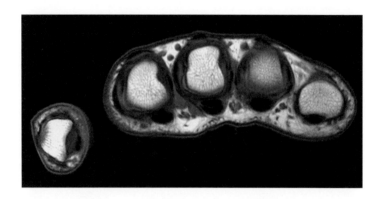

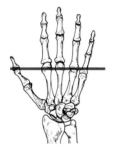

手背側

橈側 ☐ 尺側

手掌側

上肢，軸位断

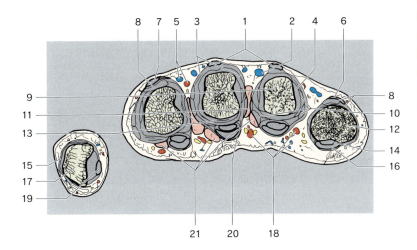

1 指伸筋(腱) Extensor digitorum muscle (tendons)
2 背側指静脈 Dorsal digital vein
3 矢状索 Sagittal ligament
4 側副靱帯 Collateral ligament
5 背側指動脈,神経 Dorsal digital artery and nerve
6 小指伸筋(腱) Extensor digiti minimi muscle(tendon)
7 示指伸筋(腱) Extensor indicis muscle (tendon)
8 指背(伸筋)腱膜展開部 Dorsal(extensor) expansion
"指背腱膜" dorsal aponeurosis
9 中手骨(体) Metacarpals(shafts)
10 骨間筋(腱) Interosseous muscle(tendon)
11 骨間筋 Interosseous muscle
12 第5基節骨(底) Proximal phalanx Ⅴ(base)
13 掌側靱帯 Palmar ligament
14 深指屈筋(腱) Flexor digitorum profundus muscle(tendons)
15 母指伸筋(腱膜) Extensor pollicis muscle (aponeurosis)
16 浅指屈筋(腱) Flexor digitorum superficialis muscle(tendon)
17 第1基節骨 Proximal phalanx Ⅰ
18 掌側指動脈,神経 Palmar digital arteries and nerves
19 長母指屈筋(腱) Flexor pollicis longus muscle (tendon)
20 指の線維鞘 Digital fibrous sheath
21 虫様筋 Lumbrical muscle

68　上　肢

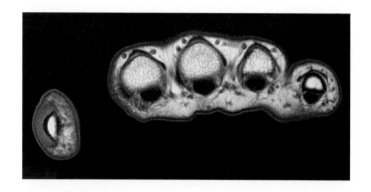

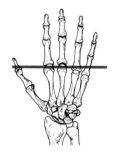

手背側

橈側 □ 尺側

手掌側

上肢，軸位断

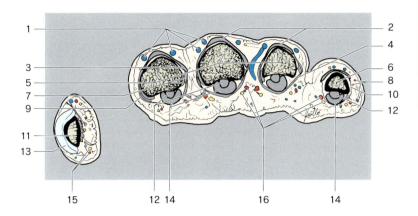

1 背側指静脈 Dorsal digital vein
2 指伸筋(腱膜) Extensor digitorum muscle (aponeurosis)
3 側副靱帯 Collateral ligament
4 指の線維鞘 Digital fibrous sheath
5 第2-4基節骨(底) Proximal phalanges Ⅱ-Ⅳ(bases)
6 第5基節骨(体) Proximal phalanx Ⅴ(shaft)
7 骨間筋(腱) Interosseous muscles(tendon)
8 背側指動脈，神経 Dorsal digital artery and nerve
9 矢状索 Sagittal ligament
10 側副靱帯 Collateral ligament
11 第1末節骨 Distal phalanx Ⅰ
12 深指屈筋(腱) Flexor digitorum profundus muscle(tendons)
13 爪体 Body of fingernail
14 浅指屈筋(腱) Flexor digitorum superficialis muscle(tendons)
15 母指の掌側指動脈，神経 Palmar digital arteries and nerves of thumb
16 掌側指動脈，神経 Palmar digital arteries and nerves

70　上　肢

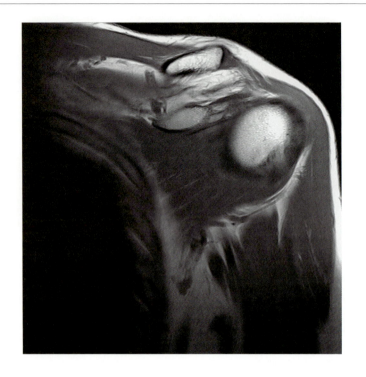

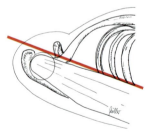

頭側

内側　□　外側

尾側

肩，冠状断　71

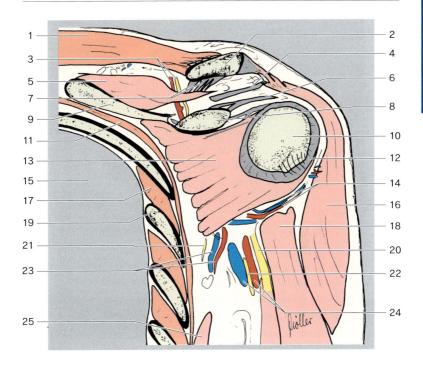

1 僧帽筋　Trapezius muscle
2 鎖骨　Clavicle
3 肩甲上動(静)脈，神経　Suprascapular artery (+vein) and nerve
4 烏口肩峰靱帯　Coracoacromial ligament
5 棘上筋　Supraspinatus muscle
6 烏口上腕靱帯　Coracohumeral ligament
7 烏口鎖骨靱帯　Coracoclavicular ligament
8 烏口突起　Coracoid process
9 肩甲骨(上縁)　Scapula (superior border)
10 上腕骨(頭)　Humerus (head)
11 前鋸筋　Serratus anterior muscle
12 関節包　Joint capsule
13 肩甲下筋　Subscapularis muscle
14 前上腕回旋動静脈　Anterior circumflex humeral artery and vein
15 肺　Lung
16 三角筋　Deltoid muscle
17 肋間筋　Intercostal muscle
18 烏口腕筋　Coracobrachialis muscle
19 肋骨　Rib
20 橈骨神経　Radial nerve
21 胸背神経　Thoracodorsal nerve
22 正中神経　Median nerve
23 肩甲下動脈　Subscapular artery and vein
24 上腕動静脈　Brachial artery and vein
25 広背筋　Latissimus dorsi muscle

72　上　肢

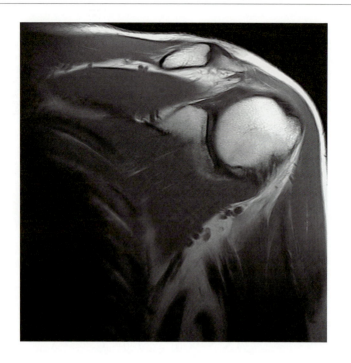

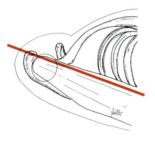

頭側

内側 □ 外側

尾側

肩, 冠状断 73

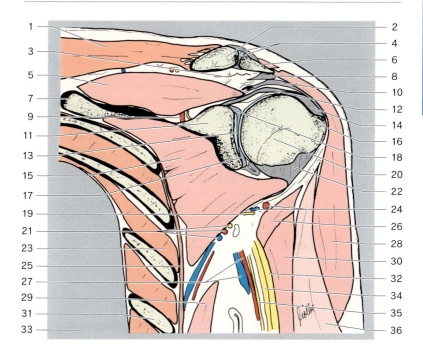

1 僧帽筋 Trapezius muscle
2 鎖骨 Clavicle
3 肩峰下包 Subacromial bursa
4 肩鎖関節 Acromioclavicular joint, 肩鎖靱帯 Acromioclavicular ligament
5 棘上筋 Supraspinatus muscle
6 肩峰 Acromion
7 肩甲骨 Scapula
8 烏口肩峰靱帯 Coracoacromial ligament
9 肩甲上動(静)脈,神経 Suprascapular artery (+vein) and nerve
10 烏口上腕靱帯 Coracohumeral ligament
11 関節窩 Glenoid
12 上腕二頭筋(長頭,腱) Biceps brachii muscle (long head, tendon)
13 肩関節(関節窩上腕関節) Glenohumeral joint
14 棘上筋(腱付着部) Supraspinatus muscle (tendon attachment)
15 肩甲下筋 Subscapularis muscle
16 大結節 Greater tubercle
17 (下方)関節唇 Glenoid labrum (inferior)
18 (上方)関節唇 Glenoid labrum (superior)
19 腋窩神経 Axillary nerve
20 上腕骨(頭) Humerus (head)
21 肩甲下動静脈,神経 Subscapular artery, vein, and nerve
22 関節上腕靱帯 Glenohumeral ligament
23 肋間筋 Intercostal muscle
24 後上腕回旋動静脈 Posterior circumflex humeral artery and vein
25 前鋸筋 Serratus anterior muscle
26 大円筋 Teres major muscle
27 腋窩動静脈 Axillary artery and vein
28 三角筋 Deltoid muscle
29 広背筋 Latissimus dorsi muscle
30 烏口腕筋 Coracobrachialis muscle
31 肋骨 Rib
32 橈骨神経 Radial nerve
33 肺 Lung
34 正中神経 Median nerve
35 尺骨神経 Ulnar nerve
36 上腕二頭筋(長頭) Biceps brachii muscle (long head)

74　上肢

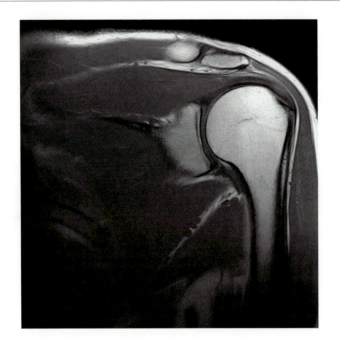

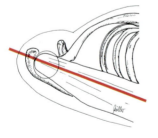

	頭側	
内側		外側
	尾側	

肩，冠状断 75

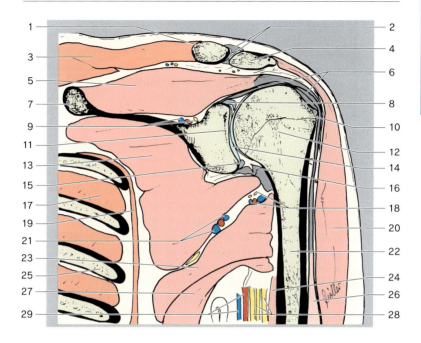

1 鎖骨 Clavicle
2 肩鎖関節 Acromioclavicular joint, 肩鎖靱帯 Acromioclavicular ligament
3 僧帽筋 Trapezius muscle
4 肩峰 Acromion
5 棘上筋 Supraspinatus muscle
6 上腕二頭筋(長頭，腱) Biceps brachii muscle (long head, tendon)
7 肩甲骨 Scapula
8 (上方)関節唇 Glenoid labrum(superior)
9 肩甲上動脈，静脈，神経 Suprascapular artery, vein, and nerve
10 大結節 Greater tubercle
11 関節窩 Glenoid
12 上腕骨(頭) Humerus(head)
13 肩甲下筋 Subscapularis muscle
14 肩関節(関節窩上腕関節) Glenohumeral joint
15 (下方)関節唇 Glenoid labrum(inferior)
16 腋窩陥凹 Axillary recess
17 肋間筋 Intercostal muscle
18 後上腕回旋動静脈 Posterior circumflex humeral artery and vein, 腋窩神経 Axillary nerve
19 前鋸筋 Serratus anterior muscle
20 三角筋 Deltoid muscle
21 肩甲下動静脈 Subscapular artery and vein
22 上腕骨(体) Humerus(shaft)
23 大円筋 Teres major muscle
24 烏口腕筋 Coracobrachialis muscle
25 肋骨 Rib
26 上腕二頭筋(長頭) Biceps brachii muscle (long head)
27 広背筋 Latissimus dorsi muscle
28 尺骨神経 Ulnar nerve, 正中神経 Median nerve, 橈骨神経 Radial nerve
29 上腕動静脈 Brachial artery and vein

76　上　肢

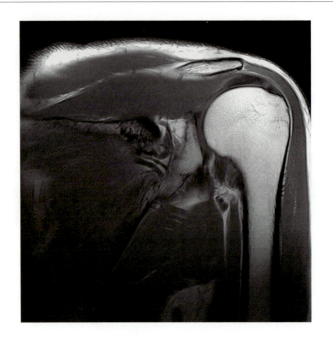

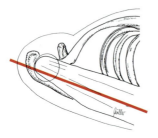

頭側
内側　　　外側
尾側

肩，冠状断

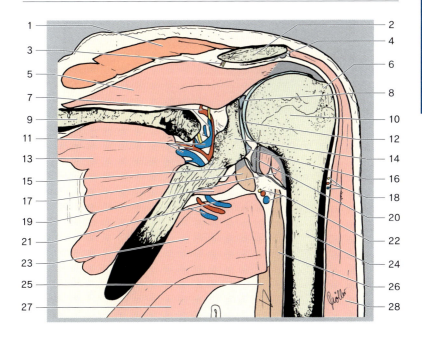

1 僧帽筋 Trapezius muscle
2 肩峰 Acromion
3 肩甲下動静脈(肩峰枝) Suprascapular artery and vein(acromial branch)
4 肩峰下包 Subacromial bursa
5 棘上筋 Supraspinatus muscle
6 大結節 Greater tubercle
7 肩甲上動静脈，神経 Suprascapular artery, vein, and nerve
8 (上方)関節唇 Glenoid labrum(superior)
9 肩甲骨 Scapula
10 上腕骨(頭) Humerus(head)
11 肩甲回旋動静脈 Circumflex scapular artery and vein
12 肩関節(関節窩上腕関節) Glenohumeral joint
13 棘下筋 Infraspinatus muscle
14 関節窩 Glenoid
15 肩甲頚 Neck of scapula
16 (下方)関節唇 Glenoid labrum(inferior)
17 上腕三頭筋(長頭，腱付着部) Triceps brachii muscle(long head, tendon attachment)
18 後上腕回旋動静脈 Posterior circumflex humeral artery and vein,
腋窩神経(筋枝) Axillary nerve(muscular branches)
19 小円筋 Teres minor muscle
20 腋窩陥凹 Axillary recess
21 肩甲下動静脈 Subscapular artery and vein
22 後上腕回旋動静脈 Posterior circumflex humeral artery and vein,
腋窩神経 Axillary nerve
23 大円筋 Teres major muscle
24 上腕骨(体) Humerus(shaft)
25 上腕三頭筋(長頭) Triceps brachii muscle(long head)
26 上腕三頭筋(外側頭) Triceps brachii muscle(lateral head)
27 広背筋 Latissimus dorsi muscle
28 三角筋 Deltoid muscle

78 上 肢

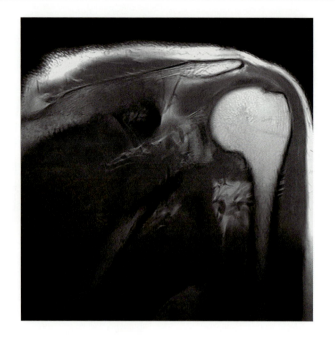

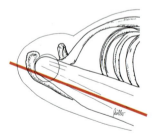

頭側
内側 　　 外側
尾側

肩，冠状断 79

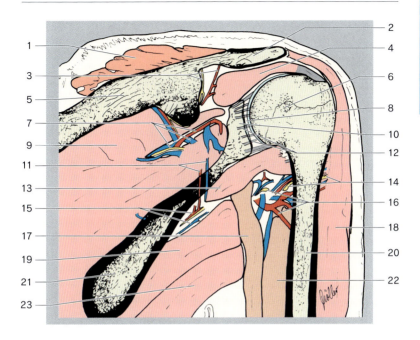

1 僧帽筋 Trapezius muscle
2 肩峰 Acromion
3 肩甲上動脈，神経(肩峰枝) Suprascapular artery and nerve (acromial branch)
4 棘上筋 Supraspinatus muscle
5 肩甲棘 Scapula (spine)
6 上腕骨(頭) Humerus (head)
7 肩甲上動静脈，神経 Suprascapular artery, vein, and nerve
8 肩関節(関節窩上腕関節) Glenohumeral joint
9 棘下筋 Infraspinatus muscle
10 関節窩 Glenoid
11 肩甲回旋動静脈 Circumflex scapular artery and vein
12 関節包 Joint capsule
13 小円筋 Teres minor muscle
14 後上腕回旋動静脈 Posterior circumflex humeral artery and vein, 腋窩神経(筋枝) Axillary nerve (muscular branches)
15 肩甲下動静脈 Subscapular artery and vein
16 後上腕回旋動静脈 Posterior circumflex humeral artery and vein, 腋窩神経 Axillary nerve
17 上腕三頭筋(長頭) Triceps brachii muscle (long head)
18 三角筋 Deltoid muscle
19 大円筋 Teres major muscle
20 上腕骨(体) Humerus (shaft)
21 肩甲骨 Scapula
22 上腕三頭筋(外側頭) Triceps brachii muscle (lateral head)
23 広背筋 Latissimus dorsi muscle

80 上肢

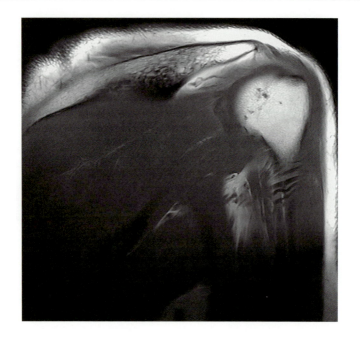

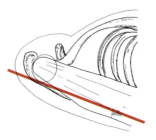

頭側
内側　　外側
尾側

肩，冠状断 *81*

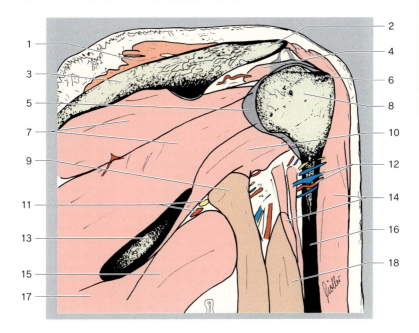

1 僧帽筋 Trapezius muscle
2 肩峰 Acromion
3 肩甲棘 Scapula(spine)
4 棘上筋 Supraspinatus muscle
5 関節包 Joint capsule
6 大結節 Greater tubercle
7 棘下筋 Infraspinatus muscle
8 上腕骨(頭) Humerus(head)
9 上腕三頭筋(長頭) Triceps brachii muscle (long head)
10 小円筋 Teres minor muscle
11 肩甲下動(静)脈,神経 Subscapular artery (+vein)and nerve
12 後上腕回旋動静脈 Posterior circumflex humeral artery and vein, 腋窩神経 Axillary nerve
13 肩甲骨 Scapula
14 三角筋 Deltoid muscle
15 大円筋 Teres major muscle
16 上腕骨(体) Humerus(shaft)
17 広背筋 Latissimus dorsi muscle
18 上腕三頭筋(外側頭) Triceps brachii muscle (lateral head)

82　上　肢

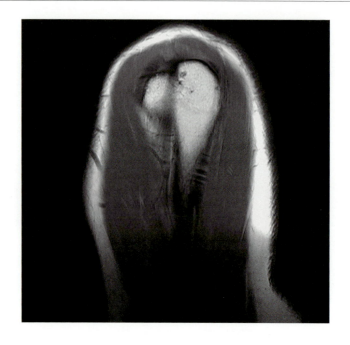

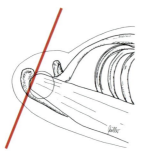

頭側
腹側　　背側
尾側

肩，矢状断 *83*

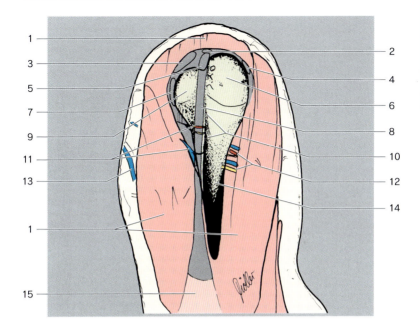

1 三角筋(肩峰部) Deltoid muscle (acromial part)
2 棘上筋(腱) Supraspinatus muscle (tendon)
3 (上)関節上腕靱帯 Glenohumeral ligament (superior)
4 棘下筋(腱) Infraspinatus muscle (tendon)
5 結節間溝(上腕二頭筋溝) Intertubercular sulcus (bicipital groove)
6 大結節 Greater tubercle
7 (中)関節上腕靱帯 Glenohumeral ligament (middle)
8 上腕二頭筋(長頭,腱) Biceps brachii muscle (long head, tendon)
9 小結節 Lesser tubercle
10 大結節稜 Crest of greater tubercle
11 前上腕回旋動静脈 Anterior circumflex humeral artery and vein
12 後上腕回旋動静脈 Posterior circumflex humeral artery and vein, 腋窩神経(枝) Axillary nerve
13 橈側皮静脈 Cephalic vein
14 上腕骨(体) Humerus (shaft)
15 上腕二頭筋(長頭) Biceps brachii muscle (long head)

84　上　肢

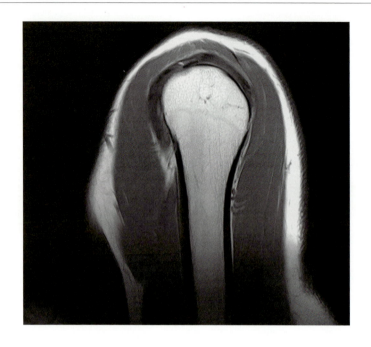

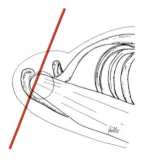

頭側

腹側　□　背側

尾側

肩，矢状断

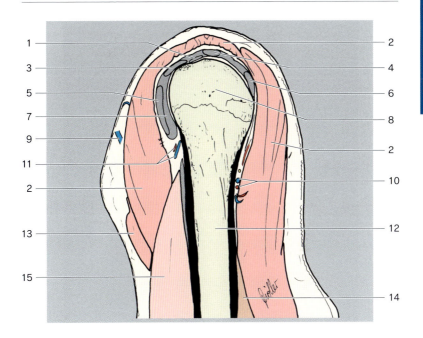

1 上腕二頭筋（長頭，腱） Biceps brachii muscle (long head, tendon)
2 三角筋（肩峰部） Deltoid muscle (acromial part)
3 （上）関節上腕靱帯 Glenohumeral ligament (superior)
4 棘上筋（腱） Supraspinatus muscle (tendon)
5 （中）関節上腕靱帯 Glenohumeral ligament (middle)
6 棘下筋（腱） Infraspinatus muscle (tendon)
7 関節包 Joint capsule
8 上腕骨（頭） Humerus (head)
9 橈側皮静脈 Cephalic vein
10 後上腕回旋動静脈 Posterior circumflex humeral artery and vein
11 前上腕回旋動静脈 Anterior circumflex humeral artery and vein
12 上腕骨（体） Humerus (shaft)
13 大胸筋 Pectoralis major muscle
14 上腕三頭筋（内側頭） Triceps brachii muscle (medial head)
15 上腕二頭筋（長頭） Biceps brachii muscle (long head)

86 上肢

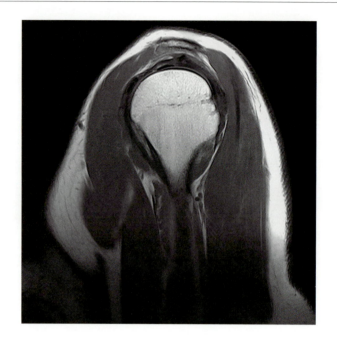

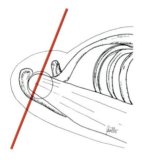

頭側

腹側 □ 背側

尾側

肩，矢状断

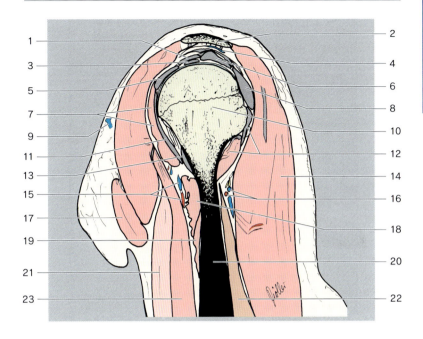

1 横上腕靱帯 Transverse humeral ligament
2 肩峰 Acromion
3 上腕二頭筋(長頭,腱) Biceps brachii muscle (long head, tendon)
4 三角筋下包 Subdeltoid bursa
5 (上)関節上腕靱帯 Glenohumeral ligament (superior)
6 棘上筋(腱) Supraspinatus muscle(tendon)
7 肩甲下筋 Subscapularis muscle
8 棘下筋(腱) Infraspinatus muscle(tendon)
9 橈側皮静脈 Cephalic vein
10 上腕骨(頭) Humerus(head)
11 (中)関節上腕靱帯 Glenohumeral ligament (middle)
12 小円筋(+腱付着部) Teres minor muscle (+tendon attachment)
13 (下)関節上腕靱帯 Glenohumeral ligament (inferior)
14 三角筋(肩峰部) Deltoid muscle(acromial part)
15 前上腕回旋動静脈 Anterior circumflex humeral artery and vein
16 後上腕回旋動静脈 Posterior circumflex humeral artery and vein
17 大胸筋 Pectoralis major muscle
18 広背筋 Latissimus dorsi muscle
19 大円筋 Teres major muscle
20 上腕骨(体) Humerus(shaft)
21 上腕二頭筋(長頭) Biceps brachii muscle (long head)
22 上腕三頭筋(内側頭) Triceps brachii muscle (medial head)
23 烏口腕筋 Coracobrachialis muscle

88　上　肢

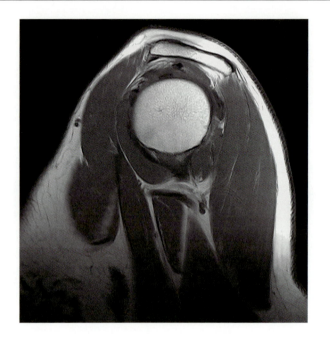

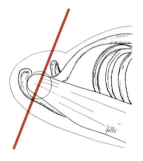

頭側
腹側 □ 背側
尾側

肩，矢状断

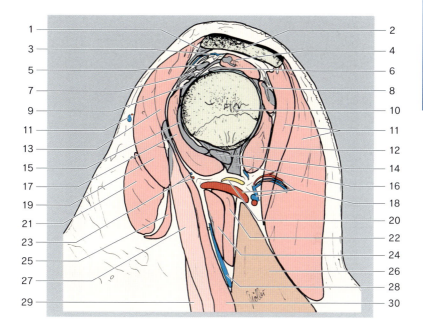

1 烏口肩峰靱帯 Coracoacromial ligament
2 肩峰 Acromion
3 肩峰下包 Subacromial bursa
4 棘上筋(+腱) Supraspinatus muscle (+tendon)
5 烏口上腕靱帯 Coracohumeral ligament
6 上腕二頭筋(長頭,腱) Biceps brachii muscle (long head, tendon)
7 横上腕靱帯 Transverse humeral ligament
8 棘下筋(+腱) Infraspinatus muscle (+tendon)
9 上関節上腕靱帯 Superior glenohumeral ligament
10 上腕骨(頭) Humerus (head)
11 橈側皮静脈 Cephalic vein
12 小円筋 Teres minor muscle
13 三角筋(肩峰部) Deltoid muscle (acromial part)
14 下関節上腕靱帯 Inferior glenohumeral ligament
15 中関節上腕靱帯 Middle glenohumeral ligament
16 大円筋(腱) Teres major muscle (tendon)
17 肩甲下筋 Subscapularis muscle
18 後上腕回旋動静脈 Posterior circumflex humeral artery and vein
19 三角筋(鎖骨部) Deltoid muscle (clavicular part)
20 腋窩神経 Axillary nerve
21 大胸筋 Pectoralis major muscle
22 大円筋 Teres major muscle
23 前上腕回旋動静脈 Anterior circumflex humeral artery and vein
24 広背筋 Latissimus dorsi muscle
25 小胸筋 Pectoralis minor muscle
26 上腕三頭筋(長頭) Triceps brachii muscle (long head)
27 上腕二頭筋(短頭+腱) Biceps brachii muscle (short head+tendon)
28 尺側皮静脈 Basilic vein
29 上腕二頭筋(長頭) Biceps brachii muscle (long head)
30 烏口腕筋 Coracobrachialis muscle

90 上　肢

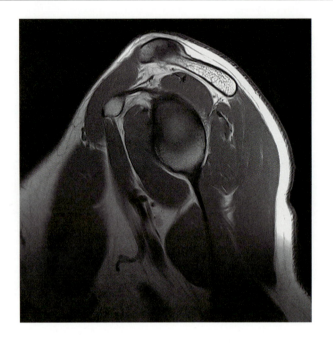

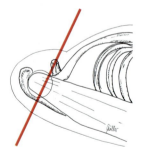

頭側

腹側　　背側

尾側

肩, 矢状断

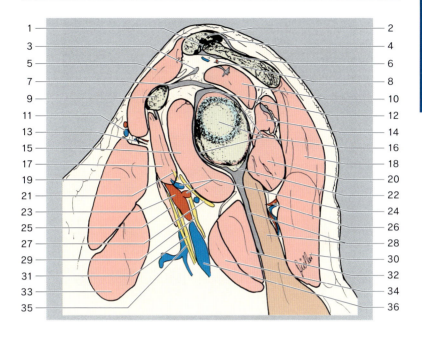

1 肩鎖関節 Acromioclavicular joint
2 鎖骨 Clavicle
3 烏口肩峰靱帯 Coracoacromial ligament
4 肩鎖靱帯 Acromioclavicular ligament
5 三角筋(鎖骨部) Deltoid muscle (clavicular part)
6 肩峰 Acromion
7 烏口上腕靱帯 Coracohumeral ligament
8 胸肩峰動脈(肩峰枝) Thoracoacromial artery (acromial branch)
9 烏口突起 Coracoid process
10 棘上筋(+腱) Supraspinatus muscle (+tendon)
11 橈側皮静脈 Cephalic vein
12 上腕二頭筋(長頭,腱付着部) Biceps brachii muscle (long head, tendon attachment)
13 胸肩峰動脈(三角筋枝) Thoracoacromial artery (deltoid branch)
14 棘下筋(+腱) Infraspinatus muscle (+tendon)
15 肩甲下筋 Subscapularis muscle
16 肩関節(関節窩上腕関節) Glenohumeral joint, 関節包 Joint capsule
17 烏口腕筋 Coracobrachialis muscle
18 三角筋(肩峰部) Deltoid muscle (acromial part)
19 大胸筋 Pectoralis major muscle
20 小円筋 Teres minor muscle
21 筋皮神経 Musculocutaneous nerve
22 関節下結節 Infraglenoid tubercle
23 上腕動脈 Brachial artery
24 後上腕回旋動静脈 Posterior circumflex humeral artery and vein
25 上腕二頭筋(短頭) Biceps brachii muscle (short head)
26 後上腕回旋動静脈(筋枝) Posterior circumflex humeral artery and vein (muscular branches)
27 腋窩神経 Axillary nerve
28 上腕三頭筋(長頭+腱) Triceps brachii muscle (long head + tendon)
29 橈骨神経 Radial nerve
30 三角筋(肩甲棘部) Deltoid muscle (spinal part)
31 尺骨神経 Ulnar nerve
32 大円筋 Teres major muscle
33 小胸筋 Pectoralis minor muscle
34 広背筋 Latissimus dorsi muscle
35 正中神経 Median nerve
36 上腕静脈 Brachial vein

92　上　肢

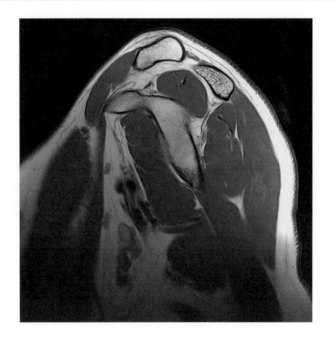

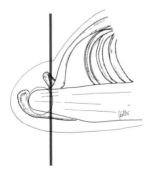

頭側

腹側　□　背側

尾側

肩，矢状断

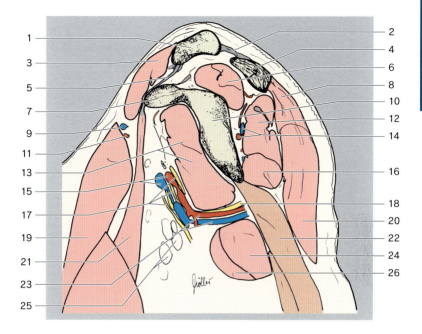

1 鎖骨 Clavicle
2 僧帽筋 Trapezius muscle
3 三角筋(鎖骨部) Deltoid muscle (clavicular part)
4 肩峰 Acromion
5 烏口鎖骨靱帯 Coracoclavicular ligament
6 棘上筋 Supraspinatus muscle
7 烏口突起 Coracoid process
8 三角筋(肩峰部) Deltoid muscle (acromial part)
9 橈側皮静脈 Cephalic vein
10 肩甲骨 Scapula
11 胸肩峰動脈(胸筋枝) Thoracoacromial artery (pectoral branch)
12 棘下筋(＋腱) Infraspinatus muscle (+tendon)
13 肩甲下筋 Subscapularis muscle
14 肩甲回旋動静脈 Circumflex scapular artery and vein
15 腋窩動静脈 Axillary artery and vein
16 小円筋 Teres minor muscle
17 腕神経叢 Brachial plexus
18 腋窩神経 Axillary nerve
19 大胸筋 Pectoralis major muscle
20 三角筋(肩甲棘部) Deltoid muscle (spinal part)
21 小胸筋 Pectoralis minor muscle
22 上腕三頭筋(長頭，腱) Triceps brachii muscle (long head, tendon)
23 後上腕回旋動静脈 Posterior circumflex humeral artery and vein
24 大円筋 Teres major muscle
25 腋窩リンパ節 Axillary lymph node
26 広背筋 Latissimus dorsi muscle

94　上　肢

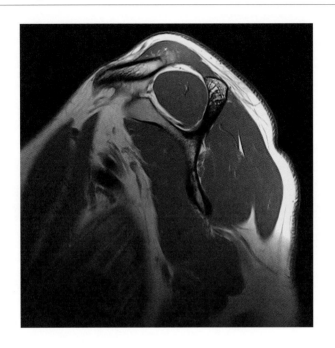

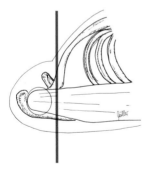

頭側

腹側　☐　背側

尾側

肩，矢状断

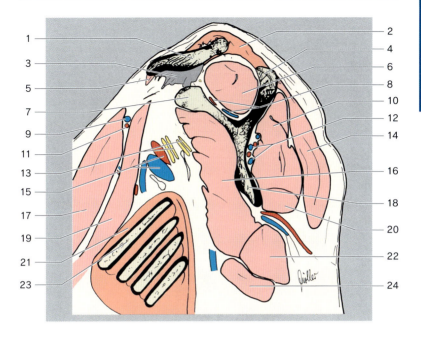

1 鎖骨 Clavicle
2 僧帽筋 Trapezius muscle
3 烏口鎖骨靱帯 Coracoclavicular ligament
4 肩峰 Acromion
5 三角筋(鎖骨部) Deltoid muscle(clavicular part)
6 棘上筋 Supraspinatus muscle
7 肩甲棘 Scapula(spine)
8 肩甲上動静脈 Suprascapular artery and vein
9 橈側皮静脈 Cephalic vein
10 棘下筋 Infraspinatus muscle
11 胸肩峰動脈(胸筋枝) Thoracoacromial artery (pectoral branch)
12 肩甲回旋動静脈 Circumflex scapular artery and vein
13 腕神経叢 Brachial plexus
14 三角筋(肩甲棘部) Deltoid muscle(spinal part)
15 腋窩動静脈 Axillary artery and vein
16 肩甲下筋 Subscapularis muscle
17 大胸筋 Pectoralis major muscle
18 肩甲骨(体) Scapula(body)
19 小胸筋 Pectoralis minor muscle
20 小円筋 Teres minor muscle
21 前鋸筋 Serratus anterior muscle
22 大円筋 Teres major muscle
23 肋骨 Ribs
24 広背筋 Latissimus dorsi muscle

96 上肢

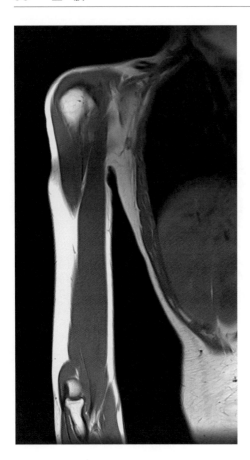

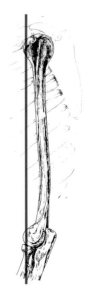

1 鎖骨 Clavicle
2 鎖骨下静脈 Subclavian vein
3 烏口突起 Coracoid process
4 内頸静脈 Internal jugular vein
5 上腕二頭筋(長頭,腱) Biceps brachii muscle (long head, tendon)

上腕, 冠状断

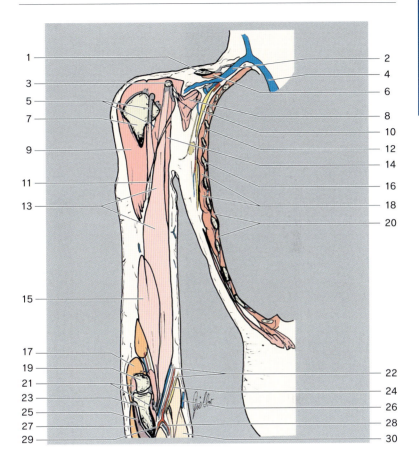

- 6 鎖骨下筋 Subclavius muscle
- 7 上腕骨(頭, 頸) Humerus (head, neck)
- 8 小胸筋 Pectoralis minor muscle
- 9 三角筋 Deltoid muscle
- 10 長胸神経 Long thoracic nerve
- 11 大胸筋(腱) Pectoralis major muscle (tendon)
- 12 肋間動静脈, 神経 Intercostal artery, vein, and nerve
- 13 上腕二頭筋(短頭) Biceps brachii muscle (short head)
- 14 烏口腕筋 Coracobrachialis muscle
- 15 上腕筋 Brachialis muscle
- 16 肋骨 Rib
- 17 腕橈骨筋 Brachioradialis muscle
- 18 前鋸筋 Serratus anterior muscle
- 19 上腕骨(小頭) Humerus (capitulum)
- 20 肋間筋 Intercostal muscles
- 21 回外筋 Supinator muscle
- 22 上腕動静脈 Brachial artery and vein
- 23 橈骨(頭) Radius (head)
- 24 正中神経 Median nerve
- 25 指伸筋 Extensor digitorum muscle
- 26 橈側皮静脈 Cephalic vein
- 27 短橈側手根伸筋 Extensor carpi radialis brevis muscle
- 28 尺骨動脈 Ulnar artery
- 29 橈骨動脈 Radial artery
- 30 円回内筋 Pronator teres muscle

98　上肢

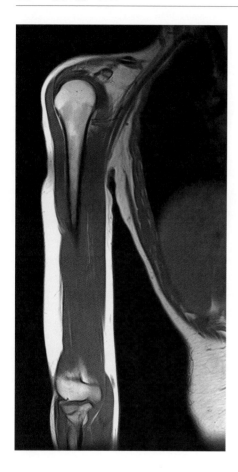

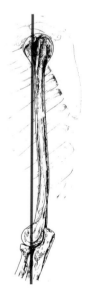

1　鎖骨　Clavicle
2　斜角筋　Scalenus muscle
3　僧帽筋　Trapezius muscle
4　鎖骨下動脈　Subclavian artery
5　棘上筋(腱)　Supraspinatus muscle(tendon)
6　鎖骨下静脈　Subclavian vein
7　烏口上腕靱帯　Coracohumeral ligament
8　鎖骨下筋　Subclavius muscle
9　上腕二頭筋(長頭, 腱)　Biceps brachii muscle (long head, tendon)
10　烏口鎖骨靱帯　Coracoclavicular ligament
11　上腕骨(頭)　Humerus(head)
12　烏口突起　Coracoid process
13　大結節　Greater tubercle
14　正中神経　Median nerve
15　前上腕回旋動静脈　Anterior circumflex humeral artery and vein
16　関節窩　Glenoid
17　三角筋　Deltoid muscle
18　腋窩動静脈　Axillary artery and vein

上腕, 冠状断 99

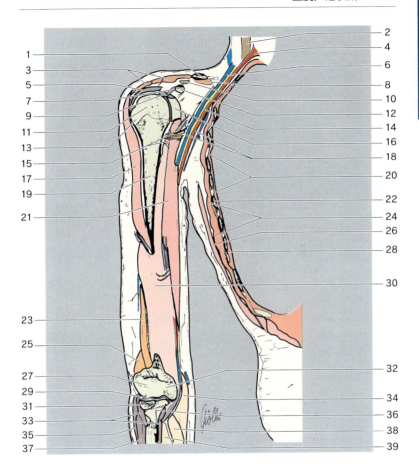

19 上腕骨(体) Humerus (shaft)
20 肋間筋 Intercostal muscles
21 烏口腕筋 Coracobrachialis muscle
22 肋骨 Rib
23 腕橈骨筋 Brachioradialis muscle
24 前鋸筋 Serratus anterior muscle
25 長橈側手根伸筋 Extensor carpi radialis longus muscle
26 広背筋 Latissimus dorsi muscle
27 上腕骨(小頭) Humerus (capitulum)
28 肋間動静脈,神経 Intercostal artery, vein, and nerve
29 腕橈関節 Humeroradial joint
30 上腕筋 Brachialis muscle
31 橈骨(頭) Radius (head)
32 上腕骨(滑車) Humerus (trochlea)
33 回外筋 Supinator muscle
34 円回内筋 Pronator teres muscle
35 尺側手根伸筋 Extensor carpi ulnaris muscle
36 尺骨 Ulna
37 指伸筋 Extensor digitorum muscle
38 橈側手根屈筋 Flexor carpi radialis muscle
39 浅指屈筋 Flexor digitorum superficialis muscle

上肢

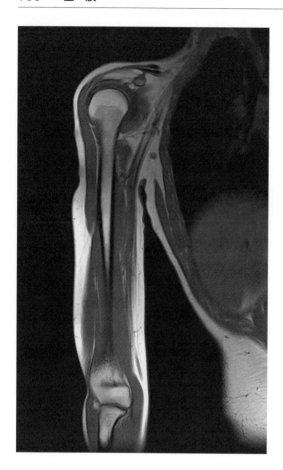

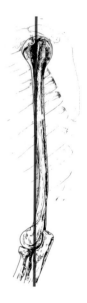

1 斜角筋 Scalenus muscle
2 腕神経叢 Brachial plexus
3 僧帽筋 Trapezius muscle
4 後神経束 Posterior(dorsal)funiculus
5 肩峰 Acromion
6 鎖骨 Clavicle
7 棘上筋(腱) Supraspinatus muscle(tendon)
8 烏口鎖骨靱帯 Coracoclavicular ligament
9 上腕二頭筋(長頭,腱) Biceps brachii muscle (long head, tendon)
10 烏口突起 Coracoid process
11 上腕骨(頭) Humerus(head)
12 関節窩 Glenoid
13 三角筋 Deltoid muscle
14 肩甲下筋 Subscapularis muscle
15 上腕骨(体) Humerus(shaft)
16 前上腕回旋動静脈 Anterior circumflex humeral artery and vein
17 烏口腕筋 Coracobrachialis muscle
18 大円筋 Teres major muscle

上腕，冠状断 101

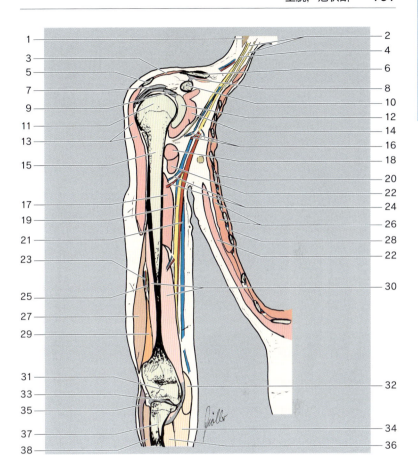

19 正中神経 Median nerve
20 肋骨 Rib
21 尺側皮静脈 Basilic vein
22 広背筋 Latissimus dorsi muscle
23 上腕深動静脈 Deep brachial artery and vein
24 肋間動静脈，神経 Intercostal artery, vein, and nerve
25 橈骨神経 Radial nerve
26 前鋸筋 Serratus anterior muscle
27 上腕三頭筋(外側頭) Triceps brachii muscle (lateral head)
28 肋間筋 Intercostal muscles
29 腕橈骨筋 Brachioradialis muscle
30 上腕筋 Brachialis muscle
31 上腕骨(滑車) Humerus (trochlea)
32 円回内筋 Pronator teres muscle
33 腕尺関節 Humeroulnar joint
34 橈側手根屈筋 Flexor carpi radialis muscle
35 尺側手根伸筋 Extensor carpi ulnaris muscle
36 浅指屈筋 Flexor digitorum superficialis muscle
37 尺骨 Ulna
38 肘筋 Anconeus muscle

102　上　肢

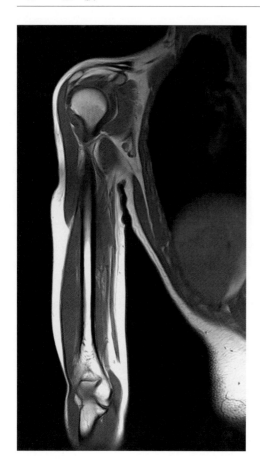

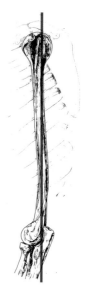

1 鎖骨 Clavicle
2 斜角筋 Scalenus muscle
3 僧帽筋 Trapezius muscle
4 鎖骨下筋 Subclavius muscle
5 烏口鎖骨靱帯 Coracoclavicular ligament
6 前鋸筋 Serratus anterior muscle
7 肩峰 Acromion
8 烏口突起 Coracoid process
9 上腕二頭筋(長頭,腱) Biceps brachii muscle (long head, tendon)
10 関節窩 Glenoid
11 棘上筋(腱) Supraspinatus muscle (tendon)
12 肩甲下筋 Subscapularis muscle
13 上腕骨(頭) Humerus (head)
14 肋間筋 Intercostal muscles
15 棘下筋 Infraspinatus muscle
16 前鋸筋 Serratus anterior muscle
17 小円筋 Teres minor muscle
18 胸背動静脈 Thoracodorsal artery and vein
19 後上腕回旋動静脈 Posterior circumflex humeral artery and vein
20 大円筋 Teres major muscle

上腕，冠状断

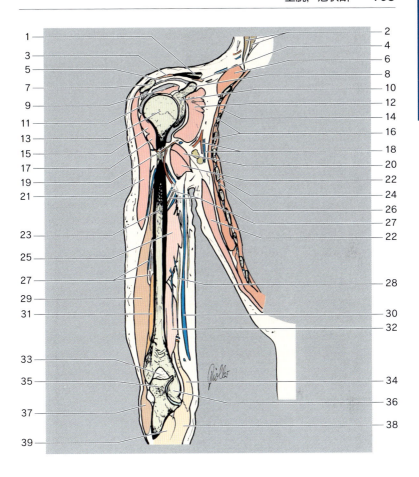

21 三角筋 Deltoid muscle
22 広背筋 Latissimus dorsi muscle
23 上腕骨(体) Humerus (shaft)
24 肋骨 Rib
25 上腕筋 Brachialis muscle
26 肋間動静脈,神経 Intercostal artery, vein, and nerve
27 上腕深動静脈 Deep brachial artery and vein
28 尺骨神経 Ulnar nerve
29 上腕三頭筋(外側頭) Triceps brachii muscle (lateral head)
30 尺側皮静脈 Basilic vein
31 腕橈骨筋 Brachioradialis muscle
32 上腕筋 Brachialis muscle
33 肘頭窩 Olecranon fossa
34 円回内筋 Pronator teres muscle
35 肘頭 Olecranon
36 上腕骨の内側上顆 Medial epicondyle of humerus
37 肘筋 Anconeus muscle
38 浅指屈筋 Flexor digitorum superficialis muscle
39 深指屈筋 Flexor digitorum profundus muscle

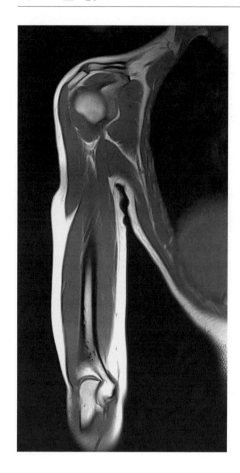

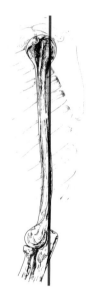

1 僧帽筋 Trapezius muscle
2 斜角筋 Scalenus muscle
3 鎖骨 Clavicle
4 肩甲下動静脈 Subscapular artery and vein
5 肩鎖関節 Acromioclavicular joint
6 前鋸筋 Serratus anterior muscle
7 肩峰 Acromion
8 棘下筋 Infraspinatus muscle
9 上腕二頭筋(長頭,腱) Biceps brachii muscle (long head, tendon)
10 肋間筋 Intercostal muscles
11 棘上筋(腱) Supraspinatus muscle (tendon)
12 関節窩 Glenoid
13 烏口突起 Coracoid process
14 肩甲下筋 Subscapularis muscle
15 上腕骨(頭) Humerus (head)

上腕，冠状断　**105**

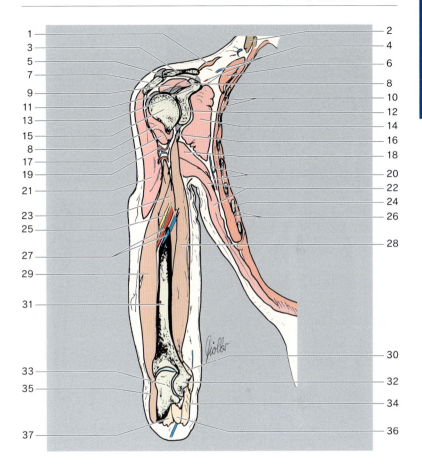

16 上腕三頭筋(長頭,腱付着部) Triceps brachii muscle (long head, tendon attachment)
17 小円筋 Teres minor muscle
18 大円筋 Teres major muscle
19 後上腕回旋動静脈 Posterior circumflex humeral artery and vein
20 胸背動静脈 Thoracodorsal artery and vein
21 三角筋 Deltoid muscle
22 広背筋 Latissimus dorsi muscle
23 上腕三頭筋(内側頭) Triceps brachii muscle (medial head)
24 肋骨 Rib
25 橈骨神経 Radial nerve
26 肋間動静脈,神経 Intercostal artery, vein, and nerve
27 上腕深動静脈 Deep brachial artery and vein
28 上腕三頭筋(長頭) Triceps brachii muscle (long head)
29 上腕三頭筋(外側頭) Triceps brachii muscle (lateral head)
30 円回内筋 Pronator teres muscle
31 上腕骨(体) Humerus (shaft)
32 上腕骨の内側上顆 Medial epicondyle of humerus
33 肘頭 Olecranon
34 浅指屈筋 Flexor digitorum superficialis muscle
35 肘筋 Anconeus muscle
36 尺側手根屈筋 Flexor carpi ulnaris muscle
37 深指屈筋 Flexor digitorum profundus muscle

106 上肢

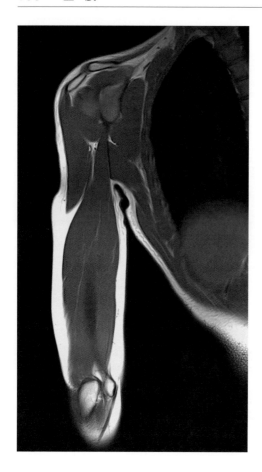

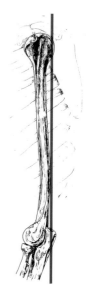

1 鎖骨 Clavicle
2 斜角筋 Scalenus muscles
3 肩鎖関節 Acromioclavicular joint
4 僧帽筋 Trapezius muscle
5 棘上筋 Supraspinatus muscle
6 前鋸筋 Serratus anterior muscle
7 肩峰 Acromion
8 棘下筋 Infraspinatus muscle
9 小円筋 Teres minor muscle
10 関節窩 Glenoid

上腕，冠状断 107

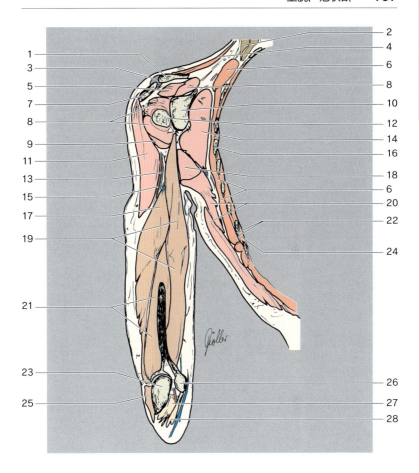

11 三角筋 Deltoid muscle
12 上腕骨(頭) Humerus (head)
13 橈骨神経 Radial nerve
14 肩甲下筋 Subscapularis muscle
15 上腕深動静脈 Deep brachial artery and vein
16 肋骨 Rib
17 上腕三頭筋(外側頭) Triceps brachii muscle (lateral head)
18 大円筋 Teres major muscle
19 上腕二頭筋(長頭) Biceps brachii muscle (long head)
20 広背筋 Latissimus dorsi muscle
21 上腕三頭筋(内側頭) Triceps brachii muscle (medial head)
22 肋間動静脈, 神経 Intercostal artery, vein, and nerve
23 肘頭 Olecranon
24 肋間筋 Intercostal muscles
25 肘筋 Anconeus muscle
26 上腕骨の内側上顆 Medial epicondyle of humerus
27 深指屈筋 Flexor digitorum profundus muscle
28 尺側手根屈筋 Flexor carpi ulnaris muscle

108　上　肢

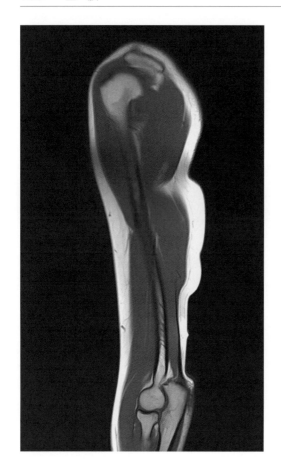

近位/頭側

腹側　　背側

遠位

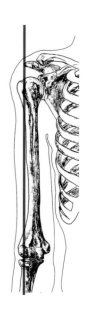

上腕, 矢状断

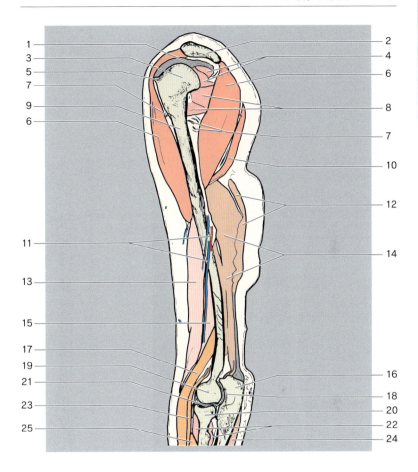

1 棘上筋(腱) Supraspinatus muscle (tendon)
2 肩峰 Acromion
3 上腕骨(頭) Humerus (head)
4 棘下筋 Infraspinatus muscle
5 大結節 Greater tubercle
6 三角筋(肩峰部) Deltoid muscle (acromial part)
7 後上腕回旋動静脈 Posterior circumflex humeral artery and vein
8 小円筋 Teres minor muscle
9 上腕骨(体) Humerus (shaft)
10 三角筋 Deltoid muscle
11 上腕深動静脈 Deep brachial artery and vein
12 上腕三頭筋(長頭) Triceps brachii muscle (long head)
13 上腕二頭筋(長頭) Biceps brachii muscle (long head)
14 上腕三頭筋(外側頭) Triceps brachii muscle (lateral head)
15 上腕筋 Brachialis muscle
16 肘頭 Olecranon
17 腕橈骨筋 Brachioradialis muscle
18 腕尺関節 Humeroulnar joint
19 上腕骨(小頭) Humerus (capitulum)
20 橈骨(頭) Radius (head)
21 腕橈関節 Humeroradial joint
22 回外筋 Supinator muscle
23 長橈側手根伸筋 Extensor carpi radialis longus muscle
24 肘筋 Anconeus muscle
25 短橈側手根伸筋 Extensor carpi radialis brevis muscle

110　上　肢

近位/頭側

腹側　　背側

遠位

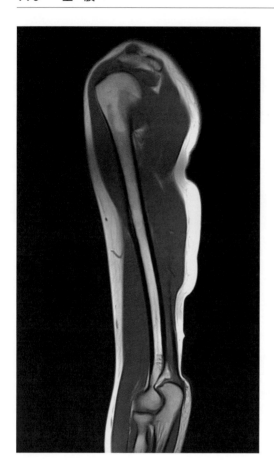

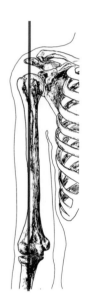

1　鎖骨　Clavicle
2　肩鎖靱帯　Acromioclavicular ligament
3　肩峰　Acromion
4　棘下筋　Infraspinatus muscle
5　棘上筋(腱)　Supraspinatus muscle(tendon)
6　上腕骨(頭)　Humerus(head)
7　上腕骨(大結節)　Humerus(greater tubercle)
8　小円筋　Teres minor muscle
9　上腕骨(頸)　Humerus(neck)

上腕，矢状断 111

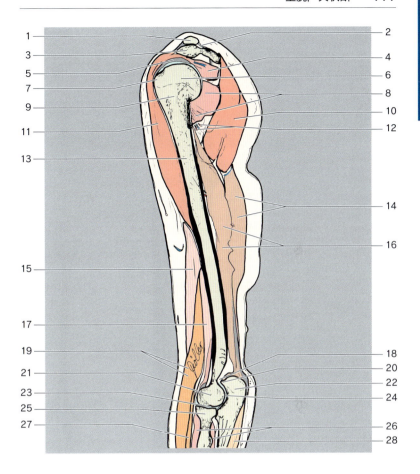

10 三角筋(肩峰部) Deltoid muscle (acromial part)
11 三角筋 Deltoid muscle
12 後上腕回旋動静脈 Posterior circumflex humeral artery and vein
13 上腕骨(体) Humerus (shaft)
14 上腕三頭筋(長頭) Triceps brachii muscle (long head)
15 上腕二頭筋(長頭) Biceps brachii muscle (long head)
16 上腕三頭筋(外側頭) Triceps brachii muscle (lateral head)
17 上腕筋 Brachialis muscle
18 肘頭窩 Olecranon fossa
19 腕橈骨筋 Brachioradialis muscle
20 鈎状突起 Coronoid process
21 上腕骨(小頭) Humerus (capitulum)
22 肘頭 Olecranon
23 腕橈関節 Humeroradial joint
24 腕尺関節 Humeroulnar joint
25 橈骨(頭) Radius (head)
26 回外筋 Supinator muscle
27 長橈側手根伸筋 Extensor carpi radialis longus muscle
28 深指屈筋 Flexor digitorum profundus muscle

112　上肢

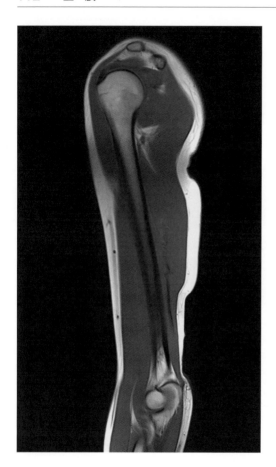

近位/頭側

腹側　□　背側

遠位

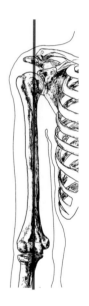

1　鎖骨　Clavicle
2　肩鎖靱帯　Acromioclavicular ligament
3　棘上筋(+腱)　Supraspinatus muscle (+tendon)
4　肩峰　Acromion
5　上腕骨(大結節)　Humerus (greater tubercle)
6　棘下筋　Infraspinatus muscle
7　上腕骨(頭)　Humerus (head)
8　小円筋　Teres minor muscle
9　三角筋　Deltoid muscle
10　三角筋(肩峰部)　Deltoid muscle (acromial part)
11　上腕骨(体)　Humerus (shaft)

上腕，矢状断 113

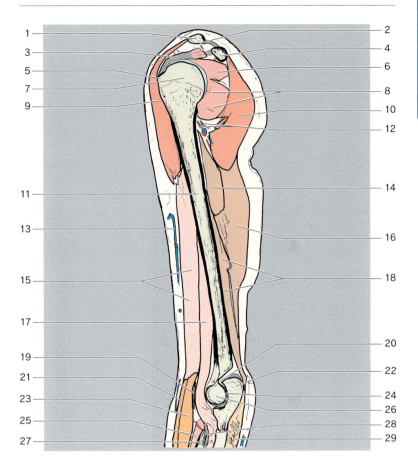

12 後上腕回旋動静脈 Posterior circumflex humeral artery and vein
13 橈側皮静脈 Cephalic vein
14 上腕三頭筋(外側頭) Triceps brachii muscle(lateral head)
15 上腕二頭筋(長頭) Biceps brachii muscle(long head)
16 上腕三頭筋(長頭) Triceps brachii muscle(long head)
17 上腕筋 Brachialis muscle
18 上腕三頭筋(内側頭) Triceps brachii muscle(medial head)
19 橈骨神経 Radial nerve
20 肘頭窩 Olecranon fossa
21 腕橈骨筋 Brachioradialis muscle
22 肘頭 Olecranon
23 長橈側手根伸筋 Extensor carpi radialis longus muscle
24 腕尺関節 Humeroulnar joint
25 回外筋 Supinator muscle
26 上腕骨(小頭) Humerus(capitulum)
27 橈骨(体) Radius(shaft)
28 上腕二頭筋(腱) Biceps brachii muscle(tendon)
29 深指屈筋 Flexor digitorum profundus muscle

114 上 肢

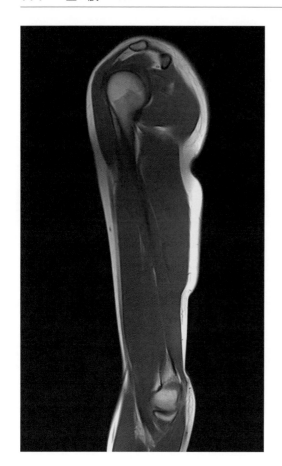

近位/頭側

腹側 　　 背側

遠位

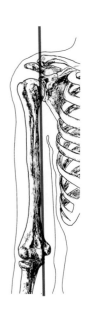

上腕, 矢状断 115

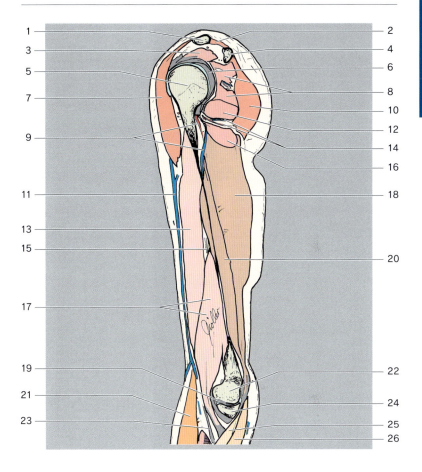

1 鎖骨 Clavicle
2 僧帽筋 Trapezius muscle
3 棘上筋(+腱) Supraspinatus muscle (+tendon)
4 肩峰 Acromion
5 上腕骨(頭) Humerus (head)
6 関節包 Joint capsule
7 三角筋 Deltoid muscle
8 棘下筋 Infraspinatus muscle
9 後上腕回旋動静脈 Posterior circumflex humeral artery and vein
10 三角筋(肩峰部) Deltoid muscle (acromial part)
11 橈側皮静脈 Cephalic vein
12 小円筋 Teres minor muscle
13 上腕二頭筋(長頭) Biceps brachii muscle (long head)
14 後上腕回旋動静脈(筋枝) Posterior circumflex humeral artery and vein (muscular branch)
15 正中神経 Median nerve
16 大円筋 Teres major muscle
17 上腕筋 Brachialis muscle
18 上腕三頭筋(長頭) Triceps brachii muscle (long head)
19 腕尺関節 Humeroulnar joint
20 上腕三頭筋(内側頭) Triceps brachii muscle (medial head)
21 腕橈骨筋 Brachioradialis muscle
22 上腕骨(滑車) Humerus (trochlea)
23 上腕二頭筋(腱) Biceps brachii muscle (tendon)
24 尺骨 Ulna
25 尺側手根屈筋 Flexor carpi ulnaris muscle
26 深指屈筋 Flexor digitorum profundus muscle

116　上肢

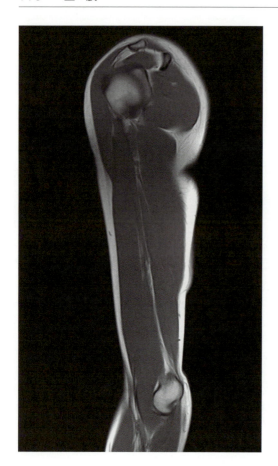

近位/頭側

腹側 □ 背側

遠位

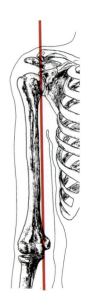

1 鎖骨 Clavicle
2 僧帽筋 Trapezius muscle
3 棘上筋(+腱) Supraspinatus muscle (+tendon)
4 肩峰 Acromion
5 関節包 Joint capsule
6 関節窩 Glenoid
7 関節唇 Glenoid labrum
8 棘下筋 Infraspinatus muscle
9 上腕骨(頭) Humerus (head)
10 三角筋(肩峰部) Deltoid muscle (acromial part)
11 三角筋 Deltoid muscle
12 小円筋 Teres minor muscle

上腕，矢状断　117

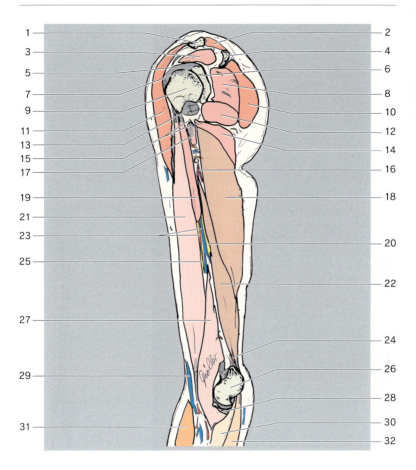

13 関節上腕靱帯 Glenohumeral ligament
14 大円筋 Teres major muscle
15 後上腕回旋動静脈 Posterior circumflex humeral artery and vein
16 後上腕回旋動静脈（筋枝）Posterior circumflex humeral artery and vein (muscular branch)
17 広背筋 Latissimus dorsi muscle
18 上腕三頭筋（長頭）Triceps brachii muscle (long head)
19 烏口腕筋 Coracobrachialis muscle
20 尺骨神経 Ulnar nerve
21 上腕二頭筋（長頭）Biceps brachii muscle (long head)
22 上腕三頭筋（内側頭）Triceps brachii muscle (medial head)
23 上腕深動静脈 Deep brachial artery and vein
24 尺側側副動静脈 Collateral ulnar artery and vein
25 正中神経 Median nerve
26 内側上顆 Medial epicondyle
27 上腕筋 Brachialis muscle
28 肘頭 Olecranon
29 肘正中皮静脈 Median cubital vein
30 尺側手根屈筋 Flexor carpi ulnaris muscle
31 腕橈骨筋 Brachioradialis muscle
32 深指屈筋 Flexor digitorum profundus muscle

118　上　肢

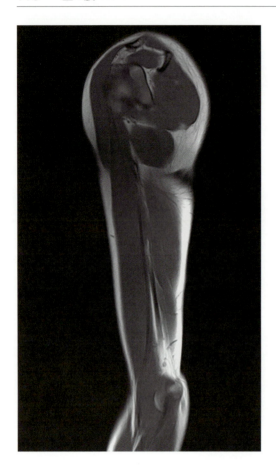

近位/頭側

腹側 □ 背側

遠位

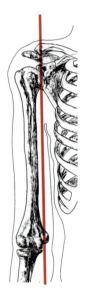

1　鎖骨　Clavicle
2　僧帽筋　Trapezius muscle
3　烏口鎖骨靱帯　Coracoclavicular ligament
4　肩峰　Acromion
5　棘上筋　Supraspinatus muscle
6　関節窩　Glenoid
7　関節包　Joint capsule
8　三角筋(肩峰部)　Deltoid muscle (acromial part)
9　三角筋　Deltoid muscle
10　棘下筋　Infraspinatus muscle
11　上腕骨(頭)　Humerus (head)
12　小円筋　Teres minor muscle

上腕，矢状断 119

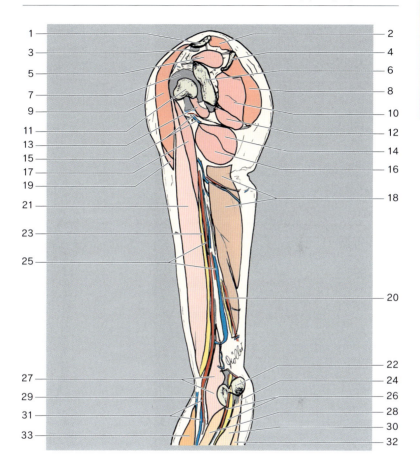

13 肩甲下筋 Subscapularis muscle
14 大円筋 Teres major muscle
15 後上腕回旋動静脈 Posterior circumflex humeral artery and vein
16 広背筋 Latissimus dorsi muscle
17 烏口腕筋 Coracobrachialis muscle
18 上腕三頭筋（長頭）Triceps brachii muscle (long head)
19 大胸筋 Pectoralis major muscle
20 尺骨神経 Ulnar nerve
21 上腕二頭筋（長頭）Biceps brachii muscle (long head)
22 上腕骨（滑車）Humerus (trochlea)
23 正中神経 Median nerve
24 屈筋群の共通頭 Common head of flexor muscles
25 上腕動静脈 Brachial artery and vein
26 尺骨神経 Ulnar nerve, 尺側側副動脈 Collateral ulnar artery
27 上腕筋 Brachialis muscle
28 浅指屈筋 Flexor digitorum superficialis muscle
29 肘正中皮静脈 Median cubital vein
30 尺側手根屈筋 Flexor carpi ulnaris muscle
31 尺骨動静脈 Ulnar artery and vein
32 深指屈筋 Flexor digitorum profundus muscle
33 腕橈骨筋 Brachioradialis muscle

120　上　肢

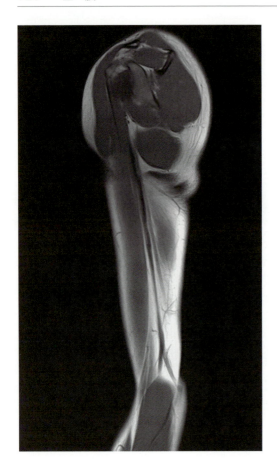

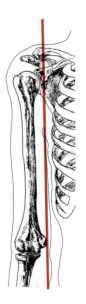

近位/頭側
腹側　背側
遠位

1　鎖骨　Clavicle
2　僧帽筋　Trapezius muscle
3　烏口突起　Coracoid process
4　棘上筋　Supraspinatus muscle
5　三角筋　Deltoid muscle
6　肩峰　Acromion

上腕，矢状断 121

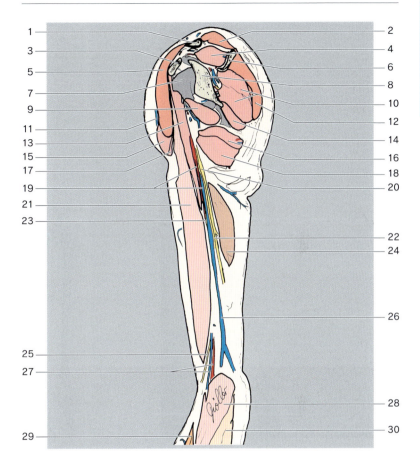

- 7 関節包 Joint capsule
- 8 肩甲骨(頸) Scapula (neck)
- 9 肩甲下筋 Subscapularis muscle
- 10 棘下筋 Infraspinatus muscle
- 11 橈側皮静脈 Cephalic vein
- 12 三角筋(肩峰部) Deltoid muscle (acromial part)
- 13 烏口腕筋 Coracobrachialis muscle
- 14 小円筋 Teres minor muscle
- 15 大胸筋 Pectoralis major muscle
- 16 大円筋 Teres major muscle
- 17 小胸筋 Pectoralis minor muscle
- 18 広背筋 Latissimus dorsi muscle
- 19 上腕動静脈 Brachial artery and vein
- 20 橈骨神経 Radial nerve
- 21 上腕二頭筋(長頭) Biceps brachii muscle (long head)
- 22 尺骨神経 Ulnar nerve
- 23 正中神経 Median nerve
- 24 上腕三頭筋(長頭) Triceps brachii muscle (long head)
- 25 内側前腕皮神経 Medial cutaneous nerve of forearm
- 26 尺側皮静脈 Basilic vein
- 27 尺骨動静脈 Ulnar artery and vein
- 28 上腕筋 Brachialis muscle
- 29 腕橈骨筋 Brachioradialis muscle
- 30 尺側手根屈筋 Flexor carpi ulnaris muscle

122 上 肢

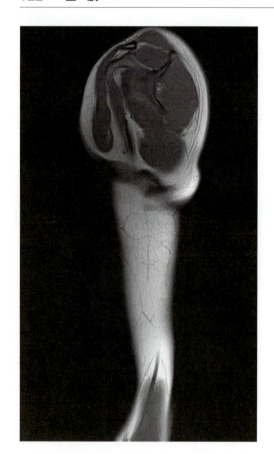

近位/頭側

腹側 　　 背側

遠位

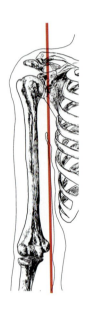

上腕，矢状断 *123*

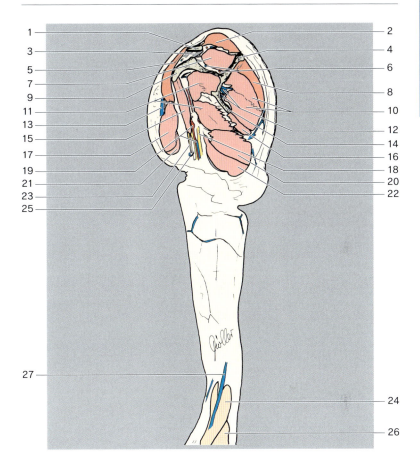

1. 鎖骨 Clavicle
2. 僧帽筋 Trapezius muscle
3. 烏口鎖骨靱帯 Coracoclavicular ligament
4. 肩峰 Acromion
5. 三角筋 Deltoid muscle
6. 肩甲上動静脈 Suprascapular artery and vein
7. 棘上筋 Supraspinatus muscle
8. 三角筋(肩峰部) Deltoid muscle (acromial part)
9. 烏口突起 Coracoid process
10. 棘下筋 Infraspinatus muscle
11. 肩甲下筋 Subscapularis muscle
12. 肩甲回旋動静脈 Circumflex scapular artery and vein
13. 橈側皮静脈 Cephalic vein
14. 肩甲骨 Scapula
15. 烏口腕筋 Coracobrachialis muscle
16. 小円筋 Teres minor muscle
17. 大胸筋 Pectoralis major muscle
18. 橈骨神経 Radial nerve
19. 上腕動静脈 Brachial artery and vein
20. 大円筋 Teres major muscle
21. 小胸筋 Pectoralis minor muscle
22. 広背筋 Latissimus dorsi muscle
23. 正中神経 Median nerve
24. 円回内筋 Pronator teres muscle
25. 尺骨神経 Ulnar nerve
26. 尺側手根屈筋 Flexor carpi ulnaris muscle
27. 尺側皮静脈 Basilic vein

124 上 肢

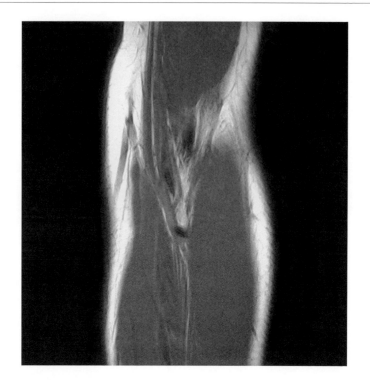

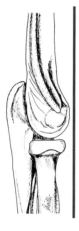

	近位	
尺側		橈側
内側		外側
	遠位	

肘，冠状断 **125**

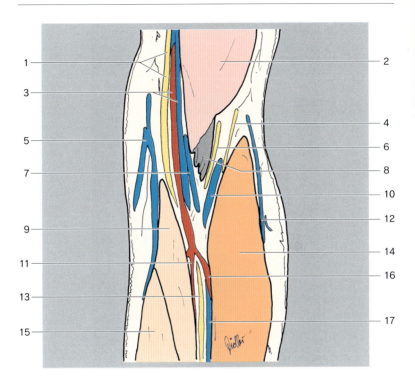

1 正中神経 Median nerve
2 上腕筋 Brachialis muscle
3 上腕動静脈 Brachial artery and vein
4 外側前腕皮神経 Lateral cutaneous nerve of forearm
5 尺側皮静脈 Basilic vein
6 橈骨神経(深枝) Radial nerve(deep branch)
7 肘正中皮静脈 Median cubital vein
8 上腕二頭筋(腱) Biceps brachii muscle (tendon)
9 円回内筋 Pronator teres muscle
10 橈側正中皮静脈 Median cephalic vein
11 尺骨動脈 Ulnar artery
12 橈側皮静脈 Cephalic vein
13 正中神経 Median nerve
14 腕橈骨筋 Brachioradialis muscle
15 橈側手根屈筋 Flexor carpi radialis muscle
16 橈骨動脈 Radial artery
17 前腕正中皮静脈 Median vein of forearm

126 上肢

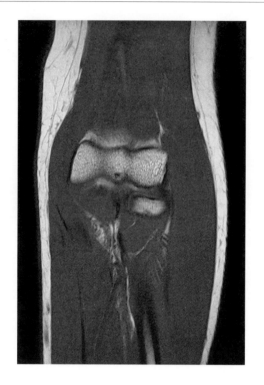

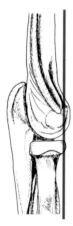

近位
尺側 ☐ 橈側
内側   外側
遠位

肘，冠状断 **127**

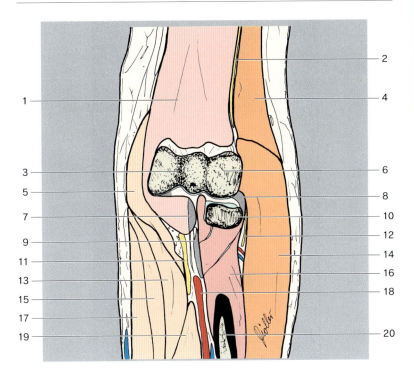

1 上腕筋 Brachialis muscle
2 橈骨神経 Radial nerve
3 上腕骨(滑車) Humerus(trochlea)
4 腕橈骨筋 Brachioradialis muscle
5 円回内筋 Pronator teres muscle
6 上腕骨(小頭) Humerus(capitulum)
7 上腕筋(腱) Brachialis muscle(tendon)
8 橈骨輪状靱帯 Anular ligament,
  外側側副靱帯 Radial collateral ligament
9 上腕二頭筋(腱) Biceps brachii muscle (tendon)
10 橈骨(頭) Radius(head)
11 正中神経 Median nerve
12 橈骨神経(深枝) Radial nerve(deep branch)
13 橈側手根屈筋 Flexor carpi radialis muscle
14 長橈側手根伸筋 Extensor carpi radialis longus muscle,
  短橈側手根伸筋 Extensor carpi radialis brevis muscle
15 長掌筋 Palmaris longus muscle
16 回外筋 Supinator muscle
17 尺側手根屈筋 Flexor carpi ulnaris muscle
18 骨間動静脈 Interosseous artery and vein
19 深指屈筋 Flexor digitorum profundus muscle
20 橈骨(体) Radius(shaft)

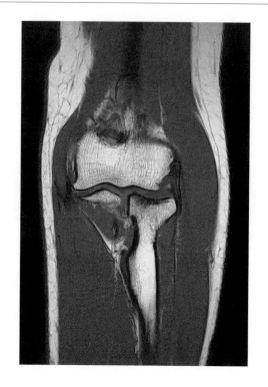

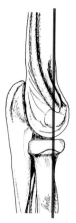

	近位	
尺側内側		橈側外側
	遠位	

肘，冠状断

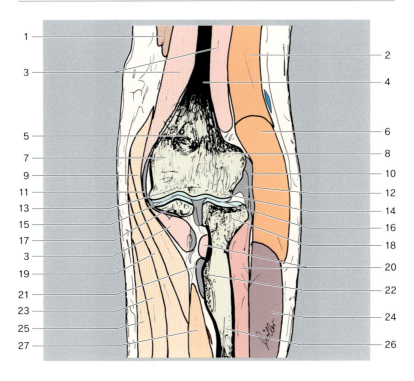

1 上腕三頭筋 Triceps brachii muscle
2 腕橈骨筋 Brachioradialis muscle
3 上腕筋 Brachialis muscle
4 上腕骨(体) Humerus(shaft)
5 鈎突窩 Coronoid fossa
6 長橈側手根伸筋 Extensor carpi radialis longus muscle
7 内側上顆 Medial epicondyle
8 外側上顆 Lateral epicondyle
9 円回内筋 Pronator teres muscle
10 前腕伸筋群の共通腱(付着部) Common extensor tendons(attachment)
11 内側側副靱帯 Medial collateral ligament
12 外側側副靱帯 Radial collateral ligament
13 上腕骨(滑車) Humerus(trochlea)
14 上腕骨(小頭) Humerus(capitulum)
15 腕尺関節 Humeroulnar joint
16 腕橈関節 Humeroradial joint
17 尺骨(鈎状突起) Ulna(coronoid process)
18 橈骨(頭) Radius(head)
19 橈側手根屈筋 Flexor carpi radialis muscle
20 回外筋 Supinator muscle
21 上腕二頭筋(腱) Biceps brachii muscle (tendon)
22 橈骨粗面 Radial tuberosity
23 長掌筋 Palmaris longus muscle
24 指伸筋 Extensor digitorum muscle
25 浅指屈筋 Flexor digitorum superficialis muscle
26 橈骨(体) Radius(shaft)
27 深指屈筋 Flexor digitorum profundus muscle

130　上　肢

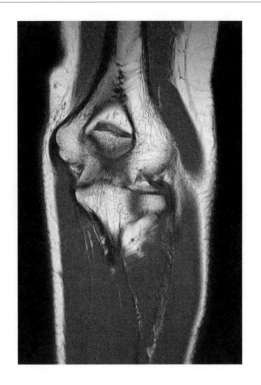

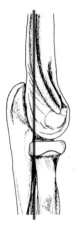

近位
尺側　　　橈側
内側　□　外側
遠位

肘，冠状断 *131*

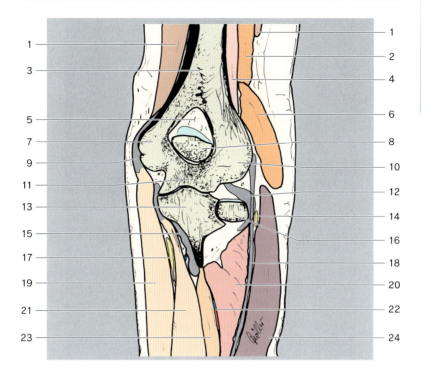

1 上腕三頭筋 Triceps brachii muscle
2 腕橈骨筋 Brachioradialis muscle
3 上腕骨(体) Humerus(shaft)
4 上腕筋 Brachialis muscle
5 肘頭窩(後脂肪体) Olecranon fossa(posterior fat body)
6 長橈側手根伸筋 Extensor carpi radialis longus muscle
7 内側上顆 Medial epicondyle
8 肘頭 Olecranon
9 前腕屈筋群の共通腱(付着部) Common flexor tendons(attachment)
10 外側上顆 Lateral epicondyle
11 上腕骨(滑車) Humerus(trochlea)
12 橈骨輪状靱帯 Anular ligament
13 尺骨(鈎状突起) Ulna(coronoid process)
14 橈骨神経(深枝) Radial nerve(deep branch)
15 上腕筋(腱付着部) Brachialis muscle (tendon attachment)
16 橈骨(頭) Radius(head)
17 尺骨神経 Ulnar nerve
18 前腕伸筋群の共通腱 Common extensor tendons
19 尺側手根屈筋 Flexor carpi ulnaris muscle
20 回外筋 Supinator muscle
21 浅指屈筋 Flexor digitorum superficialis muscle
22 総骨間動静脈 Common interosseous artery and vein
23 深指屈筋 Flexor digitorum profundus muscle
24 指伸筋 Extensor digitorum muscle

132　上　肢

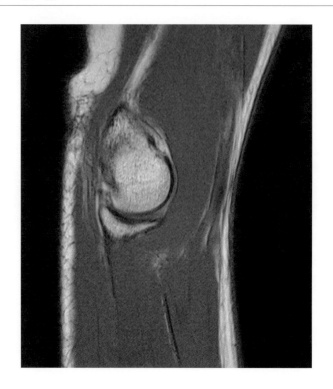

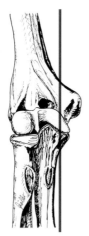

```
        近位
背側  □  腹側
        遠位
```

肘，矢状断

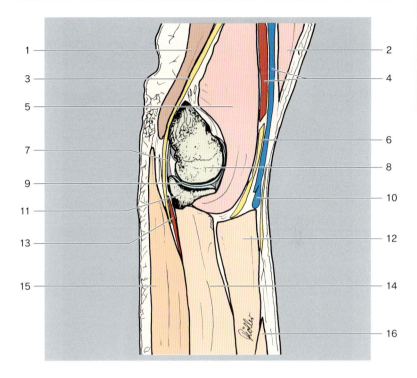

1 上腕三頭筋 Triceps brachii muscle
2 上腕二頭筋 Biceps brachii muscle
3 尺骨神経 Ulnar nerve
4 上腕動静脈 Brachial artery and vein
5 上腕筋 Brachialis muscle
6 正中神経 Median nerve
7 内側側副靱帯の後部（＋肘関節の関節包後部）
   Collateral ulnar ligament, posterior part
   (＋posterior capsule of the elbow joint)
8 上腕骨（滑車）Humerus (trochlea)
9 腕尺関節 Humeroulnar joint
10 肘正中皮静脈 Median cubital vein
11 肘頭 Olecranon
12 円回内筋 Pronator teres muscle
13 尺骨反回動脈 Ulnar recurrent artery
14 浅指屈筋 Flexor digitorum superficialis muscle
15 深指屈筋 Flexor digitorum profundus muscle
16 橈側手根屈筋 Flexor carpi radialis muscle

上 肢

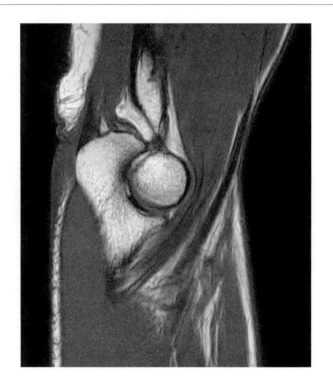

近位

背側 □ 腹側

遠位

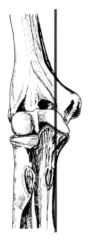

肘，矢状断　**135**

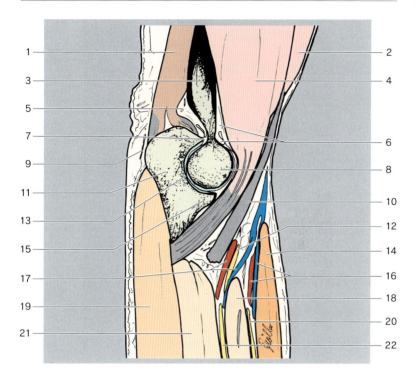

1 上腕三頭筋　Triceps brachii muscle
2 上腕二頭筋　Biceps brachii muscle
3 上腕骨　Humerus
4 上腕筋　Brachialis muscle
5 肘の後脂肪体　Posterior fat body of elbow
6 前脂肪体　Anterior fat body, 鈎突窩　Coronoid fossa
7 肘頭窩　Olecranon fossa
8 上腕骨(滑車)　Humerus(trochlea)
9 肘頭滑液包　Olecranon bursa
10 上腕二頭筋(腱)　Biceps brachii muscle (tendon)
11 肘頭　Olecranon
12 尺骨神経　Ulnar nerve
13 滑車切痕　Trochlear notch
14 腕橈骨筋　Brachioradialis muscle
15 鈎状突起　Coronoid process
16 橈骨動静脈　Radial artery and vein
17 尺骨動静脈　Ulnar artery and vein
18 円回内筋　Pronator teres muscle
19 深指屈筋　Flexor digitorum profundus muscle
20 橈骨神経　Radial nerve
21 浅指屈筋　Flexor digitorum superficialis muscle
22 正中神経　Median nerve

136　上　肢

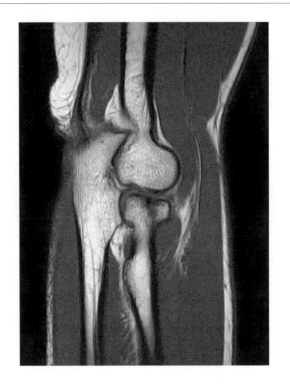

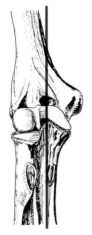

近位

背側　　腹側

遠位

肘，矢状断 **137**

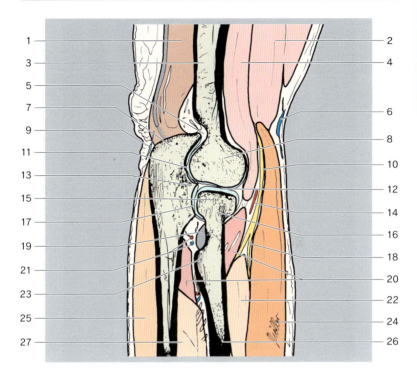

1 上腕三頭筋 Triceps brachii muscle
2 上腕二頭筋 Biceps brachii muscle
3 上腕骨(体) Humerus(shaft)
4 上腕筋 Brachialis muscle
5 肘頭窩 Olecranon fossa
6 橈側皮静脈 Cephalic vein
7 肘頭 Olecranon
8 上腕骨(小頭) Humerus(capitulum)
9 肘頭滑液包 Olecranon bursa
10 橈骨神経 Radial nerve
11 滑車切痕 Trochlear notch
12 腕橈関節 Humeroradial joint
13 鈎状突起 Coronoid process
14 上腕深動脈 Deep brachial artery
15 橈骨(頭) Radius(head)
16 橈骨(頸) Radius(neck)
17 上橈尺関節 Proximal radioulnar joint
18 橈骨神経(浅枝) Radial nerve(superficial branch)
19 上腕二頭筋(腱付着部) Biceps brachii muscle(tendon attachment)
20 回外筋 Supinator muscle
21 骨間動静脈 Interosseous artery and vein
22 浅指屈筋 Flexor digitorum superficialis muscle
23 橈骨粗面 Radial tuberosity
24 腕橈骨筋 Brachioradialis muscle
25 深指屈筋 Flexor digitorum profundus muscle
26 橈骨(体) Radius(shaft)
27 円回内筋(尺骨頭) Pronator teres muscle (ulnar head)

138　上　肢

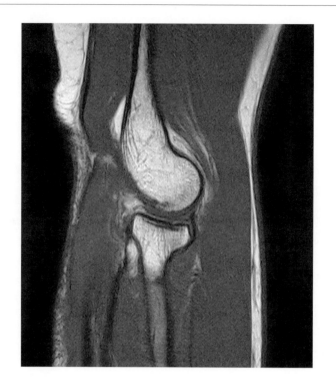

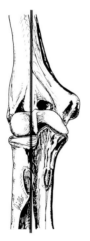

近位

背側 ☐ 腹側

遠位

肘，矢状断 **139**

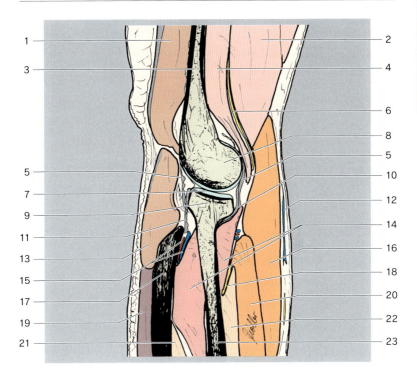

1 上腕三頭筋 Triceps brachii muscle
2 上腕二頭筋 Biceps brachii muscle
3 上腕骨(体) Humerus (shaft)
4 上腕筋 Brachialis muscle
5 関節包 Joint capsule
6 橈骨神経 Radial nerve
7 腕橈関節 Humeroradial joint
8 上腕骨(小頭) Humerus (capitulum)
9 橈骨(頭) Radius (head)
10 橈骨輪状靱帯 Anular ligament of radius
11 外側側副靱帯 Radial collateral ligament
12 橈側皮静脈 Cephalic vein
13 肘筋 Anconeus muscle
14 回外筋 Supinator muscle
15 骨間動静脈 Interosseous artery and vein
16 腕橈骨筋 Brachioradialis muscle
17 尺骨(体) Ulna (shaft)
18 橈骨神経(深枝) Radial nerve (deep branch)
19 尺側手根伸筋 Extensor carpi ulnaris muscle
20 長橈側手根伸筋 Extensor carpi radialis longus muscle
21 円回内筋(尺骨頭) Pronator teres muscle (ulnar head)
22 浅指屈筋(橈骨頭) Flexor digitorum superficialis muscle (radial head)
23 橈骨体 Radius (shaft)

140　上　肢

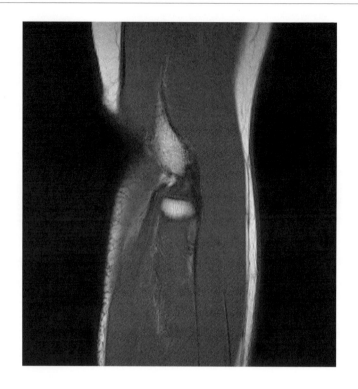

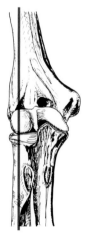

近位

背側　腹側

遠位

肘，矢状断 141

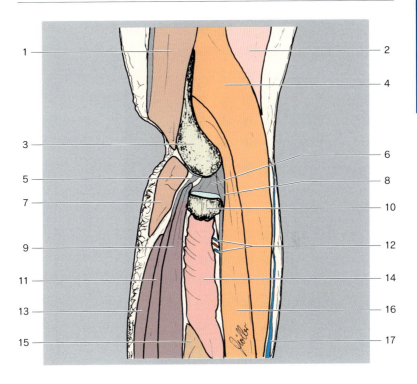

1 上腕三頭筋 Triceps brachii muscle
2 上腕筋 Brachialis muscle
3 上腕骨(小頭) Humerus (capitulum)
4 腕橈骨筋 Brachioradialis muscle
5 関節包 Joint capsule
6 外側側副靱帯 Radial collateral ligament
7 肘筋 Anconeus muscle
8 橈骨輪状靱帯 Anular ligament of radius
9 指伸筋 Extensor digitorum muscle
10 橈骨(頭) Radius (head)
11 小指伸筋 Extensor digiti minimi muscle
12 前骨間動静脈 Anterior interosseous artery and veins
13 尺側手根伸筋 Extensor carpi ulnaris muscle
14 回外筋 Supinator muscle
15 長母指外転筋 Abductor pollicis longus muscle
16 長橈側手根伸筋 Extensor carpi radialis longus muscle
17 橈側皮静脈 Cephalic vein

142 上 肢

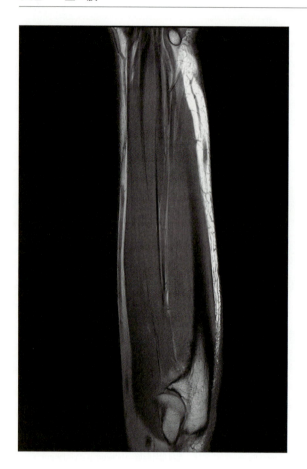

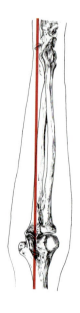

前腕，矢状断 **143**

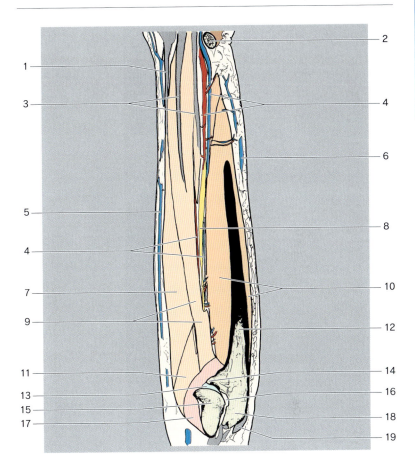

1 橈側手根屈筋(腱) Flexor carpi radialis muscle (tendon)
2 豆状骨 Pisiform
3 浅指屈筋(+腱) Flexor digitorum superficialis muscle (+tendon)
4 尺骨動静脈 Ulnar artery and vein
5 橈側皮静脈 Cephalic vein
6 尺側皮静脈 Basilic vein
7 橈側手根屈筋 Flexor carpi radialis muscle
8 尺骨神経 Ulnar nerve
9 浅指屈筋 Flexor digitorum superficialis muscle
10 深指屈筋 Flexor digitorum profundus muscle
11 円回内筋 Pronator teres muscle
12 尺骨(体) Ulna (shaft)
13 腕尺関節 Humeroulnar joint
14 鈎状突起 Coronoid process
15 上腕骨(滑車) Humerus (trochlea)
16 滑車切痕 Trochlear notch
17 上腕筋 Brachialis muscle
18 肘頭 Olecranon
19 上腕三頭筋(腱付着部) Triceps brachii muscle (tendon attachment)

上 肢

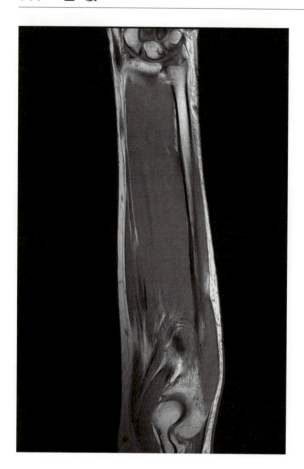

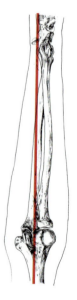

遠位
橈側　　尺側
腹側　　背側
近位

1 **有頭骨** Capitate
2 **有鈎骨** Hamate
3 **舟状骨** Scaphoid
4 **三角骨** Triquetrum
5 **月状骨** Lunate
6 **三角線維軟骨** Triangular fibrocartilage
7 **橈骨** Radius
8 **尺骨** Ulna

前腕，矢状断 145

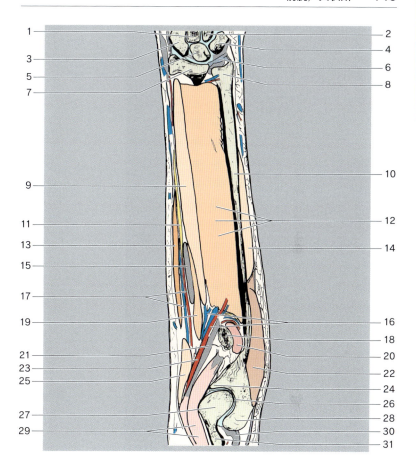

9 浅指屈筋 Flexor digitorum superficialis muscle
10 尺骨(体) Ulna (shaft)
11 正中神経 Median nerve
12 深指屈筋 Flexor digitorum profundus muscle
13 腕橈骨筋 Brachioradialis muscle
14 尺側手根屈筋 Flexor carpi ulnaris muscle
15 円回内筋(腱) Pronator teres muscle (tendon)
16 尺骨動静脈 Ulnar artery and vein
17 橈骨動静脈 Radial artery and veins
18 橈骨粗面 Radial tuberosity
19 長母指屈筋 Flexor pollicis longus muscle
20 回外筋 Supinator muscle
21 上腕二頭筋(腱) Biceps brachii muscle (tendon)
22 肘筋 Anconeus muscle
23 上腕動脈 Brachial artery
24 鈎状突起 Coronoid process
25 円回内筋 Pronator teres muscle
26 腕尺関節 Humeroulnar joint
27 上腕骨(滑車) Humerus (trochlea)
28 肘頭 Olecranon
29 上腕筋 Brachialis muscle
30 上腕三頭筋(腱) Triceps brachii muscle (tendon)
31 上腕骨(体) Humerus (shaft)

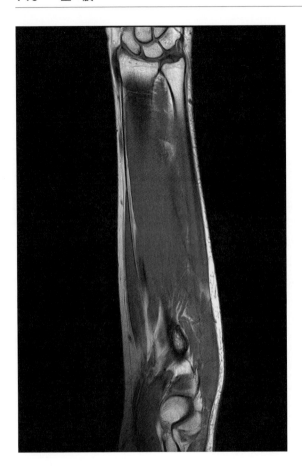

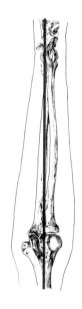

1 有頭骨 Capitate
2 有鈎骨 Hamate
3 舟状骨 Scaphoid
4 三角骨 Triquetrum
5 月状骨 Lunate
6 関節円板 Disk equivalent
7 長母指外転筋（腱）Abductor pollicis longus muscle(tendon),
   腕橈骨筋（腱）Brachioradialis muscle(tendon)
8 内側手根側副靱帯 Ulnar collateral ligament of wrist joint
9 橈骨 Radius
10 三角線維軟骨 Triangular fibrocartilage
11 橈側皮静脈 Cephalic vein
12 尺骨 Ulna
13 尺側手根伸筋 Extensor carpi ulnaris muscle
14 方形回内筋 Pronator quadratus muscle
15 浅指屈筋 Flexor digitorum superficialis muscle
16 示指伸筋（＋腱）Extensor indicis muscle (+tendon)

前腕，矢状断

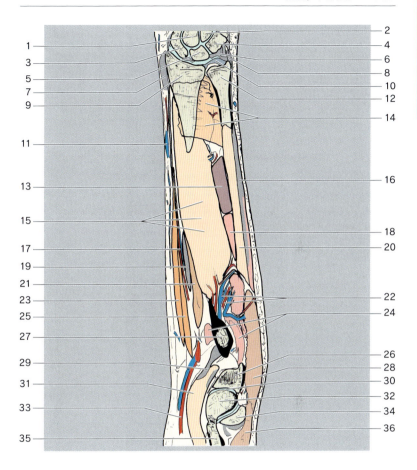

17 橈骨動静脈 Radial artery and veins
18 長母指伸筋 Extensor pollicis longus muscle
19 円回内筋(腱) Pronator teres muscle (tendon)
20 尺側手根屈筋 Flexor carpi ulnaris muscle
21 長母指屈筋 Flexor pollicis longus muscle
22 尺骨動静脈 Ulnar artery and vein
23 腕橈骨筋 Brachioradialis muscle
24 回外筋 Supinator muscle
25 長橈側手根伸筋 Extensor carpi radialis longus muscle
26 (上)橈尺関節 Radioulnar joint
27 橈骨粗面 Radial tuberosity
28 肘筋 Anconeus muscle
29 上腕二頭筋(腱) Biceps brachii muscle (tendon)
30 腕尺関節 Humeroulnar joint
31 上腕筋 Brachialis muscle
32 上腕骨(滑車) Humerus (trochlea)
33 上腕動脈 Brachial artery
34 肘頭 Olecranon
35 上腕骨(体) Humerus (shaft)
36 上腕三頭筋(＋腱) Triceps brachii muscle (+tendon)

148　上　肢

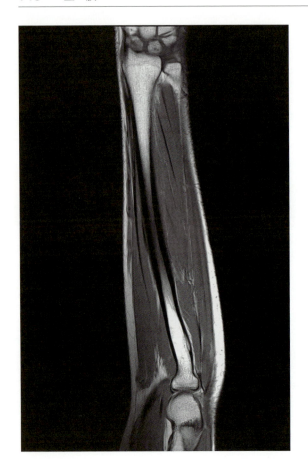

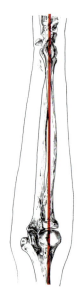

1　**小菱形骨** Trapezoid
2　**有鈎骨** Hamate
3　**有頭骨** Capitate
4　**三角骨** Triquetrum
5　**舟状骨** Scaphoid
6　**尺骨** Ulna
7　**月状骨** Lunate

前腕，矢状断 **149**

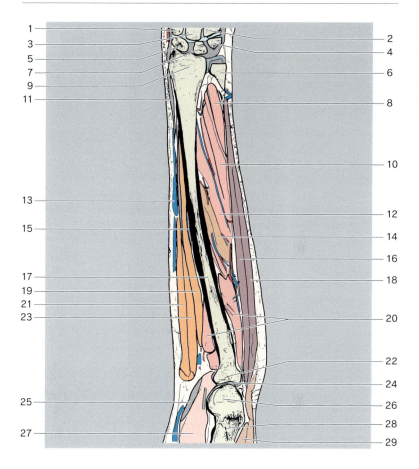

- 8 示指伸筋 Extensor indicis muscle
- 9 橈骨 Radius
- 10 短母指伸筋 Extensor pollicis brevis muscle
- 11 長母指屈筋(腱) Flexor pollicis longus muscle (tendon)
- 12 長母指伸筋 Extensor pollicis longus muscle
- 13 橈側皮静脈 Cephalic vein
- 14 長母指外転筋 Abductor pollicis longus muscle
- 15 円回内筋(腱) Pronator teres muscle (tendon)
- 16 小指伸筋 Extensor digiti minimi muscle
- 17 橈骨(体) Radius (shaft)
- 18 尺側手根伸筋 Extensor carpi ulnaris muscle
- 19 短橈側手根伸筋 Extensor carpi radialis brevis muscle
- 20 回外筋 Supinator muscle
- 21 腕橈骨筋 Brachioradialis muscle
- 22 橈骨(頭) Radius (head)
- 23 長橈側手根伸筋 Extensor carpi radialis longus muscle
- 24 腕橈関節 Humeroradial joint
- 25 上腕二頭筋(腱) Biceps brachii muscle (tendon)
- 26 上腕骨(小頭) Humerus (capitulum)
- 27 上腕筋 Brachialis muscle
- 28 上腕骨(体) Humerus (shaft)
- 29 上腕三頭筋 Triceps brachii muscle

150　上　肢

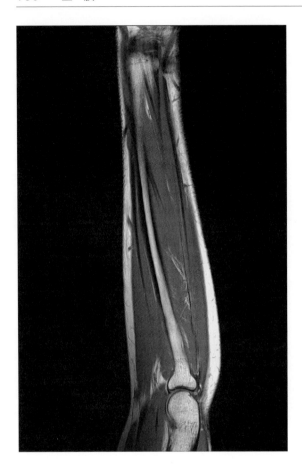

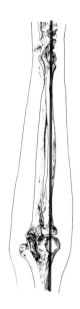

1 **関節包** Joint capsule,
  背側橈骨手根靱帯 Dorsal radiocarpal ligament
2 **小指伸筋(腱)** Extensor digiti minimi muscle (tendon)
3 **橈骨** Radius
4 **尺骨** Ulna
5 **長母指伸筋(＋腱)** Extensor pollicis longus muscle (+tendon)
6 **示指伸筋(＋腱)** Extensor indicis muscle (+tendon)

前腕，矢状断 *151*

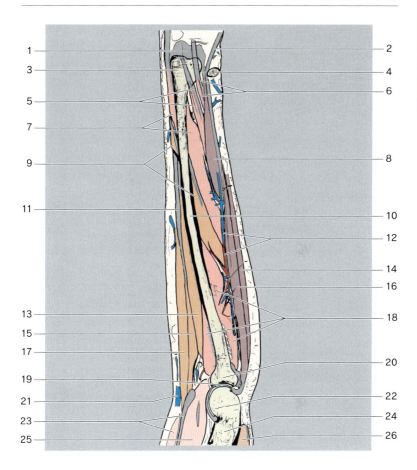

7 短母指伸筋 Extensor pollicis brevis muscle
8 指伸筋 Extensor digitorum muscle
9 長母指外転筋 Abductor pollicis longus muscle
10 橈骨(体) Radius (shaft)
11 長橈側手根伸筋(腱) Extensor carpi radialis longus muscle (tendon)
12 後骨間動静脈 Posterior interosseous artery and vein
13 短橈側手根伸筋 Extensor carpi radialis brevis muscle
14 尺側手根伸筋 Extensor carpi ulnaris muscle
15 長橈側手根伸筋 Extensor carpi radialis longus muscle
16 小指伸筋 Extensor digiti minimi muscle
17 腕橈骨筋 Brachioradialis muscle
18 回外筋 Supinator muscle
19 腕橈関節 Humeroradial joint
20 橈骨(頭) Radius (head)
21 肘正中皮静脈 Median cubital vein
22 上腕骨(小頭) Humerus (capitulum)
23 上腕二頭筋(+腱) Biceps brachii muscle (+tendon)
24 上腕骨(体) Humerus (shaft)
25 上腕筋 Brachialis muscle
26 上腕三頭筋(+腱) Triceps brachii muscle (+tendon)

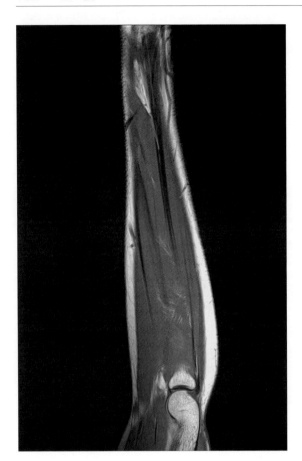

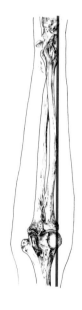

前腕，矢状断 **153**

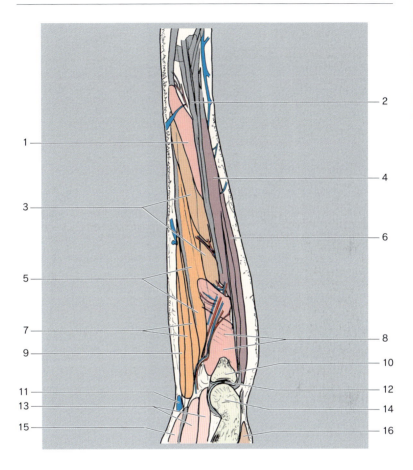

1 **短母指伸筋** Extensor pollicis brevis muscle
2 **指伸筋（腱）** Extensor digitorum muscle （tendon）
3 **長母指外転筋** Abductor pollicis longus muscle
4 **指伸筋（＋腱）** Extensor digitorum muscle （＋tendon）
5 **短橈側手根伸筋** Extensor carpi radialis brevis muscle
6 **小指伸筋** Extensor digiti minimi muscle
7 **長橈側手根伸筋** Extensor carpi radialis longus muscle
8 **回外筋** Supinator muscle
9 **腕橈骨筋** Brachioradialis muscle
10 **橈骨（頭）** Radius（head）
11 **肘正中皮静脈** Median cubital vein
12 **腕橈関節** Humeroradial joint
13 **上腕筋** Brachialis muscle
14 **上腕骨（小頭）** Humerus（capitulum）
15 **上腕二頭筋（＋腱）** Biceps brachii muscle （＋tendon）
16 **上腕三頭筋** Triceps brachii muscle

154   上肢

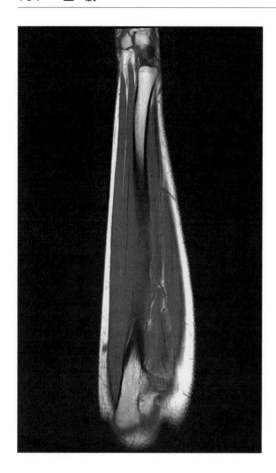

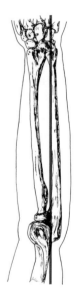

1 **小指外転筋** Abductor digiti minimi muscle
2 **三角骨** Triquetrum
3 **豆状骨** Pisiform
4 **尺骨茎状突起** Ulnar styloid process
5 **掌側尺骨手根靱帯** Palmar ulnocarpal ligament
6 **尺骨** Ulna
7 **尺骨神経** Ulnar nerve

前腕，冠状断

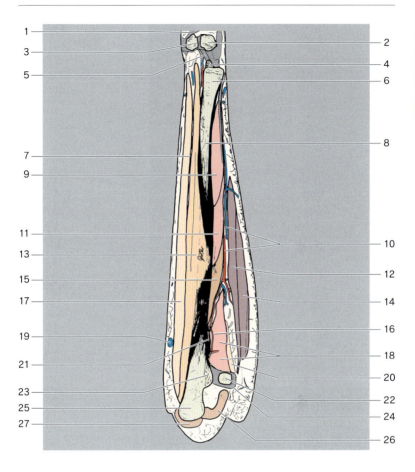

8 **尺骨(体)** Ulna (shaft)
9 **示指伸筋** Extensor indicis muscle
10 **後骨間動静脈** Posterior interosseous artery and vein
11 **短母指伸筋** Extensor pollicis brevis muscle
12 **小指伸筋** Extensor digiti minimi muscle
13 **深指屈筋** Flexor digitorum profundus muscle
14 **指伸筋** Extensor digitorum muscle
15 **長母指外転筋** Abductor pollicis longus muscle
16 **反回骨間動静脈** Recurrent interosseous artery and vein
17 **尺側手根屈筋** Flexor carpi ulnaris muscle
18 **回外筋** Supinator muscle
19 **尺側皮静脈** Basilic vein
20 **尺側手根伸筋** Extensor carpi ulnaris muscle
21 **上腕筋(付着部)** Brachialis muscle (attachment)
22 **橈骨(頭)** Radius (head)
23 **橈骨粗面** Radial tuberosity
24 **橈骨輪状靱帯** Anular ligament
25 **肘頭** Olecranon
26 **肘筋** Anconeus muscle
27 **上腕三頭筋** Triceps brachii muscle

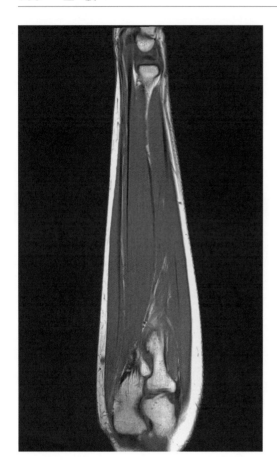
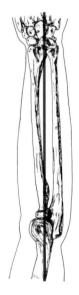

1 **尺骨静脈** Ulnar vein
2 **有鈎骨** Hamate
3 **深指屈筋(腱)** Flexor digitorum profundus muscle (tendon)
4 **三角骨** Triquetrum
5 **尺骨神経** Ulnar nerve
6 **小指伸筋(腱)** Extensor digiti minimi muscle (tendon)
7 **方形回内筋** Pronator quadratus muscle
8 **尺骨** Ulna
9 **前骨間動静脈** Anterior interosseous artery and vein
10 **小指伸筋** Extensor digiti minimi muscle
11 **示指伸筋** Extensor indicis muscle

前腕，冠状断 157

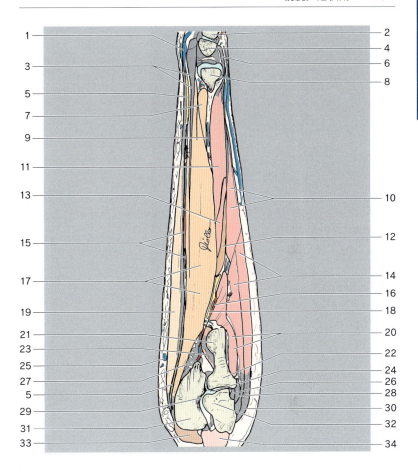

12 長母指外転筋 Abductor pollicis longus muscle
13 短母指伸筋 Extensor pollicis brevis muscle
14 指伸筋(＋腱) Extensor digitorum muscle (＋tendon)
15 尺骨動静脈 Ulnar artery and vein
16 骨間動静脈 Interosseous artery and vein
17 深指屈筋 Flexor digitorum profundus muscle
18 正中神経 Median nerve
19 尺側手根屈筋 Flexor carpi ulnaris muscle
20 回外筋 Supinator muscle
21 橈骨粗面 Radial tuberosity
22 橈骨(頭) Radius (head)
23 上腕二頭筋(＋腱) Biceps brachii muscle (＋tendon)
24 腕橈関節 Humeroradial joint
25 尺側皮静脈 Basilic vein
26 橈骨輪状靱帯 Anular ligament
27 上腕筋(付着部) Brachialis muscle (attachment)
28 外側側副靱帯 Radial collateral ligament
29 腕尺関節 Humeroulnar joint
30 伸筋群の共通腱(付着部) Common extensor tendon (attachment)
31 肘頭 Olecranon
32 上腕骨(小頭) Humerus (capitulum)
33 上腕三頭筋(＋腱) Triceps brachii muscle (＋tendon)
34 上腕筋 Brachialis muscle

158　上肢

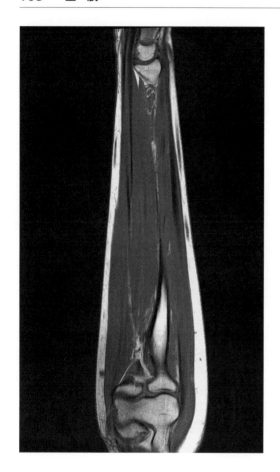

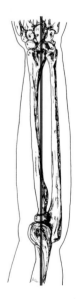

1　**正中神経** Median nerve
2　**有頭骨** Capitate
3　**手関節** Wrist joint
4　**月状骨** Lunate
5　**深指屈筋(腱)** Flexor digitorum profundus muscle(tendon)
6　**橈骨** Radius
7　**浅指屈筋(腱)** Flexor digitorum superficialis muscle(tendon)
8　**示指伸筋** Extensor indicis muscle
9　**方形回内筋** Pronator quadratus muscle
10　**後骨間動静脈** Posterior interosseous artery and vein

前腕，冠状断 159

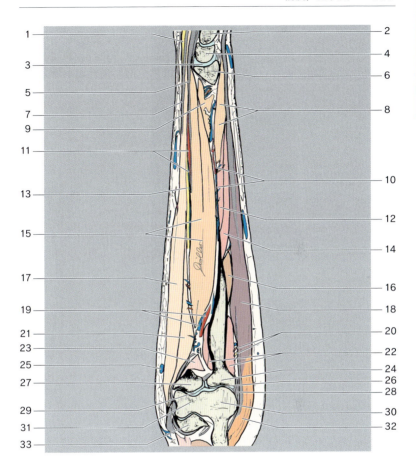

11 尺骨動静脈 Ulnar artery and vein
12 短母指伸筋 Extensor pollicis brevis muscle
13 尺骨神経 Ulnar nerve
14 長母指伸筋 Extensor pollicis longus muscle
15 深指屈筋 Flexor digitorum profundus muscle
16 長母指外転筋 Abductor pollicis longus muscle
17 尺側手根屈筋 Flexor carpi ulnaris muscle
18 指伸筋 Extensor digitorum muscle
19 前骨間動静脈 Anterior interosseous artery and vein
20 橈骨神経（深枝）Radial nerve (deep branch), 橈側反回動脈 Radial recurrent artery
21 浅指屈筋 Flexor digitorum superficialis muscle
22 回外筋 Supinator muscle
23 上腕筋 Brachialis muscle
24 橈骨（頭）Radius (head)
25 尺側皮静脈 Basilic vein
26 腕橈関節 Humeroradial joint
27 肘頭 Olecranon
28 外側側副靱帯 Radial collateral ligament
29 腕尺関節 Humeroulnar joint
30 上腕骨（小頭）Humerus (capitulum)
31 上腕骨（滑車）Humerus (trochlea)
32 短橈側手根伸筋 Extensor carpi radialis brevis muscle
33 鈎状突起 Coronoid process

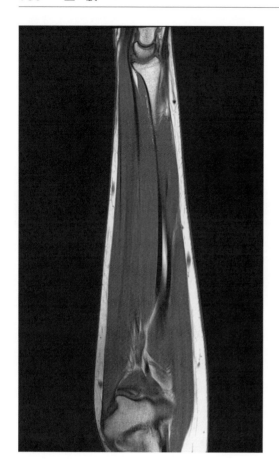

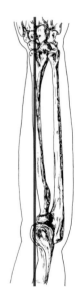

1 **有頭骨** Capitate
2 **指伸筋(腱)** Extensor digitorum muscle (tendon)
3 **浅指屈筋(腱)** Flexor digitorum superficialis muscle (tendon)
4 **月状骨** Lunate
5 **手関節** Wrist joint
6 **橈骨** Radius
7 **深指屈筋(腱)** Flexor digitorum profundus muscle (tendon)
8 **前骨間動静脈** Anterior interosseous artery and vein
9 **方形回内筋** Pronator quadratus muscle
10 **短母指伸筋** Extensor pollicis brevis muscle

前腕，冠状断

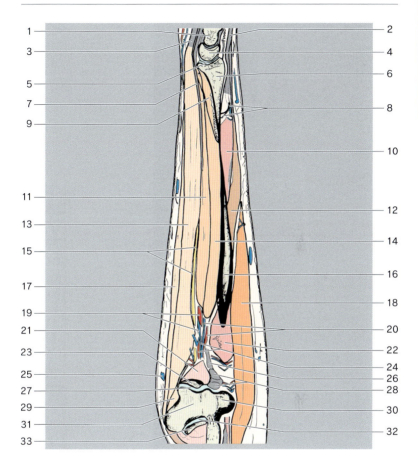

11 深指屈筋 Flexor digitorum profundus muscle
12 母指外転筋 Abductor pollicis muscle
13 浅指屈筋 Flexor digitorum superficialis muscle
14 長母指屈筋 Flexor pollicis longus muscle
15 正中神経 Median nerve
16 橈骨(体) Radius (shaft)
17 長掌筋 Palmaris longus muscle
18 長橈側手根伸筋 Extensor carpi radialis longus muscle,
短橈側手根伸筋 Extensor carpi radialis brevis muscle
19 尺骨動静脈 Ulnar artery and vein
20 後骨間動静脈 Posterior interosseous artery and vein
21 上腕筋 Brachialis muscle
22 回外筋 Supinator muscle
23 肘頭 Olecranon
24 橈骨動静脈 Radial artery and veins
25 尺側皮静脈 Basilic vein
26 上腕二頭筋(腱) Biceps brachii muscle (tendon)
27 腕尺関節 Humeroulnar joint
28 橈骨輪状靱帯 Anular ligament
29 円回内筋 Pronator teres muscle
30 上腕骨(小頭) Humerus (capitulum)
31 上腕骨(滑車) Humerus (trochlea)
32 肘頭窩 Olecranon fossa
33 鈎状突起 Coronoid process

162 上 肢

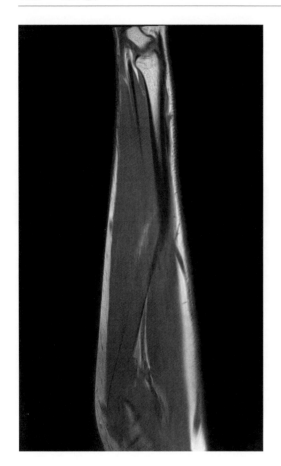

遠位
手掌側 □ 手背側
尺側   橈側
近位

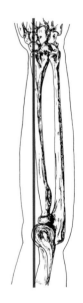

前腕，冠状断 163

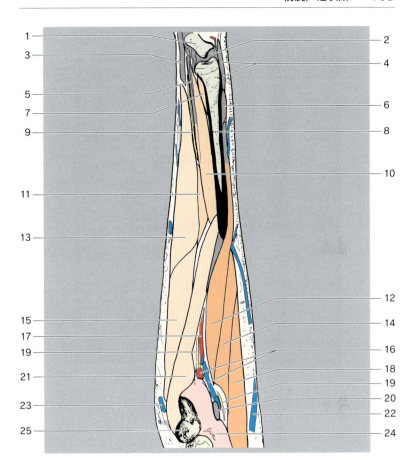

1 舟状骨 Scaphoid
2 手関節 Wrist joint
3 橈側手根屈筋(腱) Flexor carpi radialis muscle (tendon)
4 短橈側手根伸筋(腱) Extensor carpi radialis brevis muscle (tendon)
5 長母指屈筋(腱) Flexor pollicis longus muscle (tendon)
6 指伸筋 Extensor digitorum muscle
7 方形回内筋 Pronator quadratus muscle
8 橈骨(体) Radius (shaft)
9 正中神経 Median nerve
10 長母指屈筋 Flexor pollicis longus muscle
11 深指屈筋 Flexor digitorum profundus muscle
12 短橈側手根伸筋 Extensor carpi radialis brevis muscle
13 浅指屈筋 Flexor digitorum superficialis muscle
14 長橈側手根伸筋 Extensor carpi radialis longus muscle
15 橈側手根屈筋 Flexor carpi radialis muscle
16 上腕動静脈 Brachial artery and vein
17 橈骨動静脈 Radial artery and veins
18 腕橈骨筋 Brachioradialis muscle
19 橈骨神経 Radial nerve
20 上腕二頭筋(腱) Biceps brachii muscle (tendon)
21 円回内筋 Pronator teres muscle
22 橈側皮静脈 Cephalic vein
23 尺側皮静脈 Basilic vein
24 上腕筋 Brachialis muscle
25 内側上顆 Medial epicondyle

164 上肢

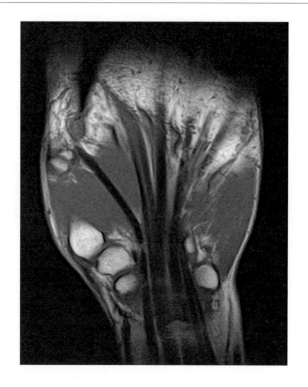

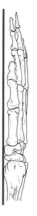

遠位
橈側 　　 尺側
近位

手，冠状断　**165**

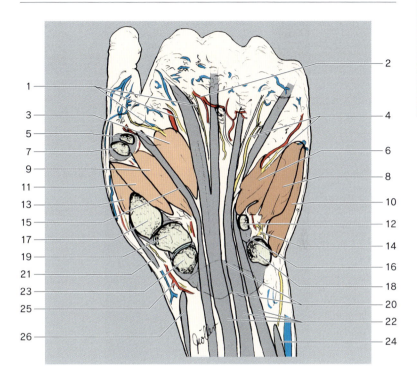

1 固有掌側指神経（正中神経）Proper palmar digital nerves(of median nerve)
2 固有掌側指動脈 Proper palmar digital arteries
3 母指内転筋（横頭）Adductor pollicis muscle (transverse head)
4 固有掌側指神経（尺骨神経）Proper palmar digital nerves(of ulnar nerve)
5 第1基節骨（底）Proximal phalanx I (base)
6 小指対立筋 Opponens digiti minimi muscle
7 第1中手骨（頭）Metacarpal I (head)
8 小指屈筋 Flexor digiti minimi muscle
9 短母指屈筋（深頭）Flexor pollicis brevis muscle(deep head)
10 小指外転筋 Abductor digiti minimi muscle
11 母指外転筋 Abductor pollicis muscle
12 有鈎骨（鈎）Hamate(hook)
13 母指対立筋 Opponens pollicis muscle
14 尺骨神経（深枝）Ulnar nerve(deep branch)
15 長母指屈筋（腱）Flexor pollicis longus muscle (tendon)
16 豆鈎靱帯 Pisohamate ligament
17 第1中手骨（底）Metacarpal I (base)
18 豆状骨 Pisiform
19 大菱形骨 Trapezium
20 掌側橈骨手根靱帯 Palmar radiocarpal ligament
21 長母指外転筋（腱付着部）Abductor pollicis longus muscle(tendon attachment)
22 深指屈筋（腱）Flexor digitorum profundus muscle(tendons)
23 舟状骨 Scaphoid
24 尺側手根屈筋 Flexor carpi ulnaris muscle
25 橈骨動脈（浅掌枝）Radial artery(superficial palmar branch)
26 腕橈骨筋（腱）Brachioradialis muscle(tendon)

166　上　肢

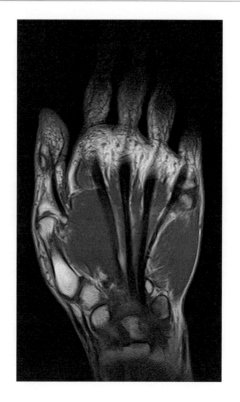

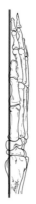

遠位

橈側　□　尺側

近位

1　**第1末節骨**　Distal phalanx I
2　**固有掌側指動脈, 神経**　Proper palmar digital arteries and nerves
3　**第1基節骨(頭)**　Proximal phalanx I (head)
4　**虫様筋**　Lumbrical muscles
5　**長母指屈筋(腱)**　Flexor pollicis longus muscle (tendon)

手，冠状断　**167**

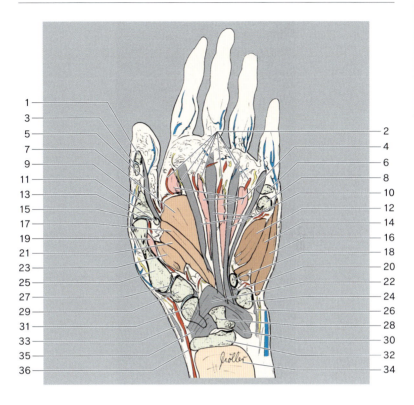

6　第5基節骨(底) Proximal phalanx V (base)
7　母指内転筋(横頭) Adductor pollicis muscle (transverse head)
8　第5中手骨(頭) Metacarpal V (head)
9　第1基節骨(底) Proximal phalanx I (base)
10　深指屈筋(腱) Flexor digitorum profundus muscle (tendons)
11　種子骨 Sesamoid bone
12　小指対立筋 Opponens digiti minimi muscle
13　第1中手指節関節 Metacarpophalangeal joint I
14　小指屈筋 Flexor digiti minimi muscle
15　関節包 Joint capsule
16　小指外転筋 Abductor digiti minimi muscle
17　母指内転筋(斜頭) Adductor pollicis muscle (oblique head)
18　有鈎骨(鈎) Hamate (hook)
19　骨間筋 Interosseous muscle
20　豆鈎靱帯 Pisohamate ligament
21　短母指屈筋 Flexor pollicis brevis muscle
22　放射性手根靱帯 Radiate carpal ligament
23　母指対立筋 Opponens pollicis muscle
24　豆状骨 Pisiform
25　第1中手骨 Metacarpal I
26　内側手根側副靱帯 Ulnar collateral ligament of wrist joint
27　第1手根中手関節 Carpometacarpal joint I
28　月状骨 Lunate
29　大菱形骨 Trapezium
30　掌側尺骨手根靱帯 Palmar ulnocarpal ligament
31　舟状骨 Scaphoid
32　橈骨 Radius
33　短母指伸筋(腱) Extensor pollicis brevis muscle (tendon)
34　方形回内筋 Pronator quadratus muscle
35　掌側橈骨手根靱帯 Palmar radiocarpal ligament
36　橈骨動脈 Radial artery

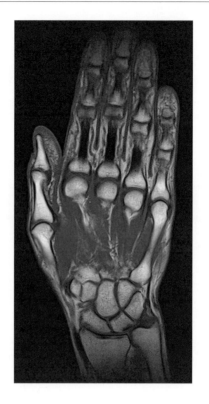

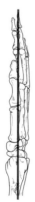

遠位

橈側 　　 尺側

近位

1 第2末節骨 Distal phalanx II
2 遠位指節間関節 Distal interphalangeal joint
3 中節骨(底) Middle phalanx (base)
4 固有掌側指神経,動脈 Proper palmar digital nerves and arteries
5 基節骨(頭) Proximal phalanx (head)
6 指屈筋(腱) Flexor digitorum muscle (tendon)
7 第1末節骨 Distal phalanx I
8 近位指節間関節 Proximal interphalangeal joint
9 第2中手骨(頭) Metacarpal II (head)
10 側副靱帯 Collateral ligament

手，冠状断　169

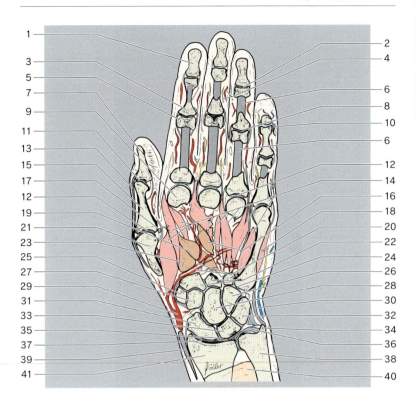

- 11 第1指節間関節 Interphalangeal joint I
- 12 中手指節関節 Metacarpophalangeal joint
- 13 長母指伸筋(腱) Extensor pollicis longus muscle(tendon)
- 14 骨間筋 Interosseous muscles
- 15 第1基節骨 Proximal phalanx I
- 16 母指内転筋(横頭) Adductor pollicis muscle (transverse head)
- 17 種子骨 Sesamoid bone
- 18 小指外転筋 Abductor digiti minimi muscle
- 19 母指内転筋(斜頭) Adductor pollicis muscle (oblique head)
- 20 深掌動脈弓 Deep palmar arch, 手掌手根動脈弓 Palmar carpal arch
- 21 第1中手骨(頭) Metacarpal I (head)
- 22 中手(底) Metacarpals(bases)
- 23 短母指屈筋 Flexor pollicis brevis muscle
- 24 手根中手関節 Carpometacarpal joint
- 25 大菱形骨 Trapezium
- 26 有鈎骨 Hamate
- 27 小菱形骨 Trapezoid
- 28 有頭骨 Capitate
- 29 橈骨動脈 Radial artery
- 30 内側手根側副靱帯 Ulnar collateral ligament of wrist joint
- 31 舟状骨 Scaphoid
- 32 三角骨 Triquetrum
- 33 月状骨 Lunate
- 34 尺骨茎状突起 Ulnar styloid process
- 35 (舟状月状)骨間靱帯 Interosseous ligament (scapholunate)
- 36 三角線維骨軟複合体(TFC) Triangular fibrocartilage complex(TFC)
- 37 手関節 Wrist joint
- 38 尺骨 Ulna
- 39 腕橈骨筋(腱) Brachioradialis muscle(tendon)
- 40 方形回内筋 Pronator quadratus muscle
- 41 橈骨 Radius

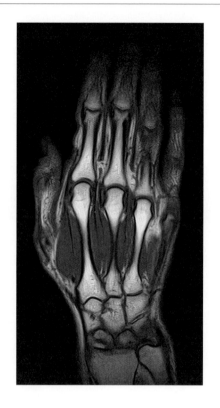

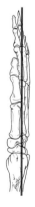

遠位

橈側 ☐ 尺側

近位

1 中節骨(底) Middle phalanx(base)
2 背側指動脈,神経 Dorsal digital arteries and nerves
3 側副靱帯 Collateral ligament
4 近位指節間関節 Proximal interphalangeal joint
5 基節骨(頭) Proximal phalanx(head)
6 中手指節関節 Metacarpophalangeal joint
7 基節骨(体) Proximal phalanx(shaft)
8 骨間筋 Interosseous muscles
9 基節骨(底) Proximal phalanx(base)
10 背側中手静脈 Dorsal metacarpal vein
11 中手骨(頭) Metacarpal(head)
12 関節包 Joint capsule

手, 冠状断 171

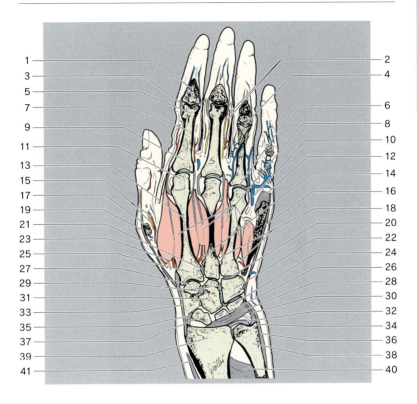

- 13 中手骨(体) Metacarpal(shaft)
- 14 背側中手動脈 Dorsal metacarpal arteries
- 15 母指の背側中手動脈,神経 Dorsal metacarpal artery and nerve of thumb
- 16 指伸筋(腱) Extensor digitorum muscle (tendon)
- 17 第1中手骨(頭) Metacarpal I (head)
- 18 背側中手動脈(貫通枝) Dorsal metacarpal arteries (perforating branches)
- 19 長母指伸筋(腱) Extensor pollicis longus muscle(tendon)
- 20 手根中手関節 Carpometacarpal joint
- 21 骨間中手靱帯 Interosseous metacarpal ligaments
- 22 有鈎骨 Hamate
- 23 橈骨動脈(背側手根枝) Radial artery (dorsal carpal branch)
- 24 三角骨 Triquetrum
- 25 第2中手骨(底) Metacarpal II (base)
- 26 月状骨 Lunate
- 27 小菱形骨 Trapezoid
- 28 背側橈骨手根靱帯 Dorsal radiocarpal ligament
- 29 骨間手根間靱帯 Interosseous intercarpal ligament
- 30 内側手根側副靱帯 Ulnar collateral ligament of wrist joint
- 31 有頭骨 Capitate
- 32 尺骨の関節円板 Ulnar articular disk
- 33 長橈側手根伸筋(腱) Extensor carpi radialis longus muscle(tendon)
- 34 尺骨茎状突起 Styloid process of ulna
- 35 外側手根側副靱帯 Radial collateral ligament of wrist joint
- 36 尺側手根伸筋(腱) Extensor carpi ulnaris muscle(tendon)
- 37 舟状骨 Scaphoid
- 38 尺骨 Ulna
- 39 橈骨 Radius
- 40 骨間膜 Interosseous membrane
- 41 腕橈骨筋(腱) Brachioradialis muscle(tendon)

172 上　肢

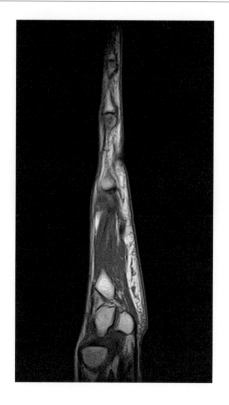

遠位

手背側 □ 手掌側

近位

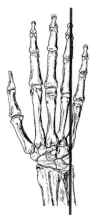

1 末節骨 Distal phalanx
2 遠位指節間関節 Distal interphalangeal joint
3 関節包 Joint capsule
4 中節骨(頭) Middle phalanx(head)
5 中節骨(底) Middle phalanx(base)
6 掌側靱帯 Palmar(collateral)ligament
7 近位指節間関節 Proximal interphalangeal joint
8 指屈筋(腱) Flexor digitorum muscle (tendon)
9 基節骨(頭) Proximal phalanx(head)
10 中手指節関節 Metacarpophalangeal joint

手，矢状断

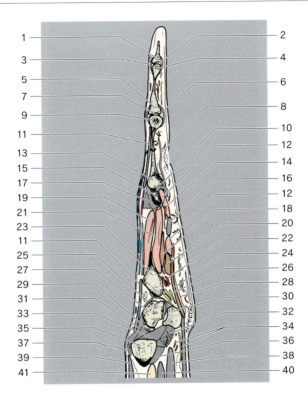

11 指伸筋(腱) Extensor digitorum muscle (tendon)
12 虫様筋 Lumbrical muscles
13 基節骨(底) Proximal phalanx (base)
14 掌側中手動脈 Palmar metacarpal artery
15 中手骨(頭) Metacarpal (head)
16 小指屈筋(腱) Flexor digiti minimi muscle (tendon)
17 側副靱帯と骨間筋の付着部 Collateral ligament and attachment of interosseous muscles
18 小指対立筋 Opponens digiti minimi muscle
19 背側骨間筋 Dorsal interosseous muscle
20 短小指屈筋 Flexor digiti minimi brevis muscle
21 掌側骨間筋 Palmar interosseous muscle
22 深掌動脈弓 Deep palmar arch
23 中手骨(底) Metacarpal V (base)
24 小指外転筋 Abductor digiti minimi muscle
25 背側手根中手靱帯 Dorsal carpometacarpal ligament
26 尺骨神経(深枝) Ulnar nerve (deep branch)
27 三角骨 Triquetrum
28 短掌筋 Palmaris brevis muscle
29 月状骨 Lunate
30 豆状骨 Pisiform
31 背側橈骨手根靱帯 Dorsal radiocarpal ligament
32 掌側尺骨手根靱帯 Palmar ulnocarpal ligament
33 三角線維軟骨 Triangular fibrocartilage complex (＋関節円板 +disk equivalent)
34 尺骨動脈, 神経 Ulnar artery and nerve
35 尺骨 Ulna
36 掌側橈尺靱帯 Palmar radioulnar ligament
37 背側橈尺靱帯 Dorsal radioulnar ligament
38 浅指屈筋(腱) Flexor digitorum superficialis muscle (tendon)
39 尺側手根伸筋(腱) Extensor carpi ulnaris muscle (tendon)
40 深指屈筋(腱) Flexor digitorum profundus muscle (tendon)
41 方形回内筋 Pronator quadratus muscle

174 上肢

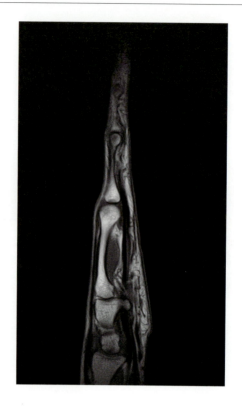

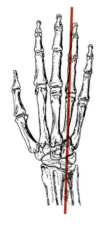

遠位
手背側 □ 手掌側
近位

1 **側副靱帯** Collateral ligament
2 **中節骨(頭)** Middle phalanx(head)
3 **背側指静脈** Dorsal digital vein
4 **掌側指静脈** Palmar digital vein
5 **中節骨(底)** Middle phalanx(base)
6 **掌側靱帯** Palmar(collateral)ligament
7 **近位指節間関節** Proximal interphalangeal joint
8 **掌側指動脈,神経** Palmar digital artery and nerve
9 **基節骨(頭)** Proximal phalanx(head)
10 **浅指屈筋(腱)** Flexor digitorum superficialis muscle(tendon)

手，矢状断 175

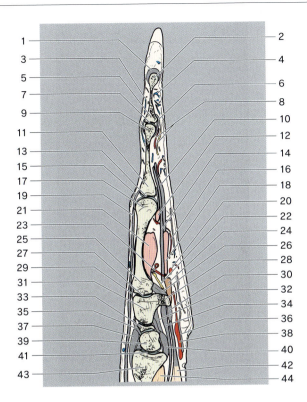

11 基節骨(底) Proximal phalanx (base)
12 掌側骨間筋 Palmar interosseous muscle
13 中手指節関節 Metacarpophalangeal joint
14 深指屈筋(腱) Flexor digitorum profundus muscle (tendon)
15 関節包 Joint capsule
16 掌側指動脈 Palmar digital artery
17 中手骨(頭) Metacarpal (head)
18 虫様筋 Lumbrical muscle
19 指伸筋(腱) Extensor digitorum muscle (tendon)
20 浅掌動脈弓 Superficial palmar arch
21 掌側骨間筋 Palmar interosseous muscle
22 尺骨神経 Ulnar nerve (deep branch)
23 深掌動脈弓 Deep palmar arch
24 短小指屈筋 Flexor digiti minimi brevis muscle
25 中手骨(底) Metacarpal (base)
26 掌側手根中手靱帯 Palmar carpometacarpal ligament
27 手根中手関節 Carpometacarpal joint
28 有鈎骨 Hamate (hook)
29 背側手根中手靱帯 Dorsal carpometacarpal ligament
30 屈筋支帯 Flexor retinaculum
31 有鈎骨 Hamate
32 掌側手根間靱帯 Palmar intercarpal ligament
33 三角骨 Triquetrum
34 指屈筋(腱) Flexor digitorum muscle (tendon)
35 背側手根間靱帯 Dorsal intercarpal ligament
36 手掌腱膜 Palmar aponeurosis
37 背側橈骨手根靱帯 Dorsal radiocarpal ligament
38 尺骨動脈 Ulnar artery
39 月状骨 Lunate
40 掌側尺骨手根靱帯 Palmar ulnocarpal ligament
41 橈骨手根関節 Radiocarpal joint
42 尺側手根屈筋 Flexor carpi ulnaris muscle
43 橈骨 Radius
44 方形回内筋 Pronator quadratus muscle

176 上肢

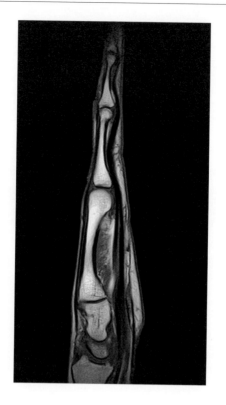

遠位

手背側 ☐ 手掌側

近位

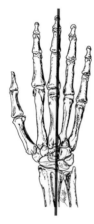

1 **末節骨** Distal phalanx
2 **中節骨(頭)** Middle phalanx(head)
3 **遠位指節間関節** Distal interphalangeal joint
4 **掌側靱帯** Palmar ligament
5 **関節包** Joint capsule
6 **掌側指動脈** Palmar digital artery
7 **中節骨(底)** Middle phalanx(base)
8 **指屈筋(腱)** Flexor digitorum muscle (tendon)
9 **近位指節間関節** Proximal interphalangeal joint
10 **基節骨(体)** Proximal phalanx(shaft)
11 **基節骨(頭)** Proximal phalanx(head)

手，矢状断

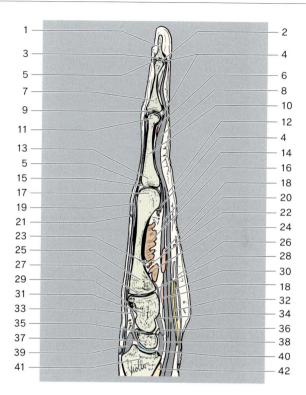

12 浅指屈筋(腱) Flexor digitorum superficialis muscle (tendon)
13 基節骨(底) Proximal phalanx (base)
14 深指屈筋(腱) Flexor digitorum profundus muscle (tendon)
15 中手指節関節 Metacarpophalangeal joint
16 母指内転筋(横頭) Adductor pollicis muscle (transverse head)
17 中手骨(頭) Metacarpal (head)
18 虫様筋 Lumbrical muscles
19 指伸筋(腱) Extensor digitorum muscle (tendon)
20 浅掌動脈弓 Superficial palmar arch
21 掌側指静脈 Palmar digital vein
22 尺骨神経(深枝) Ulnar nerve (deep branch)
23 深掌動脈弓 Deep palmar arch
24 母指内転筋(深頭) Adductor pollicis muscle (deep head)
25 中手骨(底) Metacarpal (base)
26 手掌腱膜 Palmar aponeurosis
27 手根中手関節 Carpometacarpal joint
28 掌側手根中手靱帯 Palmar carpometacarpal ligament
29 背側手根中手靱帯 Dorsal carpometacarpal ligament
30 屈筋支帯 Flexor retinaculum
31 有頭骨 Capitate
32 正中神経 Median nerve
33 背側手根間靱帯 Dorsal intercarpal ligament
34 掌側手根間靱帯 Palmar intercarpal ligament
35 (舟状有頭)手根間関節 Intercarpal (scapho-capitate) joint
36 月状骨 Lunate
37 舟状骨 Scaphoid
38 掌側橈骨手根靱帯 Palmar radiocarpal ligament
39 背側橈骨手根靱帯 Dorsal radiocarpal ligament
40 手関節 Wrist joint
41 橈骨 Radius
42 方形回内筋 Pronator quadratus muscle

178　上肢

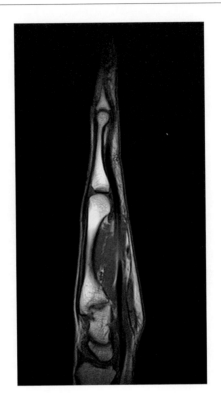

遠位

手背側 □ 手掌側

近位

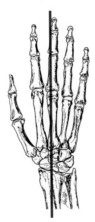

1 **側副靱帯（遠位指節間関節）** Collateral ligament (distal interphalangeal joint)
2 **近位指節間関節** Proximal interphalangeal joint
3 **中節骨（底）** Middle phalanx (base)
4 **掌側靱帯** Palmar ligament
5 **基節骨（頭）** Proximal phalanx (head)
6 **指屈筋（腱）** Flexor digitorum muscle (tendon)
7 **関節包** Joint capsule
8 **中手指節関節** Metacarpophalangeal joint

手，矢状断   179

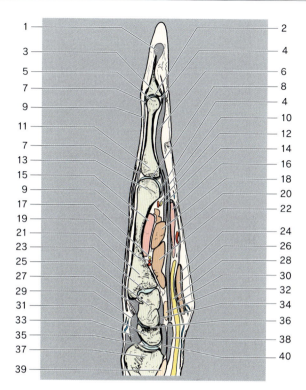

9	指伸筋(腱) Extensor digitorum muscle (tendon)	24	手掌腱膜 Palmar aponeurosis
10	浅指屈筋(腱) Flexor digitorum superficialis muscle(tendon)	25	有頭骨 Capitate
11	基節骨(底) Proximal phalanx(base)	26	短母指外転筋 Abductor pollicis brevis muscle
12	総掌側指動脈 Common palmar digital arteries	27	背側手根中手靱帯 Dorsal carpometacarpal ligament
13	中手骨(頭) Metacarpal(head)	28	正中神経 Median nerve
14	深指屈筋(腱) Flexor digitorum profundus muscle(tendon)	29	背側手根間靱帯 Dorsal intercarpal ligament
15	骨間筋 Interosseous muscle	30	屈筋支帯 Flexor retinaculum
16	虫様筋 Lumbrical muscles	31	舟状骨 Scaphoid
17	尺骨神経(深枝) Ulnar nerve(deep branch)	32	短母指屈筋(深頭) Flexor pollicis brevis muscle (deep head)
18	母指内転筋(横頭) Adductor pollicis muscle (transverse head)	33	背側橈骨手根靱帯 Dorsal radiocarpal ligament
19	深掌動脈弓 Deep palmar arch	34	掌側手根間靱帯 Palmar intercarpal ligament
20	浅掌動脈弓 Superficial palmar arch	35	橈骨手根関節 Radiocarpal joint
21	中手骨(底) Metacarpal(base)	36	(舟状有頭)手根間関節 Intercarpal(scapho-capitate)joint
22	母指内転筋(斜頭) Adductor pollicis muscle (oblique head)	37	橈骨 Radius
23	手根中手関節 Carpometacarpal joint	38	長母指屈筋(腱) Flexor pollicis longus muscle (tendon)
		39	方形回内筋 Pronator quadratus muscle
		40	掌側橈骨手根靱帯 Palmar radiocarpal ligament

180 上肢

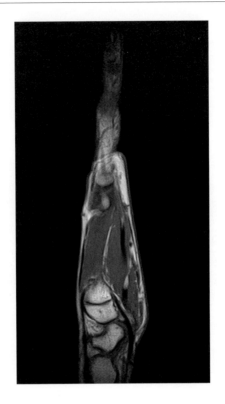

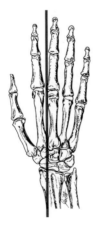

遠位

手背側 □ 手掌側

近位

1 **背側指静脈** Dorsal digital vein
2 **総掌側指動脈** Common palmar digital artery
3 **基節骨(底)** Proximal phalanx (base)
4 **虫様筋** Lumbrical muscles
5 **側副靱帯(中手指節関節)** Collateral ligament (metacarpophalangeal joint)
6 **母指内転筋(横頭)** Adductor pollicis muscle (transverse head)
7 **中手骨(頭)** Metacarpal (head)
8 **手掌腱膜** Palmar aponeurosis
9 **骨間筋** Interosseous muscle

手，矢状断

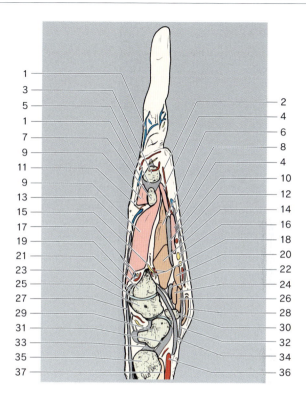

- 10 指屈筋(腱) Flexor digitorum muscle (tendon)
- 11 背側指動脈 Dorsal digital artery
- 12 浅掌動脈弓 Superficial palmar arch
- 13 指伸筋(腱) Extensor digitorum muscle (tendon)
- 14 母指内転筋(斜頭) Adductor pollicis muscle (oblique head)
- 15 尺骨神経(深枝) Ulnar nerve (deep branch)
- 16 総掌側指神経(正中神経) Common palmar digital nerve (of median nerve)
- 17 背側指動脈, 神経 Dorsal digital arteries and nerves
- 18 深掌動脈弓 Deep palmar arch
- 19 第2中手骨(底) Metacarpal II (base)
- 20 短母指屈筋(浅頭) Flexor pollicis brevis muscle (superficial head)
- 21 第3中手骨(底) Metacarpal III (base)
- 22 長母指屈筋(腱) Flexor pollicis longus muscle (tendon)
- 23 手根中手関節 Carpometacarpal joint
- 24 短母指屈筋(深頭) Flexor pollicis brevis muscle (deep head)
- 25 小菱形骨 Trapezoid
- 26 母指対立筋 Opponens pollicis muscle
- 27 短橈側手根伸筋 Extensor carpi radialis brevis muscle
- 28 短母指外転筋 Abductor pollicis brevis muscle
- 29 舟状骨 Scaphoid
- 30 有鈎骨(鈎) Hamate (hook)
- 31 掌側橈骨手根靱帯 Palmar radiocarpal ligament
- 32 屈筋支帯 Flexor retinaculum
- 33 外側手根側副靱帯 Radial collateral ligament of wrist joint
- 34 橈側手根屈筋 Flexor carpi radialis muscle
- 35 橈骨 Radius
- 36 橈骨動脈 Radial artery
- 37 方形回内筋 Pronator quadratus muscle

182　上　肢

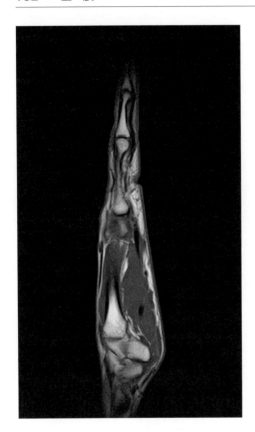

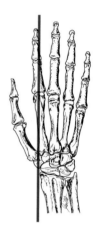

遠位

手背側　　手掌側

近位

1　末節骨　Distal phalanx
2　掌側靭帯　Palmar(collateral)ligament
3　遠位指節間関節　Distal interphalangeal joint
4　指屈筋(腱)　Flexor digitorum muscle(tendon)
5　中節骨(頭)　Middle phalanx(head)
6　固有掌側指動脈　Proper palmar digital artery
7　指伸筋(腱)　Extensor digitorum muscle(tendon)
8　固有掌側指神経　Proper palmar digital nerves
9　中節骨(底)　Middle phalanx(base)
10　指屈筋(腱)　Flexor digitorum muscle(tendon)
11　側副靭帯　Collateral ligament
12　虫様筋　Lumbrical muscles
13　基節骨(頭)　Proximal phalanx(head)
14　母指内転筋(横頭)　Adductor pollicis muscle (transverse head)
15　背側指動脈　Dorsal digital artery
16　総掌側指神経　Common palmar digital nerve
17　基節骨(底)　Proximal phalanx(base)
18　浅掌動脈弓　Superficial palmar arch
19　中手骨(頭)　Metacarpal(head)
20　正中神経　Median nerve
21　側副靭帯　Collateral ligament
22　母指内転筋(斜頭)　Adductor pollicis muscle (oblique head)
23　指動脈(貫通枝)　Digital artery(perforating branch)
24　掌側中手動脈　Palmar metacarpal artery
25　背側指静脈　Dorsal digital vein

手，矢状断

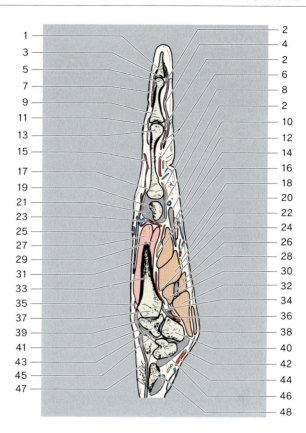

26 短母指屈筋(浅頭) Flexor pollicis brevis muscle (superficial head)
27 背側骨間筋 Dorsal interosseous muscles
28 長母指屈筋(腱) Flexor pollicis longus muscle (tendon)
29 掌側骨間筋 Palmar interosseous muscles
30 短母指屈筋(深頭) Flexor pollicis brevis muscle (deep head)
31 第2指の指伸筋(腱) Extensor digitorum II muscle (tendon)
32 母指対立筋 Opponens pollicis muscle
33 第2中手骨(体) Metacarpal II (shaft)
34 掌側手根中手靱帯 Palmar carpometacarpal ligament
35 背側中手動脈 Dorsal metacarpal artery
36 深掌動脈弓 Deep palmar arch
37 第2中手骨(底) Metacarpal II (base)
38 短母指外転筋 Abductor pollicis brevis muscle
39 手根中手関節 Carpometacarpal joint
40 大菱形骨(結節) Trapezium (tubercle)
41 背側手根中手副靱帯 Dorsal carpometacarpal ligament
42 外側手根側副靱帯 Radial collateral ligament of wrist joint
43 小菱形骨 Trapezoid
44 橈骨動脈(浅掌枝) Radial artery (superficial palmar branch)
45 背側手根間靱帯 Dorsal intercarpal ligament
46 舟状骨 Scaphoid
47 長橈側手根伸筋(腱) Extensor carpi radialis longus muscle (tendon)
48 橈骨(茎状突起) Radius (styloid process)

色分けコード：下肢　　**185**

■ 動脈

■ 神経

■ 静脈

□ 骨

□ 脂肪組織

□ 軟骨

■ 腱

■ 半月板, 関節唇など

■ 液体

■ 腸管

骨盤と大腿の筋:

縫工筋
大腿筋膜張筋
腸骨筋
腸腰筋
腰筋
大殿筋, 中殿筋, 小殿筋
腹直筋
外腹斜筋, 内腹斜筋
梨状筋
双子筋
大腿方形筋
内閉鎖筋
半腱様筋
半膜様筋
大腿二頭筋

内転筋群:
外閉鎖筋
恥骨筋
長内転筋, 短内転筋, 大内転筋
薄筋

大腿四頭筋:
大腿直筋
外側広筋, 内側広筋, 中間広筋

膝窩筋

下腿の筋:

伸筋群:
前脛骨筋
長趾伸筋
長母趾伸筋

腓骨筋群:
短腓骨筋
長腓骨筋

屈筋群:
後脛骨筋
長趾屈筋
長母趾屈筋

下腿三頭筋:
腓腹筋
ヒラメ筋
足底筋

足の筋:

短趾伸筋
短母趾伸筋

背側骨間筋, 底側骨間筋
短趾屈筋
足底方形筋
虫様筋

母趾の筋:
短母趾屈筋
母趾外転筋
母趾内転筋

小趾(第5趾)の筋:
小趾外転筋
小趾屈筋
小趾対立筋

注：下肢の指については趾を使ったが，趾のかわりに指を使うこともある.

186　下 肢

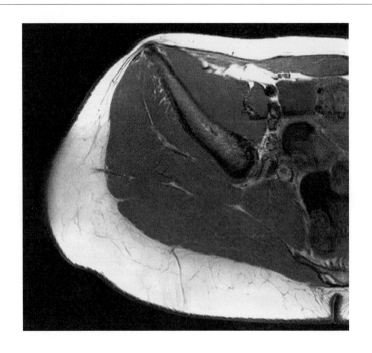

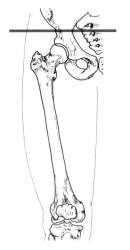

腹側

外側 ☐ 内側

背側

下肢，軸位断

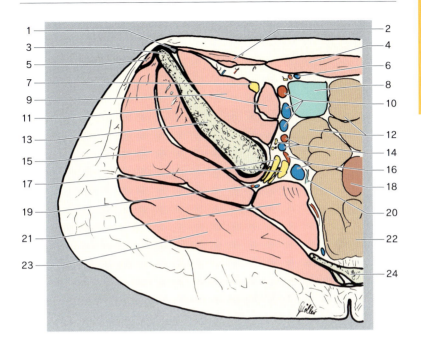

1 鼠径靭帯 Inguinal ligament
2 内腹斜筋 Internal oblique muscle, 腹横筋 Transversus abdominis muscle
3 前上腸骨棘 Anterior superior iliac spine
4 腹直筋 Rectus abdominis muscle
5 大腿筋膜張筋 Tensor fasciae latae muscle
6 下腹壁動静脈 Inferior epigastric artery and vein
7 大腿神経 Femoral nerve
8 膀胱 Urinary bladder
9 腸腰筋 Iliopsoas muscle
10 外腸骨動静脈 External iliac artery and veins
11 小殿筋 Gluteus minimus muscle
12 小腸 Small intestine
13 腸骨 Ilium
14 閉鎖動静脈，神経 Obturator artery, vein, and nerve
15 中殿筋 Gluteus medius muscle
16 内腸骨動静脈 Internal iliac artery and vein
17 仙骨神経叢 Sacral plexus
18 子宮 Uterus
19 上殿動静脈 Superior gluteal artery and vein
20 尿管 Ureter
21 梨状筋 Piriformis muscle
22 S状結腸 Sigmoid colon
23 大殿筋 Gluteus maximus muscle
24 仙骨 Sacrum

188　下　肢

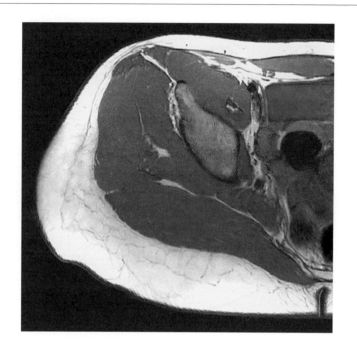

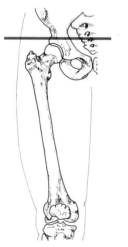

腹側
外側　内側
背側

下肢，軸位断   189

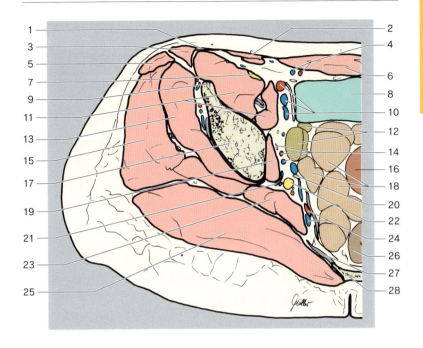

1 鼠径靱帯 Inguinal ligament
2 内腹斜筋 Internal oblique muscle, 腹横筋 Transversus abdominis muscle
3 縫工筋 Sartorius muscle
4 下腹壁動静脈 Inferior epigastric artery and vein
5 大腿筋膜張筋 Tensor fasciae latae muscle
6 腹直筋 Rectus abdominis muscle
7 大腿神経 Femoral nerve
8 膀胱 Urinary bladder
9 下前腸骨棘 Inferior anterior iliac spine
10 外腸骨動静脈 External iliac artery and veins
11 腸腰筋 Iliopsoas muscle
12 卵巣 Ovary, 卵管 Uterine tube
13 小殿筋 Gluteus minimus muscle
14 閉鎖動静脈，神経 Obturator artery, vein, and nerve
15 中殿筋 Gluteus medius muscle
16 子宮 Uterus
17 腸骨 Ilium
18 小腸 Small intestine
19 内閉鎖筋 Obturator internus muscle
20 尿管 Ureter
21 上殿動静脈 Superior gluteal artery and vein
22 腰仙骨神経叢 Lumbosacral plexus
23 梨状筋 Piriformis muscle
24 内腸骨動静脈 Internal iliac artery and vein
25 大殿筋 Gluteus maximus muscle
26 直腸 Rectum
27 仙結節靱帯 Sacrotuberous ligament
28 仙骨 Sacrum

190　下　肢

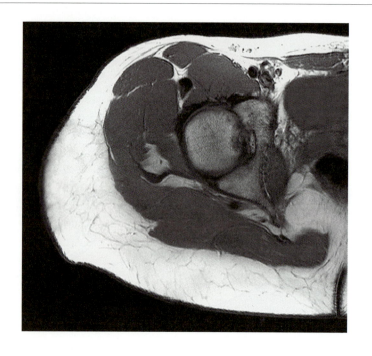

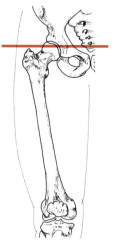

腹側

外側 □ 内側

背側

下肢，軸位断　　191

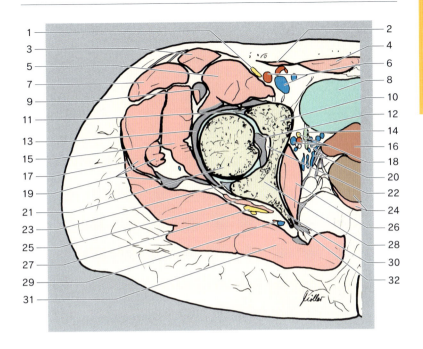

1 大腿神経 Femoral nerve
2 内腹斜筋 Internal oblique muscle, 腹横筋 Transversus abdominis muscle
3 縫工筋 Sartorius muscle
4 腹直筋 Rectus abdominis muscle
5 腸腰筋 Iliopsoas muscle
6 外腸骨動静脈 External iliac artery and vein
7 大腿筋膜張筋 Tensor fasciae latae muscle
8 膀胱 Urinary bladder
9 大腿直筋(腱) Rectus femoris muscle(tendon)
10 恥骨(上枝) Pubis(superior ramus)
11 前方関節唇 Anterior acetabular labrum
12 大腿骨頭靱帯 Ligament of head of femur
13 腸骨大腿靱帯 Iliofemoral ligament
14 尿管 Ureter
15 小殿筋 Gluteus minimus muscle
16 子宮 Uterus
17 腸脛靱帯 Iliotibial tract
18 閉鎖動静脈，神経 Obturator artery, vein, and nerve
19 中殿筋(+腱) Gluteus medius muscle(+tendon)
20 子宮静脈叢 Uterine venous plexus
21 大腿骨(頭) Femur(head)
22 寛骨臼窩 Acetabular fossa
23 後方関節唇 Posterior acetabular labrum
24 直腸 Rectum, 肛門挙筋 Levator ani muscle
25 梨状筋 Piriformis muscle
26 内閉鎖筋 Obturator internus muscle
27 坐骨神経 Sciatic nerve
28 坐骨 Ischium
29 上殿動静脈 Superior gluteal artery and vein
30 坐骨棘 Ischial spine
31 大殿筋 Gluteus maximus muscle
32 仙結節靱帯 Sacrotuberous ligament

192 下 肢

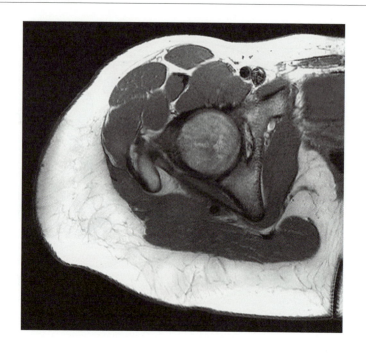

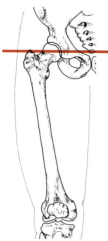

腹側
外側 □ 内側
背側

下肢，軸位断

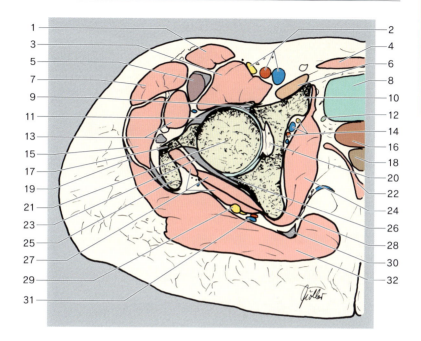

1 縫工筋 Sartorius muscle
2 大腿動静脈,神経 Femoral artery, vein, and nerve
3 腸腰筋 Iliopsoas muscle
4 腹直筋 Rectus abdominis muscle
5 大腿直筋（＋腱）Rectus femoris muscle (+tendon)
6 恥骨筋 Pectineus muscle
7 大腿筋膜張筋 Tensor fasciae latae muscle
8 膀胱 Urinary bladder
9 前方関節唇 Anterior acetabular labrum
10 恥骨（上枝）Pubis (superior ramus)
11 腸骨大腿靱帯 Iliofemoral ligament
12 尿管 Ureter
13 小殿筋（＋腱）Gluteus minimus muscle (+tendon)
14 閉鎖動静脈,神経 Obturator artery, vein, and nerve
15 中殿筋（＋腱）Gluteus medius muscle (+tendon)
16 腟 Vagina
17 大腿骨（頸）Femur (neck)
18 直腸 Rectum
19 腸脛靱帯 Iliotibial tract
20 寛骨臼窩 Acetabular fossa
21 大腿骨（頭）Femur (head)
22 肛門挙筋 Levator ani muscle
23 坐骨大腿靱帯 Ischiofemoral ligament, 関節包靱帯 Capsular ligament
24 内閉鎖筋 Obturator internus muscle
25 大転子 Greater trochanter
26 後方関節唇 Posterior acetabular labrum
27 下双子筋 Gemellus inferior muscle
28 坐骨 Ischium
29 坐骨神経 Sciatic nerve
30 仙結節靱帯 Sacrotuberous ligament
31 上殿動脈,神経 Superior gluteal artery and nerve
32 大殿筋 Gluteus maximus muscle

194 下　肢

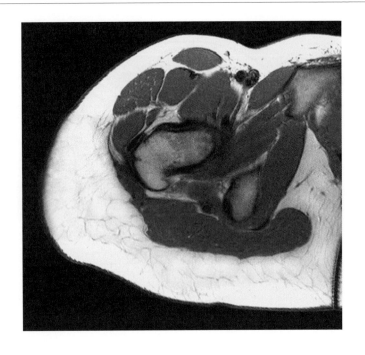

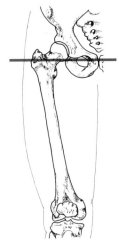

腹側

外側 □ 内側

背側

下肢，軸位断 195

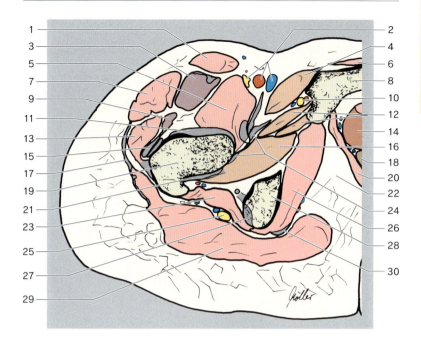

1 縫工筋 Sartorius muscle
2 大腿動静脈, 神経 Femoral artery, vein, and nerve
3 大腿直筋(＋腱) Rectus femoris muscle (＋tendon)
4 恥骨筋 Pectineus muscle
5 腸腰筋 Iliopsoas muscle
6 腹直筋 Rectus abdominis muscle
7 大腿筋膜張筋 Tensor fasciae latae muscle
8 恥骨(下枝) Pubis (inferior ramus)
9 外側広筋 Vastus lateralis muscle
10 閉鎖神経(前枝) Obturator nerve (anterior branch)
11 腸骨大腿靱帯 Iliofemoral ligament
12 短内転筋 Adductor brevis muscle
13 中殿筋(＋腱) Gluteus medius muscle (＋tendon)
14 腟 Vagina
15 小殿筋(＋腱) Gluteus minimus muscle (＋tendon)
16 外閉鎖筋 Obturator externus muscle
17 腸脛靱帯 Iliotibial tract
18 直腸 Rectum
19 大腿骨 Femur
20 肛門挙筋 Levator ani muscle
21 坐骨大腿靱帯 Ischiofemoral ligament
22 坐骨直腸窩 Ischiorectal fossa
23 大腿方形筋 Quadratus femoris muscle
24 恥骨大腿靱帯 Pubofemoral ligament
25 坐骨神経 Sciatic nerve
26 内閉鎖筋 Obturator internus muscle
27 大腿背側筋群の腱付着部 Tendon attachment of dorsal thigh muscles
28 坐骨結節 Ischial tuberosity
29 大殿筋 Gluteus maximus muscle
30 仙結節靱帯 Sacrotuberous ligament

196 下肢

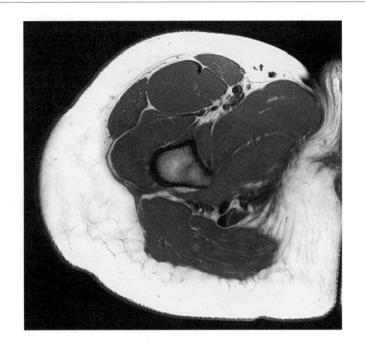

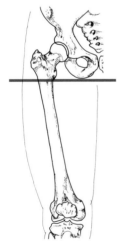

腹側

外側 ☐ 内側

背側

下肢，軸位断

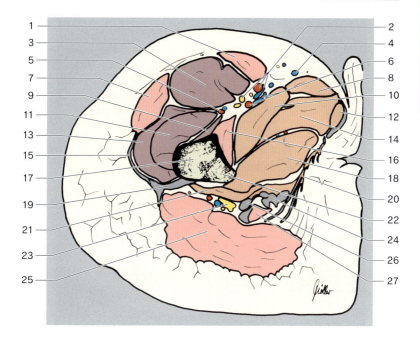

1 縫工筋 Sartorius muscle
2 大腿動静脈, 神経 Femoral artery, vein, and nerve
3 大腿直筋 Rectus femoris muscle
4 大伏在静脈 Great saphenous vein
5 外側大腿回旋動静脈 Lateral circumflex femoral artery and vein
6 大腿深動静脈 Deep artery and vein of thigh
7 大腿筋膜張筋 Tensor fasciae latae muscle
8 長内転筋 Adductor longus muscle
9 内側広筋 Vastus medialis muscle
10 恥骨筋 Pectineus muscle
11 中間広筋 Vastus intermedius muscle
12 薄筋 Gracilis muscle
13 外側広筋 Vastus lateralis muscle
14 短内転筋 Adductor brevis muscle
15 腸脛靱帯 Iliotibial tract
16 腸腰筋 Iliopsoas muscle
17 大腿骨 Femur
18 大内転筋 Adductor magnus muscle
19 外側大腿筋間中隔 Lateral femoral intermuscular septum
20 内閉鎖筋 Obturator internus muscle
21 大腿方形筋 Quadratus femoris muscle
22 小転子 Lesser trochanter
23 坐骨神経 Sciatic nerve
24 半膜様筋(腱) Semimembranosus muscle (tendon)
25 大殿筋 Gluteus maximus muscle
26 大腿二頭筋(腱) Biceps femoris muscle (tendon)
27 半腱様筋(腱) Semitendinosus muscle (tendon)

下 肢

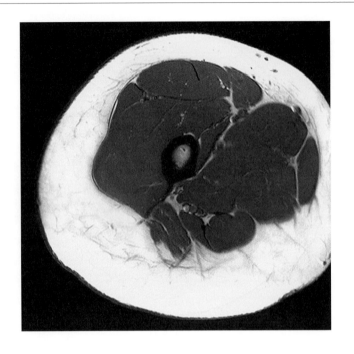

腹側
外側　内側
背側

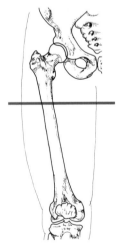

下肢, 軸位断

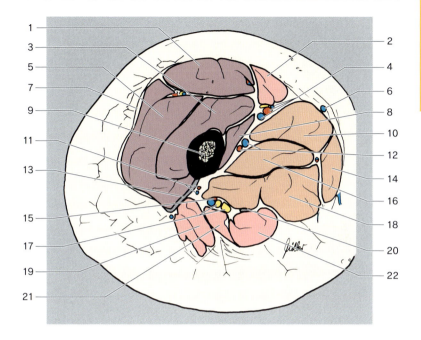

1 **大腿直筋** Rectus femoris muscle
2 **縫工筋** Sartorius muscle
3 **中間広筋** Vastus intermedius muscle
4 **大腿動静脈, 神経** Femoral artery, vein, and nerve
5 **外側広筋** Vastus lateralis muscle
6 **大伏在静脈** Great saphenous vein
7 **腸脛靱帯** Iliotibial tract
8 **内側広筋** Vastus medialis muscle
9 **大腿骨** Femur
10 **長内転筋** Adductor longus muscle
11 **貫通動静脈** Perforating artery(+vein) 大腿深動静脈の枝
12 **大腿深動静脈** Deep artery and vein of thigh
13 **外側大腿筋間中隔** Lateral femoral intermuscular septum
14 **薄筋** Gracilis muscle
15 **坐骨神経と伴行する動静脈** Artery and vein to sciatic nerve
16 **短内転筋** Adductor brevis muscle
17 **坐骨神経** Sciatic nerve
18 **大内転筋** Adductor magnus muscle
19 **大殿筋** Gluteus maximus muscle
20 **半膜様筋(腱)** Semimembranosus muscle (tendon)
21 **大腿二頭筋** Biceps femoris muscle
22 **半腱様筋** Semitendinosus muscle

200　下　肢

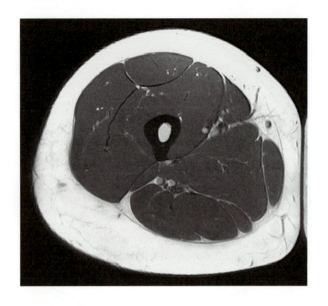

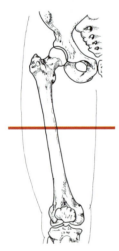

腹側

外側 □ 内側

背側

下肢，軸位断 **201**

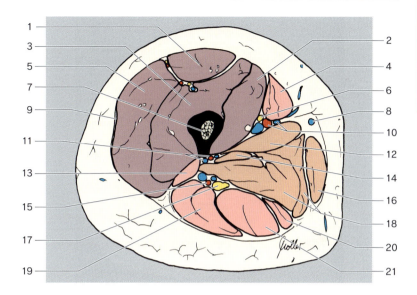

1 大腿直筋 Rectus femoris muscle
2 内側広筋 Vastus medialis muscle
3 中間広筋 Vastus intermedius muscle
4 縫工筋 Sartorius muscle
5 外側広筋 Vastus lateralis muscle
6 伏在神経 Saphenous nerve
7 大腿骨 Femur
8 大伏在静脈 Great saphenous vein
9 腸脛靱帯 Iliotibial tract
10 大腿動静脈 Femoral artery and vein
11 大腿深動静脈 Deep artery and vein of thigh
12 長内転筋 Adductor longus muscle
13 大腿二頭筋(短頭) Biceps femoris muscle (short head)
14 短内転筋 Adductor brevis muscle
15 坐骨神経と伴行する動脈 Artery to sciatic nerve
16 薄筋 Gracilis muscle
17 坐骨神経 Sciatic nerve
18 大内転筋 Adductor magnus muscle
19 大腿二頭筋(長頭) Biceps femoris muscle (long head)
20 半膜様筋 Semimembranosus muscle
21 半腱様筋 Semitendinosus muscle

202　下　肢

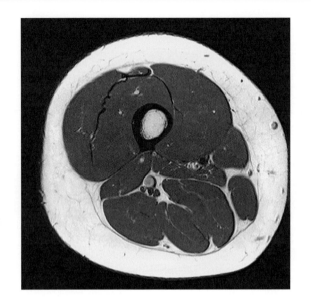

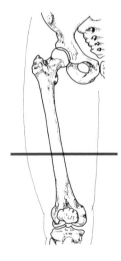

腹側

外側　内側

背側

下肢，軸位断　203

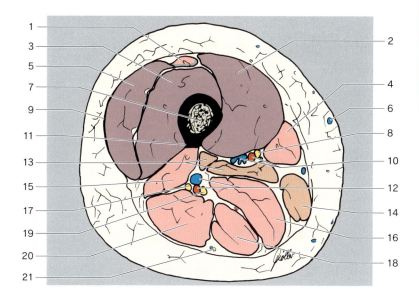

1 大腿直筋（＋腱）Rectus femoris muscle （＋tendon）
2 内側広筋 Vastus medialis muscle
3 中間広筋 Vastus intermedius muscle
4 縫工筋 Sartorius muscle
5 外側広筋 Vastus lateralis muscle
6 大伏在静脈 Great saphenous vein
7 大腿骨 Femur
8 伏在神経 Saphenous nerve
9 腸脛靱帯 Iliotibial tract
10 大腿動静脈 Femoral artery and vein
11 粗線 Linea aspera
12 貫通動静脈 Perforating artery and vein 大腿深動静脈の枝
13 大内転筋 Adductor magnus muscle
14 薄筋 Gracilis muscle
15 大腿二頭筋（短頭）Biceps femoris muscle (short head)
16 半膜様筋 Semimembranosus muscle
17 総腓骨神経 Common fibular nerve
18 半腱様筋 Semitendinosus muscle
19 脛骨神経 Tibial nerve
20 大腿二頭筋（長頭）Biceps femoris muscle (long head)
21 後大腿皮神経 Posterior femoral cutaneous nerve

204 下肢

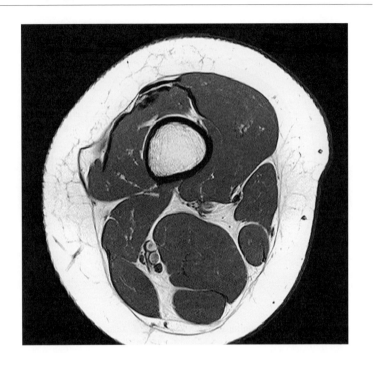

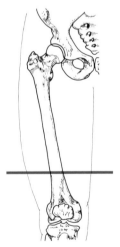

腹側

外側　　内側

背側

下肢，軸位断　**205**

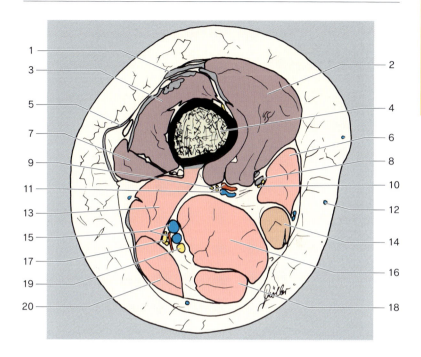

1 大腿直筋(腱) Rectus femoris muscle (tendon)
2 内側広筋 Vastus medialis muscle
3 中間広筋 Vastus intermedius muscle
4 大腿骨 Femur
5 腸脛靭帯 Iliotibial tract
6 縫工筋 Sartorius muscle
7 外側広筋 Vastus lateralis muscle
8 大内転筋(腱) Adductor magnus muscle (tendon)
9 大腿神経(筋枝) Femoral nerve (muscular branch)
10 伏在神経 Saphenous nerve
11 大腿動静脈 Femoral artery and vein
12 大伏在静脈 Great saphenous vein
13 大腿二頭筋(短頭) Biceps femoris muscle (short head)
14 薄筋 Gracilis muscle
15 貫通動静脈 Perforating artery and vein
　 大腿深動静脈の枝
16 半膜様筋 Semimembranosus muscle
17 総腓骨神経 Common fibular nerve
18 半腱様筋 Semitendinosus muscle
19 脛骨神経 Tibial nerve
20 大腿二頭筋(長頭) Biceps femoris muscle (long head)

206 下肢

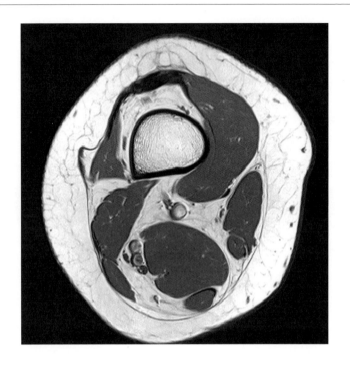

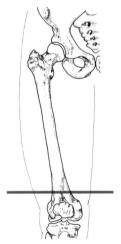

腹側

外側 内側

背側

下肢，軸位断 **207**

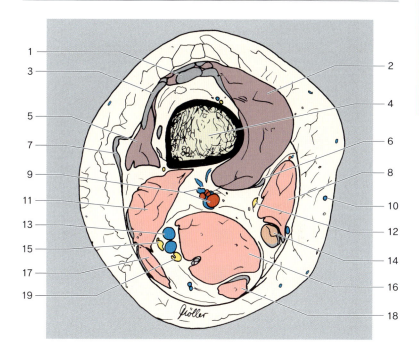

1 大腿直筋（腱）Rectus femoris muscle（tendon）
2 内側広筋 Vastus medialis muscle
3 中間広筋（＋腱）Vastus intermedius muscle（+tendon）
4 大腿骨 Femur
5 外側広筋 Vastus lateralis muscle
6 大内転筋（腱）Adductor magnus muscle（tendon）
7 腸脛靱帯 Iliotibial tract
8 縫工筋 Sartorius muscle
9 大腿動静脈 Femoral artery and vein
10 大伏在静脈 Great saphenous vein
11 大腿二頭筋（短頭）Biceps femoris muscle（short head）
12 伏在神経 Saphenous nerve
13 貫通静脈 Perforating vein
大腿深静脈の枝
14 薄筋 Gracilis muscle
15 総腓骨神経 Common fibular nerve
16 半膜様筋 Semimembranosus muscle
17 大腿二頭筋（長頭）Biceps femoris muscle（long head）
18 半腱様筋 Semitendinosus muscle
19 脛骨神経 Tibial nerve

208　下 肢

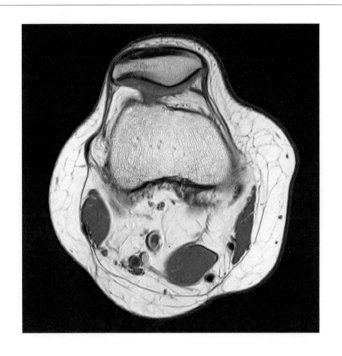

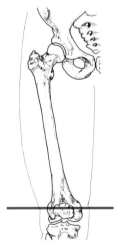

腹側

外側　☐　内側

背側

下肢，軸位断　　**209**

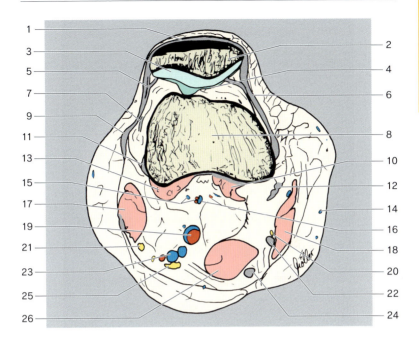

1 膝蓋靱帯 Patellar ligament
2 膝蓋骨 Patella
3 膝蓋骨後面軟骨 Retropatellar cartilage
4 大腿膝蓋関節 Femoropatellar joint
5 外側膝蓋支帯 Lateral patellar retinaculum
6 内側膝蓋支帯 Medial patellar retinaculum
7 外側広筋(腱) Vastus lateralis muscle(tendon)
8 大腿骨 Femur
9 腸脛靱帯 Iliotibial tract
10 腓腹筋(内側頭,腱) Gastrocnemius muscle (medial head, tendon)
11 膝窩筋(腱) Popliteus muscle(tendon)
12 大内転筋(腱) Adductor magnus muscle (tendon)
13 腓腹筋(外側頭) Gastrocnemius muscle (lateral head)
14 大伏在静脈 Great saphenous vein
15 外側上膝動静脈 Superior lateral genicular artery and vein
16 内側上膝動静脈 Superior medial genicular artery and vein
17 大腿二頭筋(+腱) Biceps femoris muscle (+tendon)
18 縫工筋 Sartorius muscle
19 膝窩動静脈 Popliteal artery and vein
20 伏在神経 Saphenous nerve
21 総腓骨神経 Common fibular nerve
22 薄筋(腱) Gracilis muscle(tendon)
23 貫通動静脈 Perforating artery(+vein)
大腿深動静脈の枝
24 半腱様筋 Semitendinosus muscle
25 脛骨神経 Tibial nerve
26 半膜様筋 Semimembranosus muscle

210 下肢

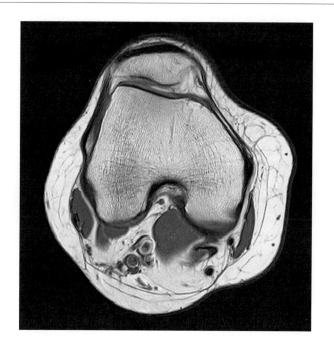

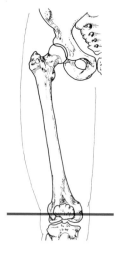

腹側
外側 　　 内側
背側

下肢, 軸位断 **211**

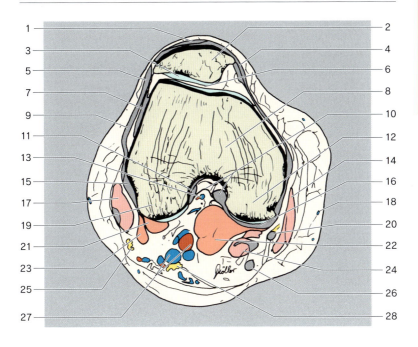

1 膝蓋靱帯 Patellar ligament
2 膝蓋骨 Patella
3 膝蓋骨後面軟骨 Retropatellar cartilage
4 内側膝蓋支帯 Medial patellar retinaculum
5 外側膝蓋支帯 Lateral patellar retinaculum
6 大腿膝蓋関節 Femoropatellar joint
7 外側側副靱帯 Lateral collateral ligament
8 大腿骨 Femur
9 腸脛靱帯 Iliotibial tract
10 関節包 Joint capsule, 後十字靱帯(付着部) Posterior cruciate ligament(attachment)
11 前十字靱帯(付着部) Anterior cruciate ligament(attachment)
12 大腿骨内側顆 Medial femoral condyle
13 中膝動脈 Middle genicular artery
14 縫工筋 Sartorius muscle
15 膝窩筋(腱) Popliteus muscle(tendon)
16 関節包 Joint capsule, 斜膝窩靱帯 Oblique popliteal ligament
17 大腿二頭筋(+腱) Biceps femoris muscle (+tendon)
18 大伏在静脈 Great saphenous vein
19 大腿骨内側顆 Medial femoral condyle
20 薄筋(腱) Gracilis muscle(tendon)
21 足底筋 Plantaris muscle
22 腓腹筋(内側頭) Gastrocnemius muscle (medial head)
23 腓腹筋(外側頭) Gastrocnemius muscle (lateral head)
24 半膜様筋(+腱) Semimembranosus muscle (+tendon)
25 総腓骨神経 Common fibular nerve
26 半腱様筋(腱) Semitendinosus muscle(tendon)
27 膝窩動静脈 Popliteal artery and vein
28 脛骨神経 Tibial nerve

212 下 肢

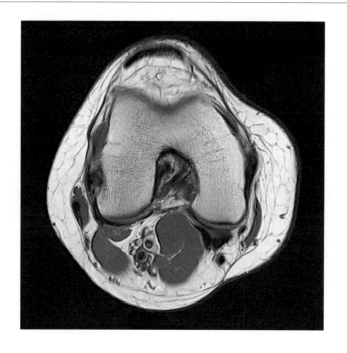

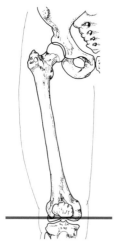

腹側
外側 □ 内側
背側

下肢，軸位断 **213**

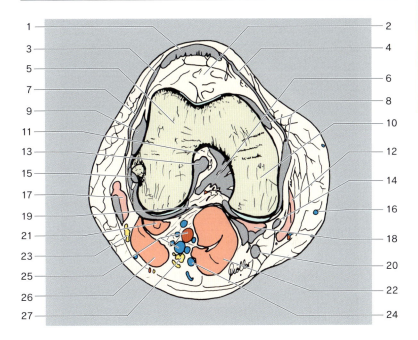

1 膝蓋靱帯 Patellar ligament
2 膝蓋下脂肪体 Infrapatellar fat body
3 外側膝蓋支帯 Lateral patellar retinaculum
4 内側膝蓋支帯 Medial patellar retinaculum
5 大腿骨外側顆 Lateral femoral condyle
6 後十字靱帯 Posterior cruciate ligament
7 腸脛靱帯 Iliotibial tract
8 内側側副靱帯 Medial collateral ligament
9 外側側副靱帯 Lateral collateral ligament
10 大腿骨内側顆 Medial femoral condyle
11 顆間窩 Intercondylar fossa
12 縫工筋 Sartorius muscle
13 前十字靱帯 Anterior cruciate ligament
14 薄筋(腱) Gracilis muscle(tendon)
15 膝窩筋(腱) Popliteus muscle(tendon)
16 大伏在静脈 Great saphenous vein
17 大腿二頭筋(＋腱) Biceps femoris muscle (＋tendon)
18 半膜様筋(＋腱) Semimembranosus muscle (＋tendon)
19 斜膝窩靱帯 Oblique popliteal ligament，関節包 Joint capsule
20 半腱様筋(腱) Semitendinosus muscle (tendon)
21 足底筋 Plantaris muscle
22 腓腹筋(内側頭) Gastrocnemius muscle (medial head)
23 総腓骨神経 Common fibular nerve
24 膝窩静脈 Popliteal vein
25 膝窩動静脈 Popliteal artery and vein
26 腓腹筋(外側頭) Gastrocnemius muscle (lateral head)
27 脛骨神経 Tibial nerve

214　下　肢

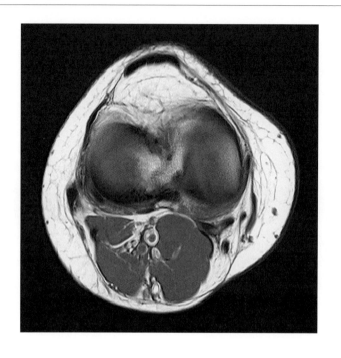

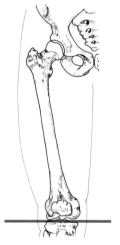

腹側

外側　☐　内側

背側

下肢，軸位断   *215*

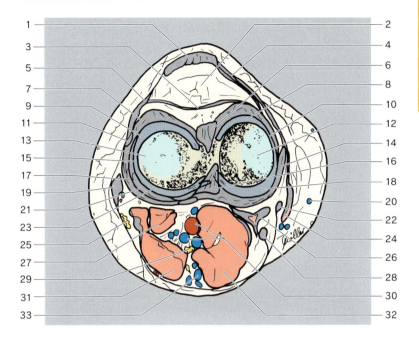

1 膝蓋靱帯 Patellar ligament
2 膝蓋下脂肪体 Infrapatellar fat body
3 横膝蓋支帯 Transverse patellar retinaculum
4 内側膝蓋支帯 Medial patellar retinaculum
5 外側膝蓋支帯 Lateral patellar retinaculum
6 前十字靱帯 Anterior cruciate ligament
7 関節包 Joint capsule
8 内側半月板(前角) Medial meniscus(anterior horn)
9 外側半月板(前角) Lateral meniscus(anterior horn)
10 内側半月板(体部) Medial meniscus(body)
11 腸脛靱帯 Iliotibial tract
12 大腿骨内側顆 Medial femoral condyle，関節軟骨 Joint cartilage
13 大腿骨外側顆 Lateral femoral condyle，関節軟骨 Joint cartilage
14 内側側副靱帯 Medial collateral ligament
15 外側半月板(体部) Lateral meniscus(body)
16 後十字靱帯 Posterior cruciate ligament
17 外側側副靱帯 Lateral collateral ligament
18 内側半月板(後角) Medial meniscus(posterior horn)
19 大腿二頭筋(腱) Biceps femoris muscle(tendon)
20 大伏在静脈 Great saphenous vein
21 膝窩筋(腱) Popliteus muscle(tendon)
22 薄筋(腱) Gracilis muscle(tendon)
23 外側半月板(後角) Lateral meniscus(posterior horn)
24 縫工筋(+腱) Sartorius muscle(+tendon)
25 総腓骨神経 Common fibular nerve
26 半膜様筋(+腱) Semimembranosus muscle (+tendon)
27 足底筋 Plantaris muscle
28 半腱様筋(腱) Semitendinosus muscle (tendon)
29 脛骨神経 Tibial nerve
30 膝窩動静脈 Popliteal artery and vein
31 腓腹筋(外側頭，腱) Gastrocnemius muscle (lateral head, tendon)
32 腓腹筋(内側頭，腱) Gastrocnemius muscle (medial head, tendon)
33 小伏在静脈 Small saphenous vein

216　下 肢

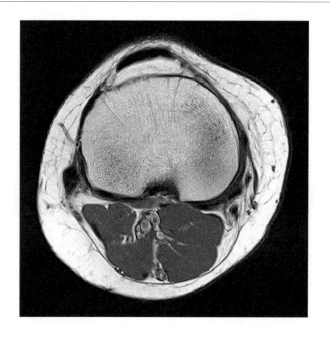

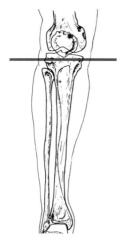

前
腹側

外側　　　内側

背側
後

下肢, 軸位断

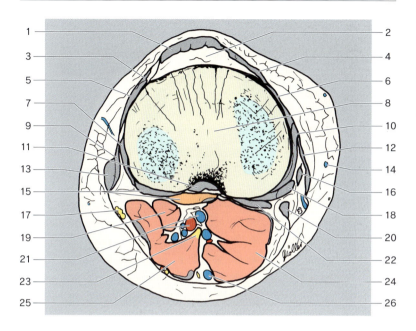

1 膝蓋靱帯 Patellar ligament
2 膝蓋下脂肪体 Infrapatellar fat body
3 外側膝蓋支帯 Lateral patellar retinaculum
4 内側膝蓋支帯 Medial patellar retinaculum
5 腸脛靱帯 Iliotibial tract
6 関節包 Joint capsule
7 外側側副靱帯 Lateral collateral ligament
8 脛骨(頭) Tibia(head)
9 外側側副靱帯 Lateral collateral ligament
10 内側側副靱帯 Medial collateral ligament
11 後十字靱帯 Posterior cruciate ligament
12 縫工筋(腱) Sartorius muscle(tendon)
13 大腿二頭筋(腱) Biceps femoris muscle (tendon)
14 大伏在静脈 Great saphenous vein
15 膝窩筋(+腱) Popliteus muscle(+tendon)
16 薄筋(腱) Gracilis muscle(tendon)
17 総腓骨神経 Common fibular nerve
18 半膜様筋(+腱) Semimembranosus muscle (+tendon)
19 足底筋 Plantaris muscle
20 半腱様筋(腱) Semitendinosus muscle(tendon)
21 膝窩動静脈 Popliteal artery and vein
22 斜膝窩靱帯と関節包 Oblique popliteal ligament and joint capsule
23 脛骨神経 Tibial nerve
24 腓腹筋(内側頭,腱) Gastrocnemius muscle (medial head, tendon)
25 腓腹筋(外側頭,腱) Gastrocnemius muscle (lateral head, tendon)
26 小伏在静脈 Small saphenous vein

218　下 肢

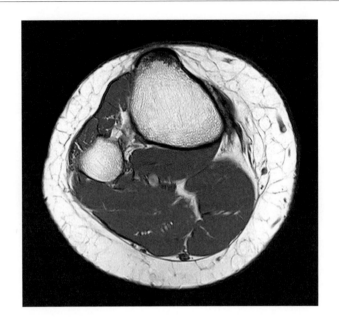

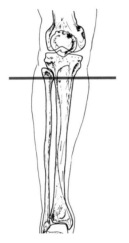

前
外側　　内側
後

下肢，軸位断 **219**

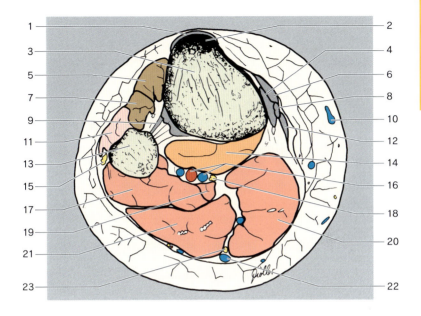

1 膝蓋靱帯 Patellar ligament
2 脛骨粗面 Tibial tuberosity
3 脛骨 Tibia
4 内側膝蓋支帯 Medial patellar retinaculum
5 前脛骨筋 Tibialis anterior muscle
6 縫工筋(腱) Sartorius muscle (tendon)
7 長趾伸筋 Extensor digitorum longus muscle
8 薄筋(腱) Gracilis muscle (tendon)
9 下腿骨間膜 Interosseous membrane of leg
10 大伏在静脈 Great saphenous vein
11 長腓骨筋 Peroneus (fibularis) longus muscle
12 半腱様筋(腱) Semitendinosus muscle (tendon)
13 腓骨(頭) Fibula (head)
14 膝窩筋 Popliteus muscle
15 総腓骨神経 Common fibular nerve
16 膝窩動静脈 Popliteal artery and vein
17 ヒラメ筋 Soleus muscle
18 脛骨神経 Tibial nerve
19 足底筋 Plantaris muscle
20 腓腹筋(内側頭) Gastrocnemius muscle (medial head)
21 腓腹筋(外側頭) Gastrocnemius muscle (lateral head)
22 小伏在静脈 Small saphenous vein
23 内側腓腹皮神経 Medial sural cutaneous nerve

220　下　肢

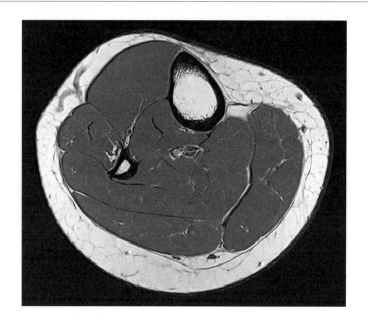

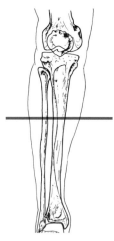

前
外側 内側
後

下肢，軸位断 *221*

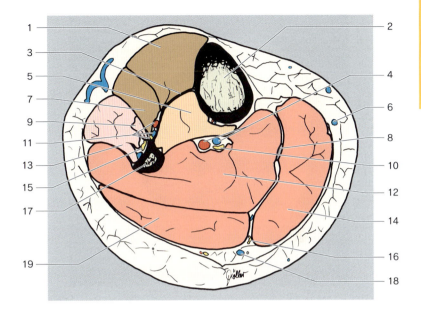

1 前脛骨筋 Tibialis anterior muscle
2 脛骨 Tibia
3 下腿骨間膜 Interosseous membrane of leg
4 脛腓動脈幹 Tibiofibular trunk
　後脛骨動静脈と腓骨動脈の共通幹
5 後脛骨筋 Tibialis posterior muscle
6 大伏在静脈 Great saphenous vein
7 長趾伸筋 Extensor digitorum longus muscle
8 足底筋(腱) Plantaris muscle (tendon)
9 短腓骨筋 Peroneus (fibularis) brevis muscle
10 脛骨神経 Tibial nerve
11 前脛骨動静脈 Anterior tibial artery and vein,
　深腓骨神経 Deep fibular nerve
12 ヒラメ筋 Soleus muscle
13 長腓骨筋 Peroneus (fibularis) longus muscle
14 腓腹筋(内側頭) Gastrocnemius muscle
　(medial head)
15 浅腓骨神経 Superficial fibular nerve
16 内側腓腹皮神経 Medial sural cutaneous nerve
17 腓骨 Fibula
18 小伏在静脈 Small saphenous vein
19 腓腹筋(外側頭) Gastrocnemius muscle
　(lateral head)

222　下　肢

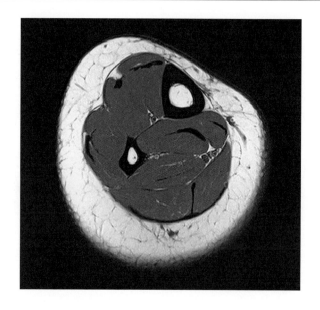

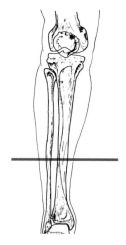

前
外側　内側
後

下肢，軸位断 **223**

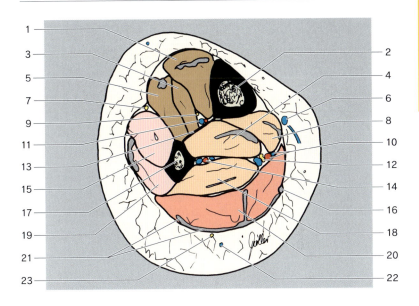

1 前脛骨筋（＋腱）Tibialis anterior muscle (＋tendon)
2 脛骨 Tibia
3 長母趾伸筋 Extensor hallucis longus muscle
4 後脛骨筋 Tibialis posterior muscle
5 長趾伸筋（＋腱）Extensor digitorum longus muscle（＋tendon）
6 大伏在静脈 Great saphenous vein
7 浅腓骨神経 Superficial fibular nerve
8 長趾屈筋（＋腱）Flexor digitorum longus muscle（＋tendon）
9 深腓骨神経 Deep fibular nerve
10 後脛骨動静脈 Posterior tibial artery and vein
11 前脛骨動静脈 Anterior tibial artery and vein
12 脛骨神経 Tibial nerve
13 下腿骨間膜 Interosseous membrane of leg
14 腓骨動静脈 Fibular artery and vein
15 短腓骨筋 Peroneus (fibularis) brevis muscle
16 足底筋（腱）Plantaris muscle（tendon）
17 腓骨 Fibula
18 長母趾屈筋 Flexor hallucis longus muscle
19 長腓骨筋（＋腱）Peroneus (fibularis) longus muscle（＋tendon）
20 ヒラメ筋 Soleus muscle
21 腓腹筋（腱）Gastrocnemius muscle
22 小伏在静脈 Small saphenous vein
23 腓腹神経 Sural nerve

下肢

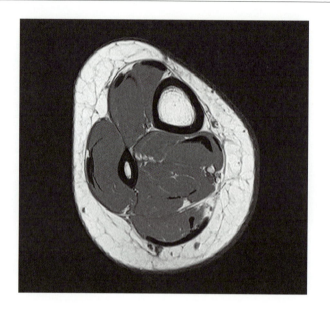

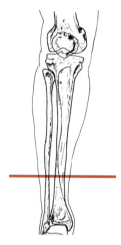

前
外側 　 内側
後

下肢，軸位断 **225**

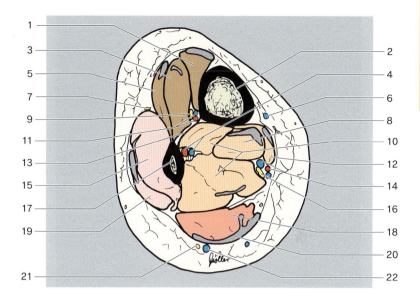

1 前脛骨筋（＋腱） Tibialis anterior muscle (+tendon)
2 脛骨 Tibia
3 長母趾伸筋 Extensor hallucis longus muscle
4 腓骨動静脈 Fibular artery and vein
5 長趾伸筋（＋腱） Extensor digitorum longus muscle(+tendon)
6 大伏在静脈 Great saphenous vein
7 浅腓骨神経 Superficial fibular nerve
8 後脛骨筋（＋腱） Tibialis posterior muscle (+tendon)
9 深腓骨神経 Deep fibular nerve
10 長母趾屈筋 Flexor hallucis longus muscle
11 前脛骨動静脈 Anterior tibial artery and vein
12 長趾屈筋（＋腱） Flexor digitorum longus muscle(+tendon)
13 下腿骨間膜 Interosseous membrane of leg
14 後脛骨動静脈 Posterior tibial artery and vein
15 短腓骨筋 Peroneus(fibularis)brevis muscle
16 脛骨神経 Tibial nerve
17 腓骨 Fibula
18 ヒラメ筋 Soleus muscle
19 長腓骨筋（＋腱） Peroneus(fibularis)longus muscle(+tendon)
20 腓腹筋（腱） Gastrocnemius muscle(tendon)，足底筋（腱） Plantaris muscle(tendon)
21 腓腹神経 Sural nerve
22 小伏在静脈 Small saphenous vein

226　下　肢

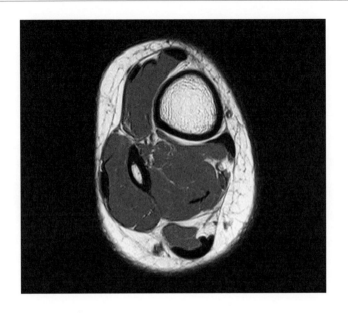

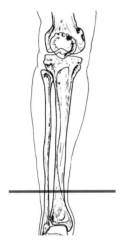

前
外側　　　内側
後

下肢, 軸位断

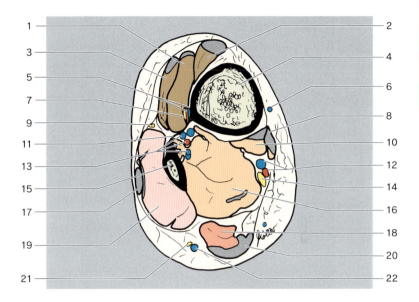

1 長母趾伸筋(+腱) Extensor hallucis longus muscle(+tendon)
2 前脛骨筋(+腱) Tibialis anterior muscle (+tendon)
3 長趾伸筋(+腱) Extensor digitorum longus muscle(+tendon)
4 脛骨 Tibia
5 前脛骨動静脈 Anterior tibial artery and vein
6 大伏在静脈 Great saphenous vein
7 深腓骨神経 Deep fibular nerve
8 長趾屈筋(+腱) Flexor digitorum longus muscle(+tendon)
9 浅腓骨神経 Superficial fibular nerve
10 後脛骨筋(+腱) Tibialis posterior muscle (+tendon)
11 下腿骨間膜 Interosseous membrane of leg
12 後脛骨動静脈 Posterior tibial artery and vein
13 腓骨動静脈 Fibular artery and veins
14 脛骨神経 Tibial nerve
15 腓骨 Fibula
16 長母趾屈筋 Flexor hallucis longus muscle
17 長腓骨筋(腱) Peroneus(fibularis)longus muscle(tendon)
18 ヒラメ筋 Soleus muscle
19 短腓骨筋 Peroneus(fibularis)brevis muscle
20 腓腹筋(腱) Gastrocnemius muscle(tendon), 足底筋(腱) Plantaris muscle(tendon)
21 腓腹神経 Sural nerve
22 小伏在静脈 Small saphenous vein

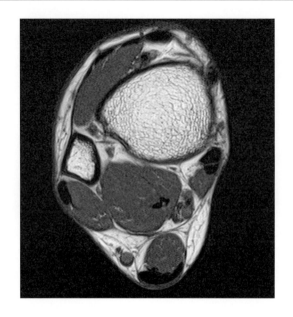

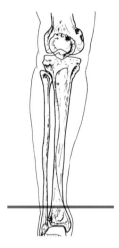

前
外側 　　 内側
後

下肢，軸位断　**229**

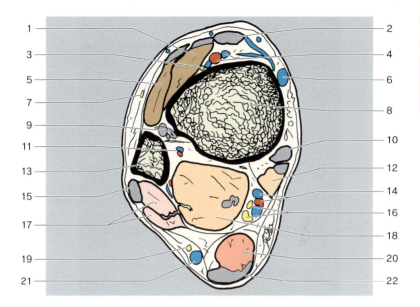

1 長母趾伸筋(＋腱) Extensor hallucis longus muscle(+tendon)
2 前脛骨筋(腱) Tibialis anterior muscle(tendon)
3 深腓骨神経 Deep fibular nerve
4 前脛骨動静脈 Anterior tibial artery and vein
5 長趾伸筋(＋腱) Extensor digitorum longus muscle(+tendon)
6 大伏在静脈 Great saphenous vein
7 浅腓骨神経 Superficial fibular nerve
8 脛骨 Tibia
9 下腿骨間膜 Interosseous membrane of leg
10 後脛骨筋(腱) Tibialis posterior muscle (tendon)
11 腓骨動静脈 Fibular artery and vein
12 長趾屈筋(＋腱) Flexor digitorum longus muscle (+tendon)
13 腓骨 Fibula
14 後脛骨動静脈 Posterior tibial artery and vein
15 長腓骨筋(腱) Peroneus(fibularis)longus muscle (tendon)
16 脛骨神経 Tibial nerve
17 短腓骨筋 Peroneus(fibularis)brevis muscle
18 長母趾屈筋 Flexor hallucis longus muscle
19 腓腹神経 Sural nerve
20 ヒラメ筋 Soleus muscle
21 小伏在静脈 Small saphenous vein
22 下腿三頭筋と足底筋の腱 Tendons of triceps surae muscle and plantaris muscle

下 肢

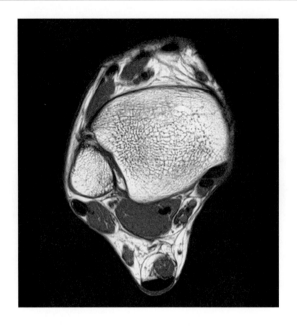

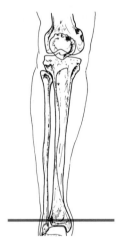

前
外側　　　内側
後

下肢，軸位断

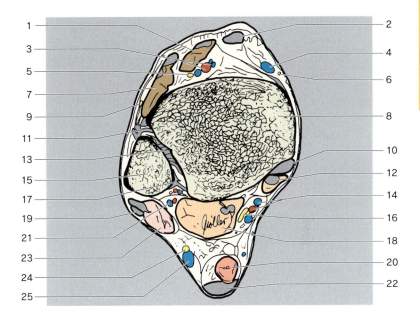

1 長母趾伸筋(＋腱) Extensor hallucis longus muscle(＋tendon)
2 前脛骨筋(腱) Tibialis anterior muscle(tendon)
3 前脛骨動静脈 Anterior tibial artery and vein
4 大伏在静脈 Great saphenous vein
5 深腓骨神経 Deep fibular nerve
6 伏在神経 Saphenous nerve
7 長趾伸筋(＋腱) Extensor digitorum longus muscle(＋tendon)
8 脛骨 Tibia
9 浅腓骨神経 Superficial fibular nerve
10 後脛骨筋(腱) Tibialis posterior muscle (tendon)
11 前脛腓靱帯 Anterior tibiofibular ligament
12 長趾屈筋(＋腱) Flexor digitorum longus muscle(＋tendon)
13 下脛腓関節 Inferior tibiofibular joint
14 後脛骨動静脈 Posterior tibial artery and vein
15 腓骨 Fibula
16 脛骨神経 Tibial nerve
17 後脛腓靱帯 Posterior tibiofibular ligament
18 長母趾屈筋(＋腱) Flexor hallucis longus muscle(＋tendon)
19 長腓骨筋(腱) Peroneus(fibularis)longus muscle(tendon)
20 ヒラメ筋 Soleus muscle
21 腓骨動静脈 Fibular artery and vein
22 下腿三頭筋と足底筋の腱 Tendons of triceps surae muscle and plantaris muscle
23 短腓骨筋(＋腱) Peroneus(fibularis)brevis muscle(＋tendon)
24 腓腹神経 Sural nerve
25 小伏在静脈 Small saphenous vein

232 下 肢

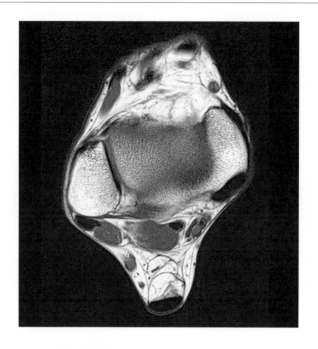

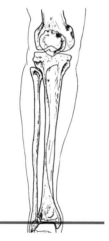

前
外側 　　　 内側
後

下肢，軸位断　233

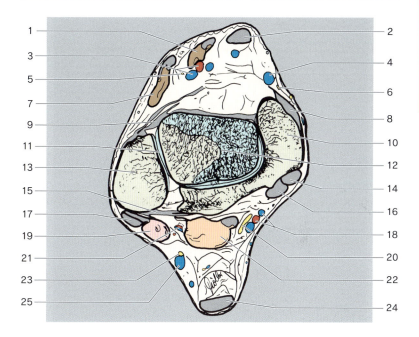

1 長母趾伸筋(＋腱) Extensor hallucis longus muscle(＋tendon)
2 前脛骨筋(腱) Tibialis anterior muscle(tendon)
3 前脛骨動静脈 Anterior tibial artery and vein
4 大伏在静脈 Great saphenous vein
5 深腓骨神経 Deep fibular nerve
6 伏在神経 Saphenous nerve
7 長趾伸筋(＋腱) Extensor digitorum longus muscle(＋tendon)
8 三角靱帯(脛舟部・前脛距部) Deltoid ligament (tibionavicular and anterior tibiotalar parts)
9 前脛腓靱帯 Anterior tibiofibular ligament
10 内果(脛骨) Medial malleolus(tibia)
11 脛腓靱帯結合 Tibiofibular syndesmosis
12 足関節 Ankle joint(距腿関節 Talocrural joint)
13 外果(腓骨) Lateral malleolus(fibula)
14 後脛骨筋(腱) Tibialis posterior muscle (tendon)
15 後脛腓靱帯 Posterior tibiofibular ligament
16 長趾屈筋(腱) Flexor digitorum longus muscle(腱)
17 長腓骨筋(腱) Peroneus(fibularis)longus muscle(tendon)
18 後脛骨動静脈 Posterior tibial artery and vein
19 短腓骨筋(＋腱) Peroneus(fibularis)brevis muscle(＋tendon)
20 脛骨神経 Tibial nerve
21 腓骨動静脈 Fibular artery and vein
22 長母趾屈筋(＋腱) Flexor hallucis longus muscle(＋tendon)
23 腓腹神経 Sural nerve
24 下腿三頭筋と足底筋の腱 Tendons of triceps surae muscle and plantaris muscle
25 小伏在静脈 Small saphenous vein

234　下　肢

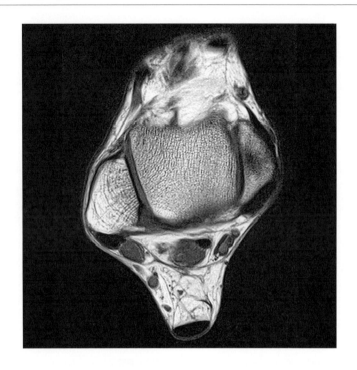

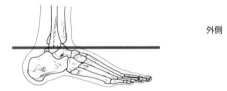

前
外側　　内側
後

下肢，軸位断 **235**

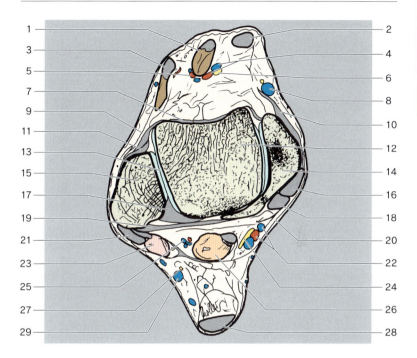

1 長母趾伸筋(腱) Extensor hallucis longus muscle(tendon)
2 前脛骨筋(腱) Tibialis anterior muscle (tendon)
3 長趾伸筋(腱) Extensor digitorum longus muscle(tendon)
4 足背動脈 Dorsalis pedis artery
5 外側足根動脈 Lateral tarsal artery
6 深腓骨神経 Deep fibular nerve
7 背側距舟靱帯 Dorsal talonavicular ligament, 関節包 Joint capsule
8 大伏在静脈 Great saphenous vein
9 伸筋支帯 Extensor retinaculum
10 三角靱帯(脛舟部・前脛距部) Deltoid ligament (tibionavicular and anterior tibiotalar parts)
11 前距腓靱帯 Anterior talofibular ligament
12 距骨 Talus
13 足関節 Ankle joint(距腿関節 Talocrural joint)
14 内果(脛骨) Medial malleolus(tibia)
15 外果(腓骨) Lateral malleolus(fibula)
16 後脛骨筋(腱) Tibialis posterior muscle (tendon)
17 後距腓靱帯 Posterior talofibular ligament
18 長趾屈筋(腱) Flexor digitorum longus muscle(tendon)
19 後脛腓靱帯 Posterior tibiofibular ligament
20 屈筋支帯 Flexor retinaculum
21 長腓骨筋(腱) Peroneus(fibularis)longus muscle(+tendon)
22 後脛骨動静脈 Posterior tibial artery and vein
23 短腓骨筋(＋腱) Peroneus(fibularis)brevis muscle(+tendon)
24 脛骨神経 Tibial nerve
25 腓骨動静脈 Fibular artery and vein
26 長母趾屈筋(＋腱) Flexor hallucis longus muscle(+tendon)
27 腓腹神経 Sural nerve
28 アキレス腱(踵骨腱) Achilles tendon(calcaneal tendon)
29 小伏在静脈 Small saphenous vein

236 下 肢

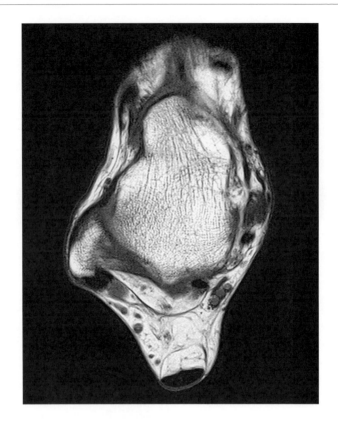

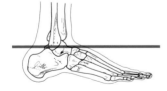

1 **長母趾伸筋(腱)** Extensor hallucis longus muscle(tendon)
2 **前脛骨筋(腱)** Tibialis anterior muscle (tendon)
3 **足背動脈** Dorsalis pedis artery
4 **背側距舟靱帯** Dorsal talonavicular ligament
5 **長趾伸筋(+腱)** Extensor digitorum longus muscle(+tendon)

下肢，軸位断 **237**

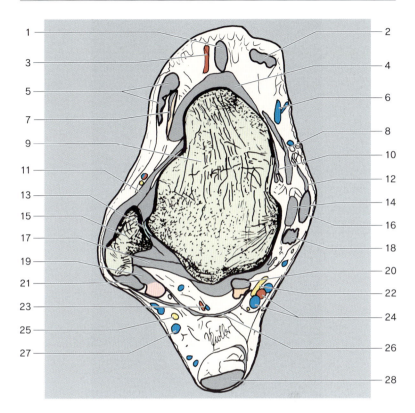

6 大伏在静脈 Great saphenous vein
7 短趾伸筋(+腱) Extensor digitorum brevis muscle(+tendon)
8 三角靱帯(脛舟部) Deltoid ligament (tibionavicular part)
9 距骨 Talus
10 三角靱帯(前脛距部) Deltoid ligament (anterior tibiotalar part)
11 前距腓靱帯 Anterior talofibular ligament
12 屈筋支帯 Flexor retinaculum
13 足関節 Ankle joint(距腿関節 Talocrural joint)
14 三角靱帯(後脛距部) Deltoid ligament (posterior tibiotalar part)
15 外果(腓骨) Lateral malleolus(fibula)
16 後脛骨筋(腱) Tibialis posterior muscle (tendon)
17 後距腓靱帯 Posterior talofibular ligament
18 長趾屈筋(腱) Flexor digitorum longus muscle(tendon)
19 短腓骨筋(+腱) Peroneus(fibularis)brevis muscle(+tendon)
20 長母趾屈筋(+腱) Flexor hallucis longus muscle(+tendon)
21 長腓骨筋(腱) Peroneus(fibularis)longus muscle(tendon)
22 脛骨神経 Tibial nerve
23 腓骨動静脈 Fibular artery and vein
24 後脛骨動静脈 Posterior tibial artery and vein
25 腓腹神経 Sural nerve
26 上腓骨筋支帯 Superior peroneal retinaculum
27 小伏在静脈 Small saphenous vein
28 アキレス腱(踵骨腱) Achilles tendon (calcaneal tendon)

238　下 肢

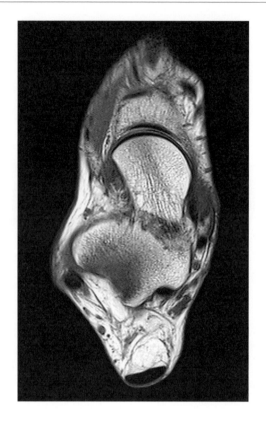

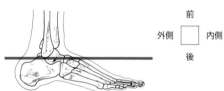

1 **足背動脈** Dorsalis pedis artery
2 **長母趾伸筋(腱)** Extensor hallucis longus muscle(tendon)
3 **背側足根靭帯** Dorsal tarsal ligaments
4 **前脛骨筋(腱)** Tibialis anterior muscle (tendon)
5 **長趾伸筋(腱)** Extensor digitorum longus muscle(tendon)

下肢，軸位断 **239**

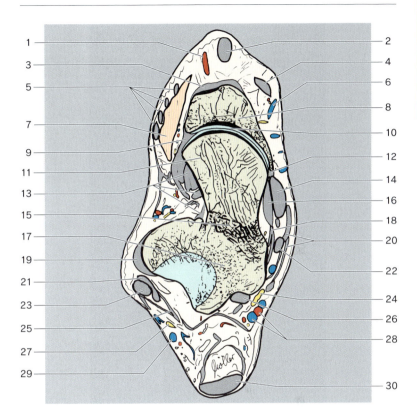

6	大伏在静脈 Great saphenous vein
7	短趾伸筋 Extensor digitorum brevis muscle
8	舟状骨 Navicular
9	背側距舟靱帯 Dorsal talonavicular ligament
10	距舟関節 Talonavicular joint
11	距骨(頭) Talus(head)
12	三角靱帯(脛舟部) Deltoid ligament(tibionavicular part)
13	骨間距踵靱帯 Talocalcaneal interosseous ligament
14	後脛骨筋(腱) Tibialis posterior muscle (tendon)
15	距骨(頸) Talus(neck)
16	三角靱帯(脛踵部) Deltoid ligament (tibiocalcaneal part)
17	距骨(体) Talus(body)
18	三角靱帯(後脛距部) Deltoid ligament (posterior tibiotalar part)
19	踵腓靱帯 Calcaneofibular ligament
20	屈筋支帯 Flexor retinaculum
21	短腓骨筋(腱) Peroneus(fibularis)brevis muscle(tendon)
22	長趾屈筋(腱) Flexor digitorum longus muscle(tendon)
23	長腓骨筋(腱) Peroneus(fibularis)longus muscle(tendon)
24	脛骨神経 Tibial nerve
25	上腓骨筋支帯 Superior fibular retinaculum
26	長母趾屈筋(腱) Flexor hallucis longus (tendon)
27	腓腹神経 Sural nerve
28	後脛骨動静脈 Posterior tibial artery and vein
29	小伏在静脈 Small saphenous vein
30	アキレス腱(踵骨腱) Achilles tendon (calcaneal tendon)

240　下肢

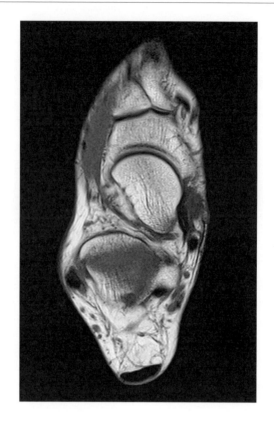

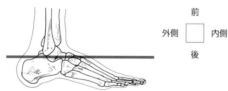

1 **足背動脈** Dorsalis pedis artery
2 **長母趾伸筋(腱)** Extensor hallucis longus muscle(tendon)
3 **中間楔状骨** Intermediate cuneiform
4 **内側楔状骨** Medial cuneiform
5 **長趾伸筋(腱)** Extensor digitorum longus muscle(tendons)
6 **前脛骨筋(腱)** Tibialis anterior muscle (tendon)

下肢，軸位断 **241**

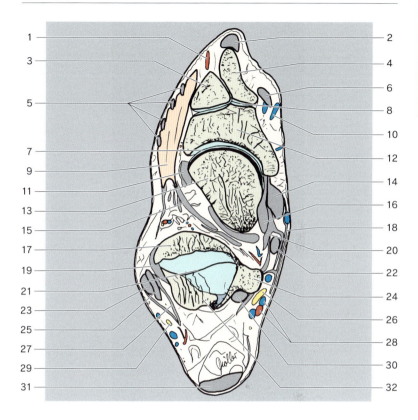

7 距舟関節 Talonavicular joint
8 楔舟関節 Cuneonavicular joint
9 短趾伸筋 Extensor digitorum brevis muscle
10 大伏在静脈 Great saphenous vein
11 二分靱帯 Bifurcate ligament
12 舟状骨 Navicular
13 距骨(頭) Talus(head)
14 後脛骨筋(腱) Tibialis posterior muscle (tendon)
15 骨間距踵靱帯 Talocalcaneal interosseous ligament
16 三角靱帯(脛踵部・脛舟部) Deltoid ligament (tibiocalcaneal and tibionavicular part)
17 距骨(体) Talus(body)
18 屈筋支帯 Flexor retinaculum
19 踵腓靱帯 Calcaneofibular ligament
20 内側距踵靱帯 Medial talocalcaneal ligament
21 距骨下(距踵)関節 Subtalar(talocalcaneal) joint
22 長趾屈筋(腱) Flexor digitorum longus muscle(tendon)
23 長腓骨筋(腱) Peroneus(fibularis)longus muscle(tendon)
24 距骨(後突起) Talus(posterior process)
25 短腓骨筋(腱) Peroneus(fibularis)brevis muscle(tendon)
26 脛骨神経 Tibial nerve
27 腓骨支帯 Peroneal retinaculum
28 後脛骨動静脈 Posterior tibial artery and vein
29 外側足背皮神経 Dorsal lateral cutaneous nerve
30 長母趾屈筋(腱) Flexor hallucis longus (tendon)
31 アキレス腱(踵骨腱) Achilles tendon (calcaneal tendon)
32 踵骨 Calcaneus

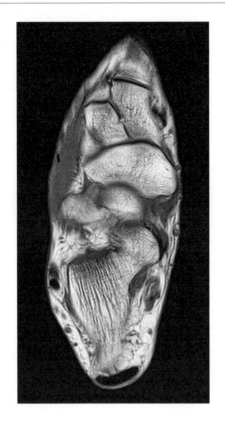

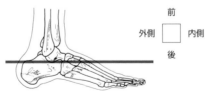

1 **長母趾伸筋(腱)** Extensor hallucis longus muscle (tendon)
2 **第1中足骨(底)** Metatarsal I (base)
3 **足背動脈** Dorsalis pedis artery
4 **第1足根中足関節** First tarsometatarsal joint
5 **第2中足骨(底)** Metatarsal II (base)

下肢，軸位断 **243**

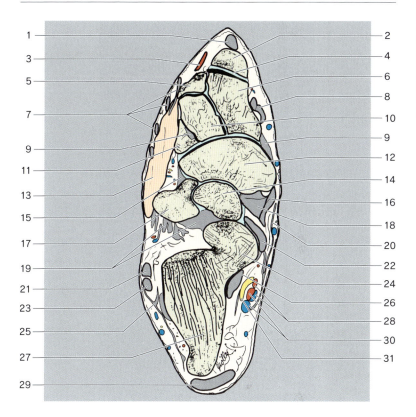

6 内側楔状骨 Medial cuneiform
7 長趾伸筋（腱）Extensor digitorum longus muscle (tendons)
8 前脛骨筋(腱) Tibialis anterior muscle (tendon)
9 背側足根靱帯 Dorsal tarsal ligaments
10 中間楔状骨 Intermediate cuneiform
11 外側楔状骨 Lateral cuneiform
12 舟状骨 Navicular
13 短趾伸筋 Extensor digitorum brevis muscle
14 距骨（頭）Talus (head)
15 二分靱帯 Bifurcate ligament
16 三角靱帯（脛舟部）Deltoid ligament (tibionavicular part)
17 踵骨 Calcaneus
18 後脛骨筋(腱) Tibialis posterior muscle (tendon)
19 骨間距踵靱帯 Talocalcaneal interosseous ligament

20 屈筋支帯 Flexor retinaculum
21 短腓骨筋(腱) Peroneus (fibularis) brevis muscle (tendon)
22 長趾屈筋(腱) Flexor digitorum longus muscle (tendon)
23 長腓骨筋(腱) Peroneus (fibularis) longus muscle (tendon)
24 踵骨（載距突起）Calcaneus (talar shelf)
25 腓骨筋支帯 Peroneal retinaculum
26 長母趾屈筋(腱) Flexor hallucis longus (tendon)
27 踵骨結節 Calcaneal tuberosity
28 内側足底動静脈 Medial plantar artery and vein
29 アキレス腱（踵骨腱）Achilles tendon (calcaneal tendon)
30 外側足底動静脈 Lateral plantar artery and vein
31 脛骨神経 Tibial nerve

244　下　肢

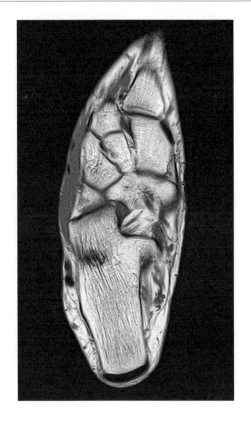

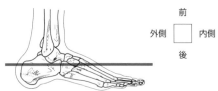

1 **長母趾伸筋(腱)** Extensor hallucis longus muscle (tendon)
2 **第1中足骨(底)** Metatarsal I (base)
3 **足背動脈** Dorsalis pedis artery
4 **第2中足骨(底)** Metatarsal II (base)
5 **背側骨間筋** Dorsal interosseous muscles
6 **骨間楔中足靱帯** Cuneometatarsal interosseous ligaments

下肢，軸位断

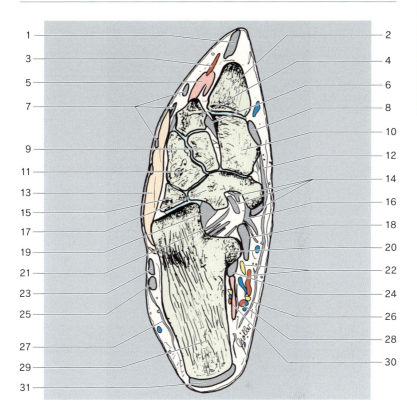

- 7 長趾伸筋(腱) Extensor digitorum longus muscle(tendons)
- 8 前脛骨筋(腱) Tibialis anterior muscle (tendon)
- 9 中間楔状骨 Intermediate cuneiform
- 10 内側楔状骨 Medial cuneiform
- 11 外側楔状骨 Lateral cuneiform
- 12 背側足根靱帯 Dorsal tarsal ligaments
- 13 短趾伸筋 Extensor digitorum brevis muscle
- 14 後脛骨筋(腱) Tibialis posterior muscle (tendon)
- 15 立方骨 Cuboid
- 16 跳躍靱帯(底側踵舟靱帯) Spring ligament (plantar calcaneonavicular ligament)
- 17 舟状骨 Navicular
- 18 長趾屈筋(腱) Flexor digitorum longus muscle(tendon)
- 19 跳躍靱帯(底側踵舟靱帯) Spring ligament (plantar calcaneonavicular ligament)
- 20 踵骨(載距突起) Calcaneus(talar shelf)
- 21 長足底靱帯 Long plantar ligament
- 22 内側足底動静脈 Medial plantar artery and vein
- 23 短腓骨筋(腱) Peroneus(fibularis)brevis muscle(tendon)
- 24 長母趾屈筋(腱) Flexor hallucis longus (tendon)
- 25 長腓骨筋(腱) Peroneus(fibularis)longus muscle(tendon)
- 26 屈筋支帯 Flexor retinaculum
- 27 腓骨筋支帯 Peroneal retinaculum
- 28 外側足底動静脈 Lateral plantar artery and vein
- 29 踵骨(踵骨結節) Calcaneus(calcaneal tuberosity)
- 30 足底方形筋 Quadratus plantae muscle
- 31 アキレス腱(踵骨腱) Achilles tendon (calcaneal tendon)

246　下 肢

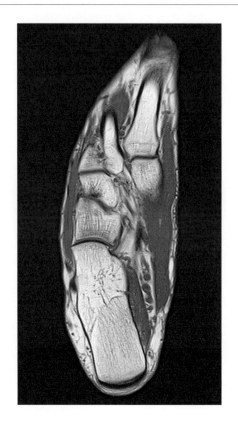

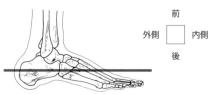

下肢，軸位断　**247**

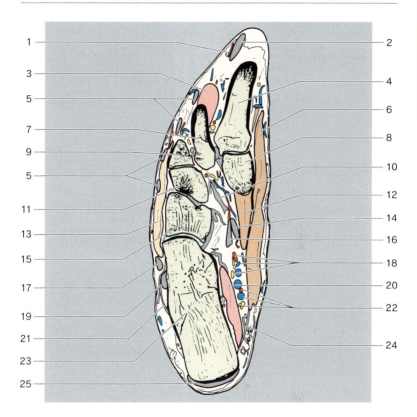

1 足背動脈 Dorsalis pedis artery
2 長母趾伸筋(腱) Extensor hallucis longus muscle (tendon)
3 背側骨間筋 Dorsal interosseous muscles
4 第1中足骨(底) Metatarsal I (base)
5 長趾伸筋(腱) Extensor digitorum longus muscle (tendons)
6 母趾外転筋 Abductor hallucis muscle
7 第2中足骨(底) Metatarsal II (base)
8 内側楔状骨 Medial cuneiform
9 第3中足骨(底) Metatarsal III (base)
10 後脛骨筋(腱) Tibialis posterior muscle (tendon)
11 外側楔状骨 Lateral cuneiform
12 短母趾屈筋 Flexor hallucis brevis muscle
13 短趾伸筋 Extensor digitorum brevis muscle
14 長母趾屈筋(腱) Flexor hallucis longus muscle (tendon)
15 立方骨 Cuboid
16 長趾屈筋(腱) Flexor digitorum longus muscle (tendon)
17 短腓骨筋(腱) Peroneus (fibularis) brevis muscle (tendon)
18 内側足底動静脈, 神経 Medial plantar artery, vein, and nerve
19 長腓骨筋(腱) Peroneus (fibularis) longus muscle (tendon)
20 足底方形筋 Quadratus plantae muscle
21 下腓骨筋支帯 Inferior fibular retinaculum
22 外側足底動静脈, 神経 Lateral plantar artery, vein, and nerve
23 踵骨 Calcaneus
24 屈筋支帯 Flexor retinaculum
25 アキレス腱(踵骨腱)(付着部) Achilles tendon (calcaneal tendon) (attachment)

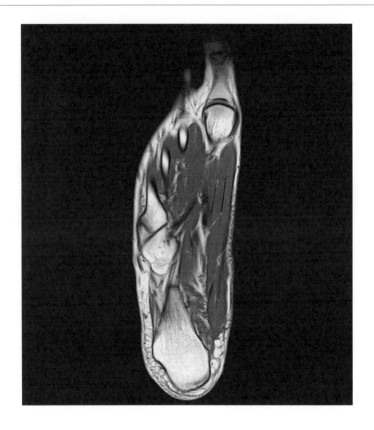

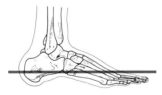

1 **長趾伸筋(腱)** Extensor digitorum longus muscle (tendons)
2 **第1基節骨** Proximal phalanx I
3 **背側骨間筋** Dorsal interosseous muscle, **底側骨間筋** Plantar interosseous muscles
4 **中足趾節関節** Metatarsophalangeal joint

下肢，軸位断 **249**

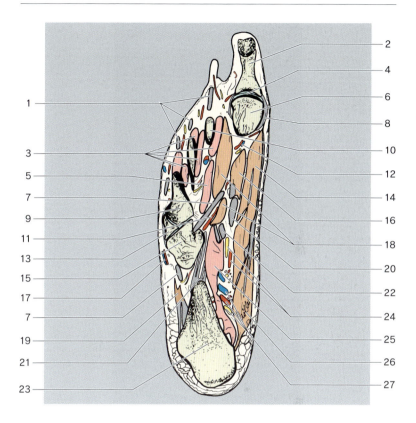

5 母趾内転筋（斜頭）Adductor hallucis muscle (oblique head)
6 第1中足骨（頭）Metatarsal I (head)
7 長腓骨筋（腱）Peroneus (fibularis) longus muscle (tendon)
8 関節包 Joint capsule
9 第4中足骨（底）Metatarsal IV (base)
10 第2中足骨 Metatarsal II
11 足底動脈弓 Plantar arch
12 底側中足動静脈, 神経 Plantar metatarsal artery, vein, and nerve
13 外側楔状骨 Lateral cuneiform
14 短母趾屈筋（内側頭）Flexor hallucis brevis muscle (medial head)
15 立方骨 Cuboid
16 短母趾屈筋（外側頭）Flexor hallucis brevis muscle (lateral head)
17 第5趾の底側趾動静脈, 神経 Fifth plantar digital artery, vein and nerve
18 母趾内転筋 Adductor hallucis muscle
19 小趾外転筋 Abductor digiti minimi muscle
20 長母趾屈筋（腱）Flexor hallucis longus muscle (tendon)
21 長足底靱帯 Long plantar ligament
22 長趾屈筋（腱）Flexor digitorum longus muscle (tendon)
23 踵骨（踵骨結節）Calcaneus (calcaneal tuberosity)
24 内側足底動脈, 神経 Medial plantar artery and nerve
25 足底方形筋 Quadratus plantae muscle
26 母趾外転筋 Abductor hallucis muscle
27 外側足底動静脈, 神経 Lateral plantar artery, vein and nerve

250 下肢

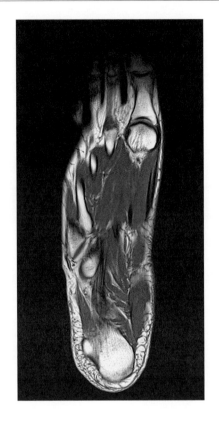

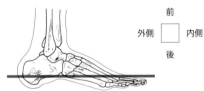

前
外側　内側
後

1 長趾伸筋（腱） Extensor digitorum longus muscle (tendon)
2 第1末節骨 Distal phalanx I
3 底側趾動脈 Plantar digital arteries
4 第1基節骨 Proximal phalanx I

下肢, 軸位断　**251**

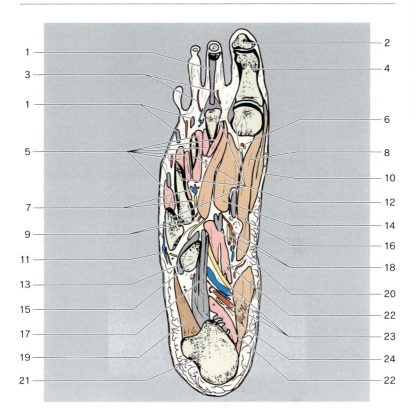

5 **背側骨間筋** Dorsal interosseous muscle,
底側骨間筋 Plantar interosseous muscles
6 **底側中足動脈, 内側足底神経** Plantar metatarsal artery, Medial plantar nerve
7 **外側足底動静脈, 神経(浅枝)** Lateral plantar artery, vein and nerve (superficial branch)
8 **短母趾屈筋(内側頭)** Flexor hallucis brevis muscle (medial head)
9 **外側足底動静脈(深枝)** Lateral plantar artery and vein (deep branch)
10 **母趾外転筋(腱)** Abductor hallucis muscle (tendon)
11 **第5趾背側趾動静脈, 神経** Fifth plantar digital artery, vein, and nerve
12 **中足骨** Metatarsals
13 **長腓骨筋(腱)** Peroneus (fibularis) longus muscle (tendon)
14 **短母趾屈筋(外側頭)** Flexor hallucis brevis muscle (lateral head)
15 **立方骨** Cuboid
16 **長母趾屈筋(腱)** Flexor hallucis longus muscle (tendon)
17 **長足底靱帯** Long plantar ligament
18 **内側足底動静脈, 神経** Medial plantar artery, vein, and nerve
19 **小趾外転筋** Abductor digiti minimi muscle
20 **長趾屈筋(腱)** Flexor digitorum longus muscle (tendon)
21 **踵骨(踵骨結節)** Calcaneus (calcaneal tuberosity)
22 **足底方形筋** Quadratus plantae muscle
23 **外側足底動静脈, 神経** Lateral plantar artery, vein, and nerve
24 **母趾外転筋** Abductor hallucis muscle

252　下 肢

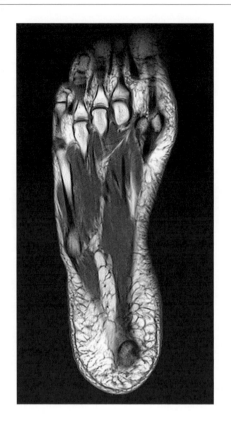

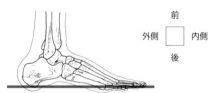

前
外側　内側
後

下肢，軸位断 **253**

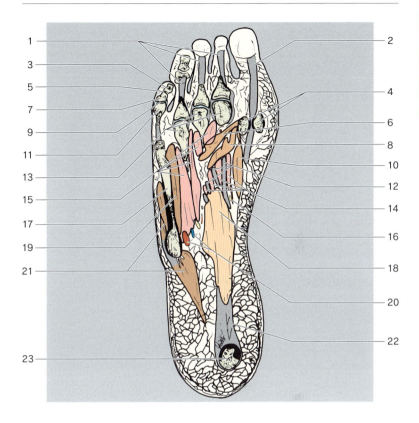

1 趾屈筋群(腱) Flexor digitorum muscles (tendons)
2 長母趾屈筋(腱) Flexor hallucis longus muscle (tendon)
3 第5末節骨 Distal phalanx V
4 種子骨 Sesamoid bones
5 第5遠位趾節間関節(DIP関節) Fifth distal interphalangeal joint (DIP)
6 母趾内転筋(横頭) Adductor hallucis muscle (transverse head)
7 第5中節骨 Middle phalanx V
8 母趾内転筋(斜頭) Adductor hallucis muscle (oblique head)
9 第5近位趾節間関節(PIP関節) Fifth proximal interphalangeal joint (PIP)
10 短母趾屈筋 Flexor hallucis brevis muscle
11 第5基節骨 Proximal phalanx V
12 長趾屈筋(腱) Flexor digitorum longus muscle (tendons)
13 中足骨(頭) Metatarsal bones (heads)
14 虫様筋 Lumbrical muscles
15 背側骨間筋 Dorsal interosseous muscle, 底側骨間筋 Plantar interosseous muscle
16 内側足底動静脈，神経(深枝) Medial plantar artery, vein, and nerve (deep branch)
17 第5中足骨 Metatarsal V
18 短趾屈筋 Flexor digitorum brevis muscle
19 短小趾屈筋 Flexor digiti minimi brevis muscle
20 外側足底動静脈 Lateral plantar artery and vein
21 小趾外転筋 Abductor digiti minimi muscle
22 足底腱膜 Plantar aponeurosis
23 踵骨(踵骨結節) Calcaneus (calcaneal tuberosity)

254　下 肢

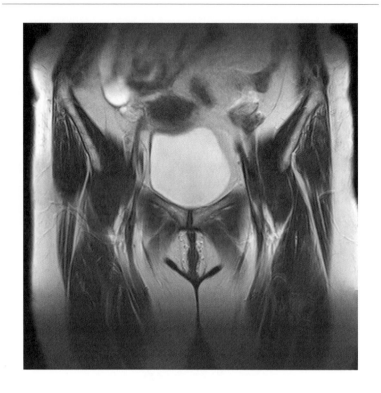

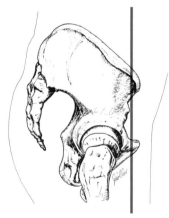

頭側
(近位)

右　　　左

尾側
(遠位)

股関節，冠状断 255

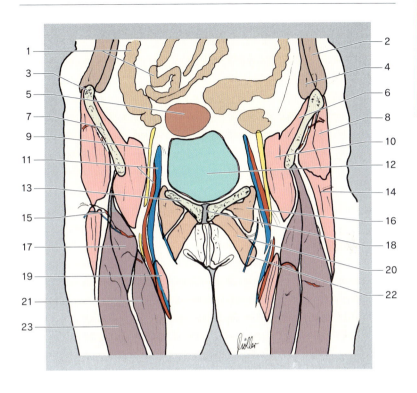

1 小腸 Small intestine
2 外腹斜筋 External oblique muscle, 内腹斜筋 Internal oblique muscle
3 前上腸骨棘 Anterior superior iliac spine
4 腹横筋 Transversus abdominis muscle
5 子宮 Uterus
6 腸骨筋 Iliacus muscle
7 腸骨 Ilium
8 中殿筋 Gluteus medius muscle
9 大腿神経 Femoral nerve
10 腸腰筋 Iliopsoas muscle
11 大腿動静脈 Femoral artery and vein
12 膀胱 Urinary bladder
13 恥骨 Pubis
14 大腿筋膜張筋 Tensor fasciae latae muscle
15 外側大腿回旋動脈（上行枝）Lateral circumflex femoral artery (ascending branch)
16 恥骨筋 Pectineus muscle
17 大腿直筋 Rectus femoris muscle
18 恥骨結合 Pubic symphysis
19 縫工筋 Sartorius muscle
20 長内転筋 Adductor longus muscle
21 内側広筋 Vastus medialis muscle
22 大伏在静脈 Great saphenous vein
23 外側広筋 Vastus lateralis muscle

256　下　肢

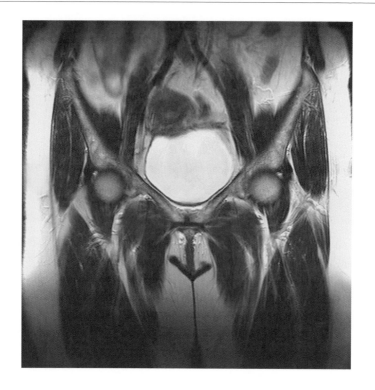

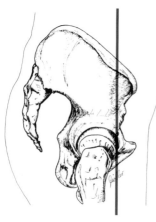

頭側
(近位)

右　　　左

尾側
(遠位)

1　下大静脈　Inferior vena cava
2　大動脈(分岐部)　Aorta(bifurcation)
3　小腸　Small intestine
4　内腹斜筋　Internal oblique muscle
5　(右)総腸骨動脈　(Right)common iliac artery
6　腹横筋　Transversus abdominis muscle

股関節，冠状断 257

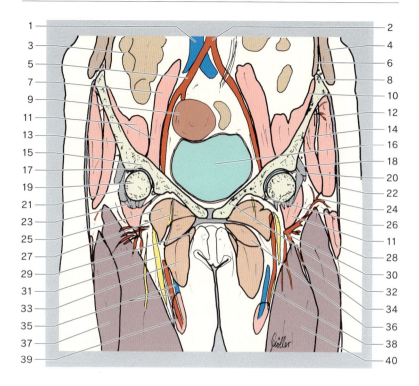

- 7 (大)腰筋 Psoas muscle
- 8 前上腸骨棘 Anterior superior iliac spine
- 9 子宮 Uterus
- 10 腸骨筋 Iliacus muscle
- 11 腸腰筋 Iliopsoas muscle
- 12 中殿筋 Gluteus medius muscle
- 13 腸骨 Ilium
- 14 小殿筋 Gluteus minimus muscle
- 15 臼蓋 Roof of acetabulum
- 16 膀胱 Urinary bladder
- 17 股関節 Hip joint
- 18 大腿直筋(腱) Rectus femoris muscle (tendon)
- 19 大腿骨(頭) Femur (head)
- 20 上方関節唇 Superior acetabular labrum
- 21 腸骨大腿靱帯(横部) Iliofemoral ligament (transverse part)
- 22 腸脛靱帯 Iliotibial tract
- 23 腸骨大腿靱帯(下行部) Iliofemoral ligament (descending part)
- 24 外側大腿回旋動脈(上行枝) Lateral circumflex femoral artery (ascending branch)
- 25 恥骨筋 Pectineus muscle
- 26 下方関節唇 Inferior acetabular labrum
- 27 閉鎖神経 Obturator nerve
- 28 大腿筋膜張筋 Tensor fasciae latae muscle
- 29 薄筋 Gracilis muscle
- 30 大腿深動脈 Deep artery of thigh
- 31 大腿神経 Femoral nerve
- 32 恥骨 Pubis
- 33 長内転筋 Adductor longus muscle
- 34 外側大腿回旋動脈(下行枝) Lateral circumflex femoral artery (descending branch)
- 35 (浅)大腿動静脈 (Superficial) Femoral artery and vein
- 36 短内転筋 Adductor brevis muscle
- 37 外側広筋 Vastus lateralis muscle
- 38 伏在神経 Saphenous nerve
- 39 縫工筋 Sartorius muscle
- 40 中間広筋 Vastus intermedius muscle

258　下 肢

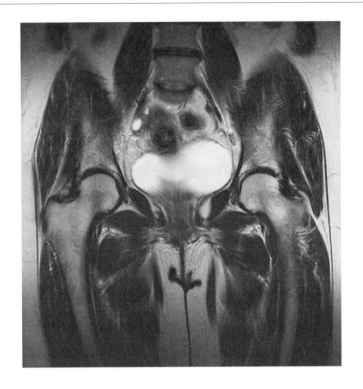

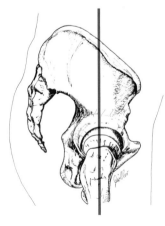

頭側
(近位)

右　　　左

尾側
(遠位)

1 **外腹斜筋** External oblique muscle,
  内腹斜筋 Internal oblique muscle
2 **第4腰椎** Fourth lumbar vertebra
3 **(大)腰筋** Psoas muscle
4 **前上腸骨棘** Anterior superior iliac spine
5 **腸骨筋** Iliacus muscle

股関節，冠状断

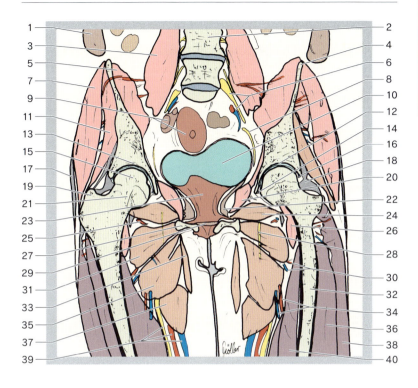

- 6 仙骨神経叢 Sacral plexus, (左)内腸骨動静脈 (Left)internal iliac artery and vein
- 7 中殿筋 Gluteus medius muscle
- 8 閉鎖神経 Obturator nerve
- 9 卵巣 Ovary, 子宮 Uterus
- 10 膀胱 Urinary bladder
- 11 小殿筋 Gluteus minimus muscle
- 12 股関節 Hip joint
- 13 臼蓋 Roof of acetabulum
- 14 下方関節唇 Inferior acetabular labrum
- 15 大腿骨(頭) Femur(head)
- 16 上方関節唇 Superior acetabular labrum
- 17 腸脛靱帯 Iliotibial tract
- 18 腸骨大腿靱帯 Iliofemoral ligament
- 19 大転子 Greater trochanter
- 20 内閉鎖筋 Obturator internus muscle
- 21 大腿骨(頸) Femur(neck)
- 22 肛門挙筋 Levator ani muscle
- 23 腟 Vagina
- 24 外閉鎖筋 Obturator externus muscle
- 25 内側大腿回旋動脈 Medial circumflex femoral artery
- 26 腸腰筋 Iliopsoas muscle
- 27 恥骨 Pubis
- 28 閉鎖神経 Obturator nerve
- 29 深会陰横筋 Deep transverse perineal muscle
- 30 外側大腿回旋動静脈(下行枝) Lateral circumflex femoral artery and vein (descending branch), 大腿神経(前皮枝) Femoral nerve(anterior cutaneous branch)
- 31 恥骨筋 Pectineus muscle
- 32 大腿骨(体) Femur(shaft)
- 33 薄筋 Gracilis muscle
- 34 大腿深動静脈 Deep artery and vein of thigh
- 35 短内転筋 Adductor brevis muscle
- 36 中間広筋 Vastus intermedius muscle
- 37 長内転筋 Adductor longus muscle
- 38 外側広筋 Vastus lateralis muscle
- 39 (浅)大腿動静脈 (Superficial)Femoral artery and vein, 伏在神経 Saphenous nerve
- 40 内側広筋 Vastus medialis muscle

260　下 肢

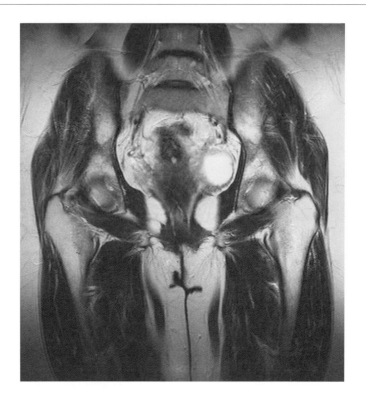

頭側
(近位)

右　　　左

尾側
(遠位)

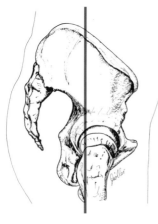

1　腰神経叢　Lumbar plexus
2　(大)腰筋　Psoas muscle
3　腸骨稜　Iliac crest
4　上殿動静脈　Superior gluteal artery and vein
5　腸骨筋　Iliacus muscle
6　仙骨　Sacrum

股関節，冠状断

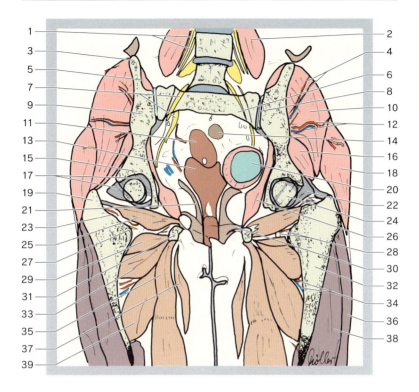

- 7 仙骨神経叢 Sacral plexus
- 8 仙腸関節 Sacroiliac joint
- 9 腸骨 Ilium
- 10 中殿筋 Gluteus medius muscle
- 11 子宮 Uterus
- 12 下殿動静脈 Inferior gluteal artery and vein
- 13 腟 Vagina
- 14 S状結腸 Sigmoid colon
- 15 臼蓋 Roof of acetabulum
- 16 小殿筋 Gluteus minimus muscle
- 17 輪帯 Zona orbicularis
- 18 大殿筋 Gluteus maximus muscle
- 19 大転子 Greater trochanter
- 20 膀胱 Urinary bladder
- 21 肛門挙筋 Levator ani muscle
- 22 坐骨大腿靱帯 Ischiofemoral ligament
- 23 転子間稜 Intertrochanteric crest
- 24 大腿骨(頭) Femur(head)
- 25 外閉鎖筋 Obturator externus muscle
- 26 内閉鎖筋 Obturator internus muscle
- 27 小転子 Lesser trochanter
- 28 内側大腿回旋動静脈 Medial circumflex femoral artery and vein
- 29 小内転筋 Adductor minimus muscle
- 30 深会陰横筋 Deep transverse perineal muscle
- 31 恥骨(下枝) Pubis(inferior ramus)
- 32 大腿骨(体) Femur(shaft)
- 33 短内転筋 Adductor brevis muscle
- 34 大腿深動静脈 Deep artery and vein of thigh
- 35 大内転筋 Adductor magnus muscle
- 36 外側広筋 Vastus lateralis muscle
- 37 薄筋 Gracilis muscle
- 38 中間広筋 Vastus intermedius muscle
- 39 長内転筋 Adductor longus muscle

262 下肢

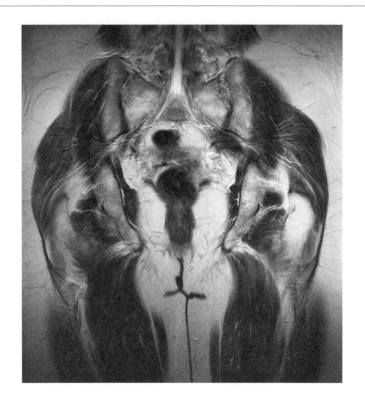

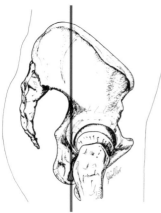

頭側
(近位)

右 　　 左

尾側
(遠位)

股関節, 冠状断 263

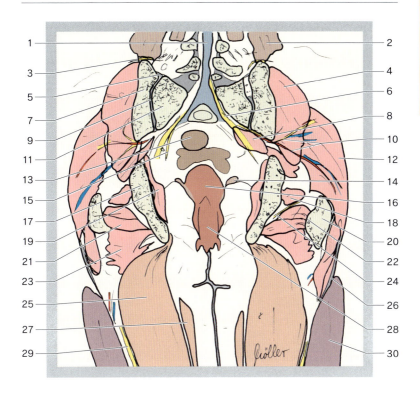

1 脊柱管 Spinal canal
2 腰腸肋筋 Iliocostalis lumborum muscle
3 上殿皮神経 Superior clunial nerves
4 中殿筋 Gluteus medius muscle
5 仙腸靱帯 Sacroiliac ligament
6 坐骨神経 Sciatic nerve
7 腸骨 Ilium
8 梨状筋 Piriformis muscle
9 仙腸関節 Sacroiliac joint
10 下殿動静脈, 神経 Inferior gluteal artery, vein, and nerve
11 仙骨(外側部) Sacrum(lateral mass)
12 大殿筋 Gluteus maximus muscle
13 S状結腸 Sigmoid colon
14 肛門挙筋 Levator ani muscle
15 陰部神経 Pudendal nerve
16 子宮 Uterus
17 坐骨 Ischium
18 上双子筋 Gemellus superior muscle
19 内閉鎖筋 Obturator internus muscle
20 大転子 Greater trochanter
21 下双子筋 Gemellus inferior muscle
22 転子間稜 Intertrochanteric crest
23 大腿方形筋 Quadratus femoris muscle
24 神経の筋枝 Muscular nerve
25 大内転筋 Adductor magnus muscle
26 腸脛靱帯 Iliotibial tract
27 薄筋 Gracilis muscle
28 腟 Vagina
29 坐骨神経 Sciatic nerve
30 外側広筋 Vastus lateralis muscle

264　下肢

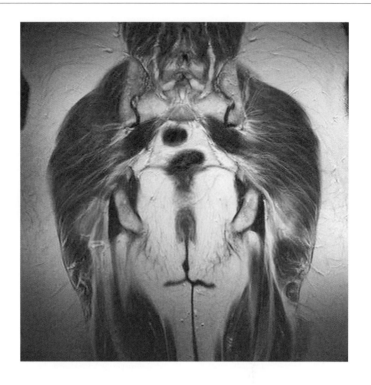

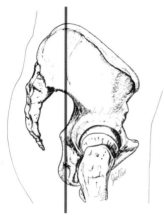

頭側
(近位)

右　　　左

尾側
(遠位)

股関節，冠状断

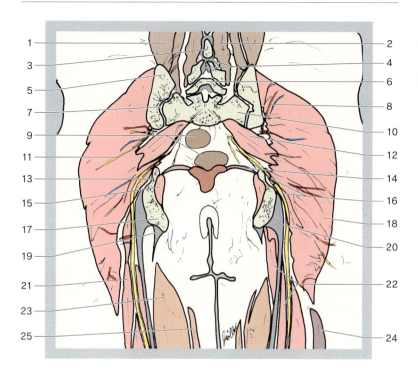

1 腰腸肋筋 Iliocostalis lumborum muscle
2 多裂筋 Multifidus muscle
3 棘突起 Spinous process
4 棘間靱帯 Interspinous ligament
5 腸骨 Ilium
6 椎弓 Vertebral arch
7 仙腸関節 Sacroiliac joint
8 上殿動静脈，神経 Superior gluteal artery, vein, and nerve
9 直腸 Rectum
10 仙骨(外側部) Sacrum (lateral mass)
11 下殿動静脈，神経 Inferior gluteal artery, vein, and nerve
12 梨状筋 Piriformis muscle
13 坐骨棘 Ischial spine
14 肛門挙筋 Levator ani muscle
15 内閉鎖筋 Obturator internus muscle
16 坐骨神経 Sciatic nerve
17 坐骨結節 Ischial tuberosity
18 大殿筋 Gluteus maximus muscle
19 大内転筋(付着部) Adductor magnus muscle (attachment)
20 半腱様筋 Semitendinosus muscle, 大腿二頭筋 Biceps femoris muscle 共通腱付着部
21 大腿二頭筋(長頭) Biceps femoris muscle (long head)
22 半腱様筋 Semitendinosus muscle
23 大内転筋 Adductor magnus muscle
24 外側広筋 Vastus lateralis muscle
25 薄筋 Gracilis muscle

266　下 肢

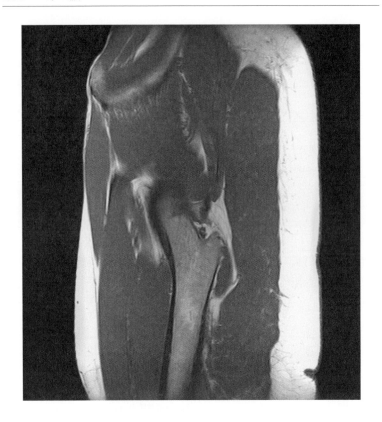

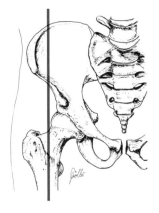

近位
腹側　　　背側
遠位

股関節, 矢状断 267

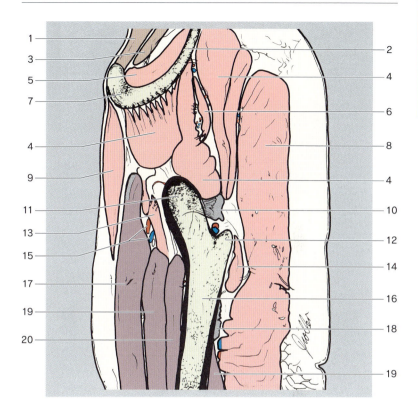

1. 外腹斜筋 External oblique muscle, 内腹斜筋 Internal oblique muscle
2. 腸骨(翼) Ilium(wing)
3. 腹横筋 Transversus abdominis muscle
4. 中殿筋 Gluteus medius muscle
5. 腸腰筋 Iliopsoas muscle
6. 小殿筋 Gluteus minimus muscle
7. 前上腸骨棘 Anterior superior iliac spine
8. 大殿筋 Gluteus maximus muscle
9. 縫工筋 Sartorius muscle
10. 内閉鎖筋 Obturator internus muscle, 双子筋 Gemellus muscles
11. 大腿骨(頸) Femur(neck)
12. 大転子 Greater trochanter
13. 腸腰筋 Iliopsoas muscle
14. 大腿方形筋 Quadratus femoris muscle
15. 外側大腿回旋動静脈 Lateral circumflex femoral artery and vein
16. 大腿骨(体) Femur(shaft)
17. 大腿直筋 Rectus femoris muscle
18. 大内転筋(腱付着部) Adductor magnus muscle(tendon attachment)
19. 中間広筋 Vastus intermedius muscle
20. 内側広筋 Vastus medialis muscle

268 下　肢

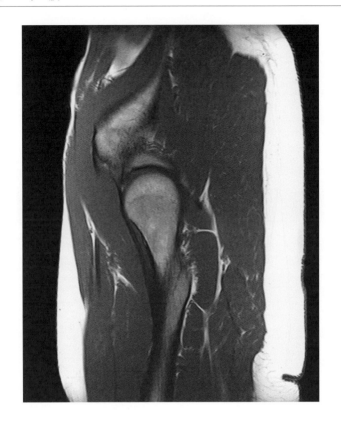

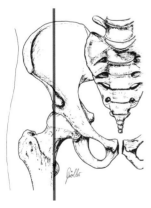

近位
腹側　　背側
遠位

股関節，矢状断 269

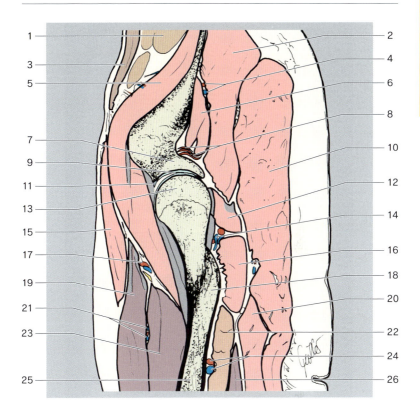

1 小腸 Small intestine
2 中殿筋 Gluteus medius muscle
3 腹直筋 Rectus abdominis muscle
4 上殿動静脈 Superior gluteal artery and vein
5 腸腰筋 Iliopsoas muscle
6 小殿筋 Gluteus minimus muscle
7 腸骨(臼蓋) Ilium(roof of acetabulum)
8 浅腸骨回旋動脈 Superficial circumflex iliac artery
9 股関節 Hip joint
10 大殿筋 Gluteus maximus muscle
11 上方関節唇 Superior acetabular labrum
12 内閉鎖筋 Obturator internus muscle.
   双子筋 Gemellus muscles
13 大腿骨(頭) Femur(head)
14 内側大腿回旋動脈 Medial circumflex femoral artery
15 縫工筋 Sartorius muscle
16 大腿方形筋 Quadratus femoris muscle
17 外側大腿回旋動脈(上行枝) Lateral circumflex femoral artery(ascending branch)
18 小転子 Lesser trochanter
19 大腿直筋 Rectus femoris muscle
20 大腿二頭筋(長頭) Biceps femoris muscle (long head)
21 外側大腿回旋動脈(下行枝) Lateral circumflex femoral artery(descending branch)
22 大内転筋 Adductor magnus muscle
23 中間広筋 Vastus intermedius muscle
24 貫通動脈 Perforating artery
25 大腿骨(体) Femur(shaft)
26 外側広筋 Vastus lateralis muscle

270 下　肢

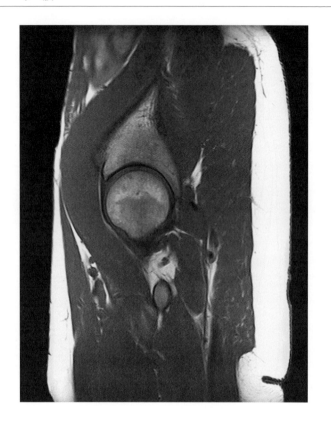

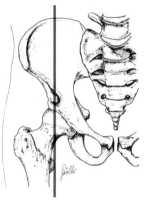

近位

腹側 □ 背側

遠位

股関節，矢状断　271

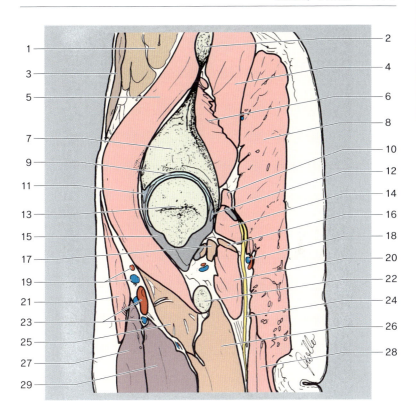

1 小腸 Small intestine
2 腸骨 Ilium
3 腹直筋 Rectus abdominis muscle
4 中殿筋 Gluteus medius muscle
5 腸腰筋 Iliopsoas muscle
6 小殿筋 Gluteus minimus muscle
7 腸骨(臼蓋) Ilium (roof of acetabulum)
8 大殿筋 Gluteus maximus muscle
9 股関節 Hip joint
10 梨状筋 Piriformis muscle
11 上方関節唇 Superior acetabular labrum
12 下方関節唇 Inferior acetabular labrum
13 大腿骨(頭) Femur (head)
14 内閉鎖筋 Obturator internus muscle, 双子筋 Gemellus muscles
15 関節包 Joint capsule
16 小内転筋 Adductor minimus muscle
17 外閉鎖筋 Obturator externus muscle
18 下殿動静脈 Inferior gluteal artery and vein
19 外側大腿回旋動脈(上行枝) Lateral circumflex femoral artery (ascending branch)
20 大腿方形筋 Quadratus femoris muscle
21 縫工筋 Sartorius muscle
22 小転子 Lesser trochanter
23 外側大腿回旋動脈(下行枝) Lateral circumflex femoral artery (descending branch)
24 坐骨神経 Sciatic nerve
25 恥骨筋 Pectineus muscle
26 大内転筋 Adductor magnus muscle
27 大腿直筋 Rectus femoris muscle
28 大腿二頭筋 Biceps femoris muscle
29 内側広筋 Vastus medialis muscle

272　下　肢

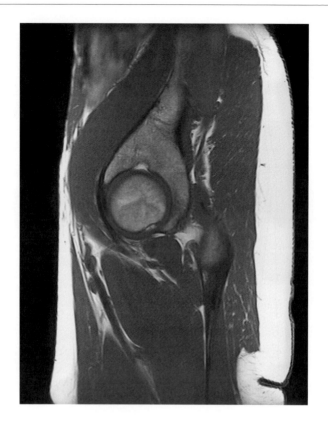

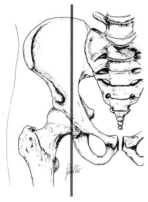

近位

腹側　　背側

遠位

1　**小腸** Small intestine
2　**中殿筋** Gluteus medius muscle
3　**腹直筋** Rectus abdominis muscle
4　**腸骨** Ilium
5　**腸腰筋** Iliopsoas muscle

股関節，矢状断 273

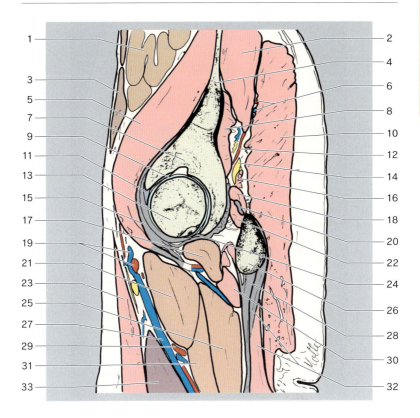

- 6 **上殿動静脈,神経** Superior gluteal artery, vein, and nerve
- 7 **腸骨(臼蓋)** Ilium (roof of acetabulum)
- 8 **小殿筋** Gluteus minimus muscle
- 9 **股関節** Hip joint
- 10 **大殿筋** Gluteus maximus muscle
- 11 **上方関節唇** Superior acetabular labrum
- 12 **上殿動静脈,下殿神経** Superior gluteal artery and vein, inferior gluteal nerve
- 13 **大腿骨(頭)** Femur (head)
- 14 **坐骨神経** Sciatic nerve
- 15 **関節包** Joint capsule
- 16 **梨状筋** Piriformis muscle
- 17 **外閉鎖筋** Obturator externus muscle
- 18 **上双子筋** Superior gemellus muscle
- 19 **外側大腿回旋動脈(上行枝)** Lateral circumflex femoris artery (ascending branch)
- 20 **内閉鎖筋(腱)** Obturator internus muscle (tendon)
- 21 **恥骨筋** Pectineus muscle
- 22 **下双子筋** Gemellus inferior muscle
- 23 **縫工筋** Sartorius muscle
- 24 **下方関節唇** Inferior acetabular labrum
- 25 **大内転筋** Adductor magnus muscle
- 26 **坐骨** Ischium
- 27 **大腿深動静脈** Deep artery and vein of thigh
- 28 **半膜様筋** Semimembranosus muscle, **半腱様筋** Semitendinosus muscle 腱付着部
- 29 **貫通動脈** Perforating arteries
- 30 **大腿方形筋** Quadratus femoris muscle
- 31 **短内転筋** Adductor brevis muscle
- 32 **大腿二頭筋(＋腱)** Biceps femoris muscle (＋tendon)
- 33 **内側広筋** Vastus medialis muscle

274　下 肢

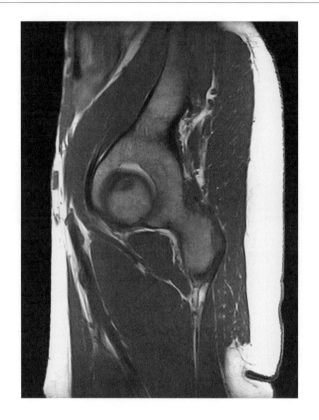

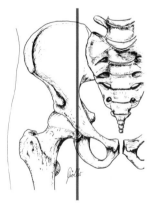

近位

腹側　　背側

遠位

股関節，矢状断 275

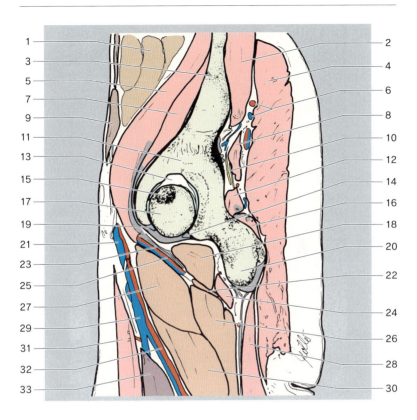

1 小腸 Small intestine
2 中殿筋 Gluteus medius muscle
3 腸骨 Ilium
4 大殿筋 Gluteus maximus muscle
5 (大)腰筋 Psoas muscle
6 上殿動静脈, 神経 Superior gluteal artery, vein, and nerve
7 腸骨筋 Iliacus muscle
8 梨状筋 Piriformis muscle
9 腹直筋 Rectus abdominis muscle
10 坐骨神経 Sciatic nerve
11 腸骨(臼蓋) Ilium (roof of acetabulum)
12 上双子筋 Gemellus superior muscle
13 寛骨臼窩 Acetabular fossa
14 下方関節唇 Inferior acetabular labrum
15 大腿骨頭窩 Fovea
16 下双子筋 Gemellus inferior muscle
17 大腿骨(頭) Femur (head)
18 外閉鎖筋 Obturator externus muscle
19 上方関節唇 Superior acetabular labrum
20 坐骨 Ischium
21 大腿動静脈 Femoral artery and vein
22 小内転筋 Adductor minimus muscle
23 坐骨大腿靱帯 Ischiofemoral ligament
24 大腿方形筋 Quadratus femoris muscle
25 外側大腿回旋動脈 Lateral circumflex femoral artery
26 大内転筋 Adductor magnus muscle
27 恥骨筋 Pectineus muscle
28 大腿二頭筋 Biceps femoris muscle
29 (浅)大腿動静脈 (Superficial) femoral artery and vein
30 短内転筋 Adductor brevis muscle
31 縫工筋 Sartorius muscle
32 大腿深動静脈 Deep artery and vein of thigh
33 内側広筋 Vastus medialis muscle

276　下 肢

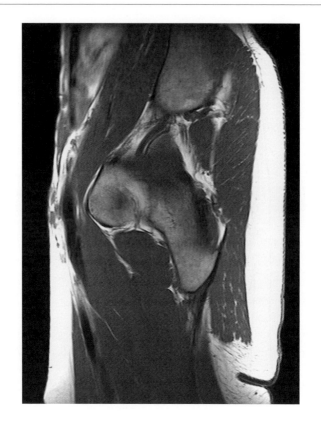

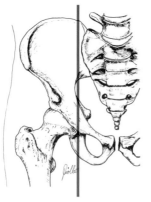

近位
腹側　　背側
遠位

股関節, 矢状断 277

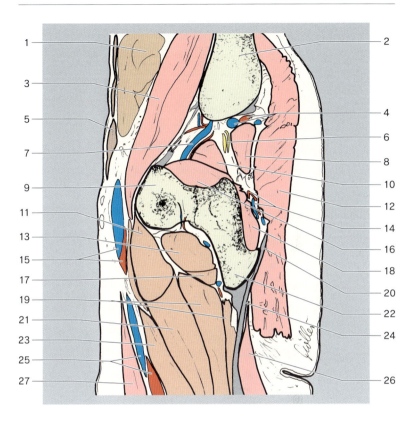

1 小腸 Small intestine
2 腸骨 Ilium
3 腸腰筋 Iliopsoas muscle
4 上殿動静脈, 神経 Superior gluteal artery, vein, and nerve
5 腹直筋 Rectus abdominis muscle
6 坐骨神経 Sciatic nerve
7 内腸骨動静脈 Internal iliac artery and vein
8 梨状筋 Piriformis muscle
9 腸骨 Ilium (joint socket)
10 上双子筋 Gemellus superior muscle
11 恥骨筋 Pectineus muscle
12 大殿筋 Gluteus maximus muscle
13 外閉鎖筋 Obturator externus muscle
14 下殿動脈, 神経 Inferior gluteal artery and nerve
15 大腿動静脈 Femoral artery and vein
16 内閉鎖筋 Obturator internus muscle
17 小内転筋 Adductor minimus muscle
18 下双子筋 Gemellus inferior muscle
19 大内転筋 Adductor magnus muscle
20 仙結節靱帯 Sacrotuberous ligament
21 短内転筋 Adductor brevis muscle
22 坐骨結節 Ischial tuberosity
23 長内転筋 Adductor longus muscle
24 大腿二頭筋 (共通腱) Biceps femoris muscle (common tendon)
25 (浅) 大腿動静脈 (Superficial) Femoral artery and vein
26 大腿二頭筋 Biceps femoris muscle
27 縫工筋 Sartorius muscle

278　下 肢

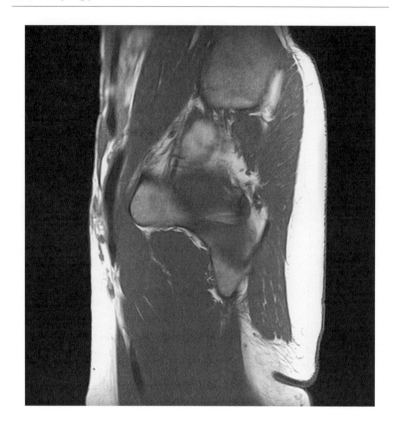

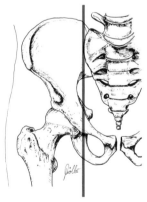

近位

腹側　　背側

遠位

股関節，矢状断 279

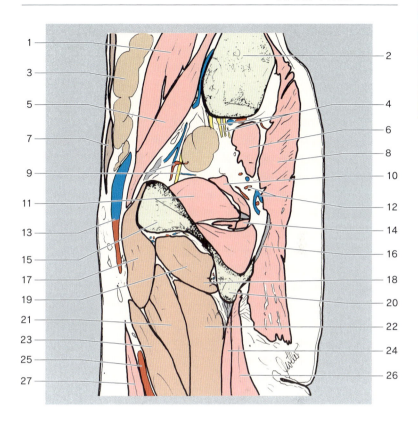

1 (大)腰筋 Psoas muscle
2 腸骨(翼) Ilium (wing)
3 小腸(回腸) Small intestine (ileum)
4 仙骨神経叢 Sacral plexus
5 腸骨筋 Iliacus muscle
6 梨状筋 Piriformis muscle
7 腹直筋 Rectus abdominis muscle
8 大殿筋 Gluteus maximus muscle
9 閉鎖動脈,神経 Obturator artery and nerve
10 上双子筋 Gemellus superior muscle
11 内閉鎖筋 Obturator internus muscle
12 上殿動静脈 Superior gluteal artery and vein, 下殿神経 Inferior gluteal nerve
13 大腿動静脈 Femoral artery and vein
14 下双子筋 Gemellus inferior muscle
15 恥骨 Pubis
16 仙結節靱帯 Sacrotuberous ligament
17 恥骨筋 Pectineus muscle
18 小内転筋 Adductor minimus muscle
19 外閉鎖筋 Obturator externus muscle
20 坐骨結節 Ischial tuberosity
21 短内転筋 Adductor brevis muscle
22 大内転筋 Adductor magnus muscle
23 長内転筋 Adductor longus muscle
24 半膜様筋 Semimembranosus muscle
25 (浅)大腿動脈 (Superficial) Femoral artery
26 半腱様筋 Semitendinosus muscle
27 縫工筋 Sartorius muscle

280 下肢

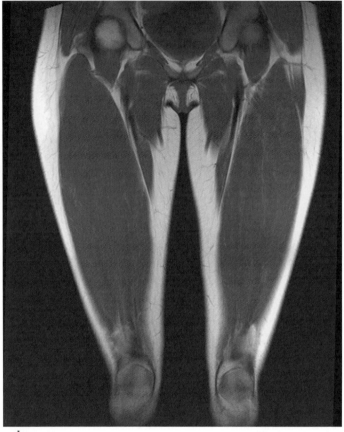

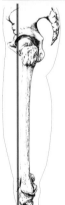

頭側

遠位

1 小殿筋 Gluteus minimus muscle
2 中殿筋 Gluteus medius muscle
3 臼蓋 Roof of acetabulum
4 腸骨大腿靱帯 Iliofemoral ligament
5 上方関節唇 Superior acetabular labrum

大腿，冠状断 **281**

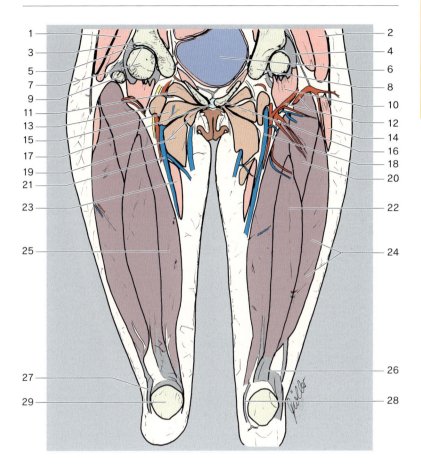

6 膀胱 Urinary bladder
7 股関節 Hip joint, 大腿骨(頭) Femur(head)
8 恥骨 Pubis
9 大転子 Greater trochanter
10 腸腰筋 Iliopsoas muscle
11 外閉鎖筋 Obturator externus muscle
12 外側大腿回旋動静脈 Lateral circumflex femoral artery and vein
13 恥骨筋 Pectineus muscle
14 大腿筋膜張筋 Tensor fasciae latae muscle
15 短内転筋 Adductor brevis muscle
16 恥骨(上枝) Pubis(superior ramus)
17 恥骨結合 Pubic symphysis
18 大腿動静脈 Femoral artery and vein
19 長内転筋 Adductor longus muscle
20 大腿直筋 Rectus femoris muscle
21 大伏在静脈 Great saphenous vein
22 中間広筋 Vastus intermedius muscle
23 縫工筋 Sartorius muscle
24 外側広筋 Vastus lateralis muscle
25 内側広筋 Vastus medialis muscle
26 大腿四頭筋腱 Quadriceps tendon
27 外側膝蓋支帯 Lateral patellar retinaculum
28 内側膝蓋支帯 Medial patellar retinaculum
29 膝蓋骨 Patella

282 下肢

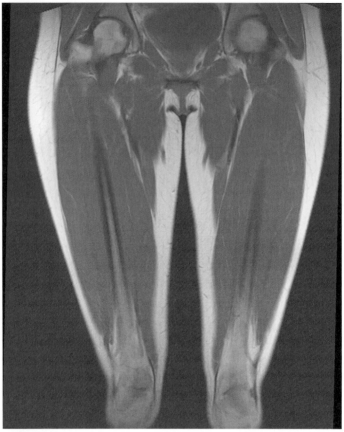

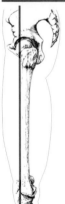

頭側

遠位

1 **中殿筋** Gluteus medius muscle
2 **小殿筋** Gluteus minimus muscle
3 **臼蓋** Roof of acetabulum
4 **膀胱** Urinary bladder
5 **股関節** Hip joint
6 **大腿骨(頭)** Femur(head)

大腿，冠状断   **283**

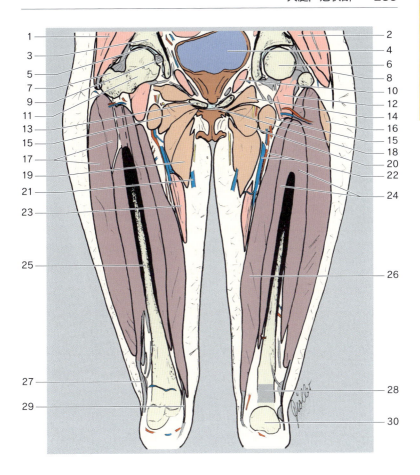

7 大転子 Greater trochanter
8 腸脛靱帯 Iliotibial tract
9 大腿骨頭靱帯 Ligament of head of femur
10 内閉鎖筋 Obturator internus muscle
11 大腿骨（頸）Femur (neck)
12 腸腰筋 Iliopsoas muscle
13 恥骨（下枝）Pubis (inferior ramus)
14 外閉鎖筋 Obturator externus muscle
15 恥骨筋 Pectineus muscle
16 大腿筋膜張筋 Tensor fasciae latae muscle
17 外側広筋 Vastus lateralis muscle
18 恥骨結合 Pubic symphysis
19 長内転筋 Adductor longus muscle
20 短内転筋 Adductor brevis muscle
21 大伏在静脈 Great saphenous vein
22 大腿動静脈 Femoral artery and vein
23 縫工筋 Sartorius muscle
24 中間広筋 Vastus intermedius muscle
25 大腿骨（体）Femur (shaft)
26 内側広筋 Vastus medialis muscle
27 外側膝蓋支帯 Lateral patellar retinaculum
28 大腿四頭筋腱 Quadriceps tendon
29 内側膝蓋支帯 Medial patellar retinaculum
30 膝蓋骨 Patella

284 下 肢

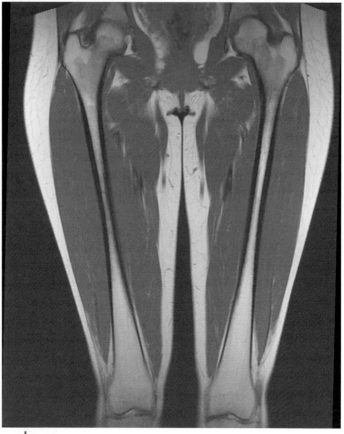

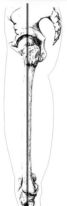

頭側

遠位

1 中殿筋 Gluteus medius muscle
2 小殿筋 Gluteus minimus muscle
3 臼蓋 Roof of acetabulum
4 股関節 Hip joint
5 大腿骨(頭) Femur (head)
6 大腿骨頭靱帯 Ligament of head of femur

大腿，冠状断 285

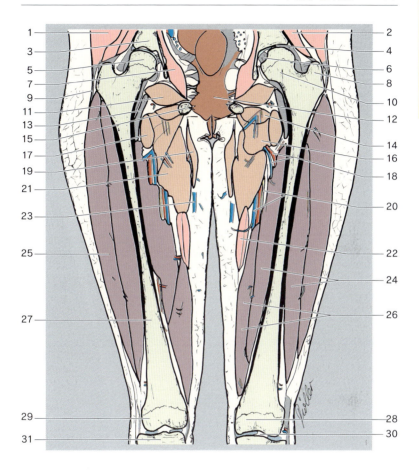

- 7 内閉鎖筋 Obturator internus muscle
- 8 大転子 Greater trochanter
- 9 腸脛靱帯 Iliotibial tract
- 10 大腿骨(頸) Femur(neck)
- 11 外閉鎖筋 Obturator externus muscle
- 12 腟 Vagina
- 13 腸腰筋(腱) Iliopsoas muscle(tendon)
- 14 小内転筋 Adductor minimus muscle
- 15 恥骨(下枝) Pubis(inferior ramus)
- 16 短内転筋 Adductor brevis muscle
- 17 恥骨筋 Pectineus muscle
- 18 大腿深動静脈 Deep femoral artery and vein
- 19 薄筋 Gracilis muscle
- 20 大腿動静脈 Femoral artery and vein, 伏在神経 Saphenous nerve
- 21 長内転筋 Adductor longus muscle
- 22 縫工筋 Sartorius muscle
- 23 大伏在静脈 Great saphenous vein
- 24 中間広筋 Vastus intermedius muscle
- 25 外側広筋 Vastus lateralis muscle
- 26 内側広筋 Vastus medialis muscle
- 27 大腿骨(体) Femur(shaft)
- 28 大腿骨内側顆 Medial femoral condyle
- 29 大腿骨外側顆 Lateral femoral condyle
- 30 膝関節 Knee joint
- 31 脛骨(頭) Tibia(head)

286 下肢

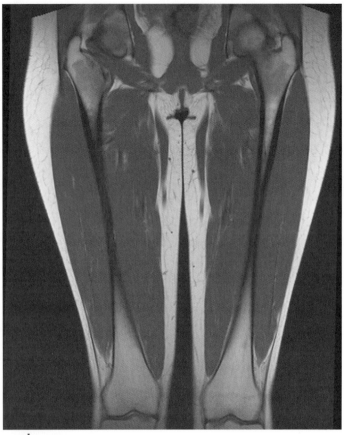

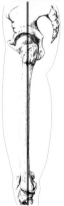

頭側

遠位

1 **中殿筋** Gluteus medius muscle
2 **小殿筋** Gluteus minimus muscle
3 **腸骨筋** Iliacus muscle
4 **臼蓋** Roof of acetabulum
5 **梨状筋** Piriformis muscle
6 **大腿骨(頭)** Femur(head)
7 **双子筋** Gemellus muscles
8 **大転子** Greater trochanter

大腿, 冠状断

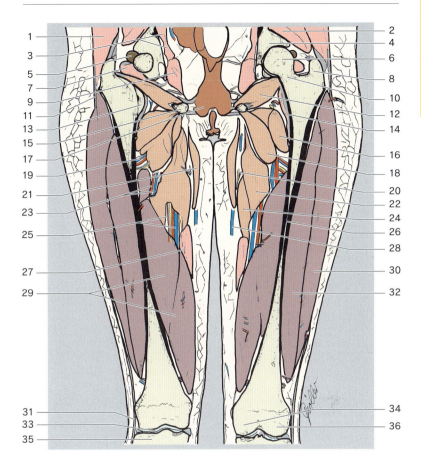

9 内閉鎖筋 Obturator internus muscle
10 大腿骨(頸) Femur (neck)
11 腸脛靱帯 Iliotibial tract
12 外閉鎖筋 Obturator externus muscle
13 小転子 Lesser trochanter
14 腸腰筋 Iliopsoas muscle
15 恥骨(下枝) Pubis (inferior ramus)
16 小内転筋 Adductor minimus muscle
17 腟 Vagina
18 短内転筋 Adductor brevis muscle
19 外側大腿回旋動静脈 Lateral circumflex femoral artery and vein
20 閉鎖神経 Obturator nerve
21 薄筋 Gracilis muscle
22 大内転筋 Adductor magnus muscle
23 大腿深動静脈 Deep femoral artery and vein
24 長内転筋 Adductor longus muscle
25 大腿動静脈 Femoral artery and vein, 伏在神経 Saphenous nerve
26 大腿骨(体) Femur (shaft)
27 縫工筋 Sartorius muscle
28 大伏在静脈 Great saphenous vein
29 内側広筋 Vastus medialis muscle
30 外側広筋 Vastus lateralis muscle
31 腸脛靱帯 Iliotibial tract
32 中間広筋 Vastus intermedius muscle
33 膝関節 Knee joint
34 大腿骨内側顆 Medial femoral condyle
35 脛骨(頭) Tibia (head)
36 大腿骨外側顆 Lateral femoral condyle

288　下 肢

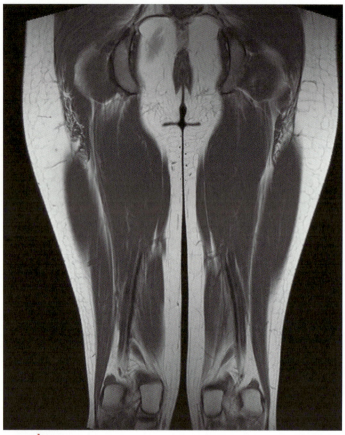

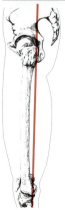

頭側

遠位

1　**大殿筋** Gluteus maximus muscle
2　**肛門挙筋** Levator ani muscle
3　**内閉鎖筋** Obturator internus muscle
4　**梨状筋** Piriformis muscle
5　**坐骨** Ischium
6　**双子筋** Gemellus muscles
7　**肛門** Anus,
　　外肛門括約筋 External anal sphincter muscle

大腿，冠状断

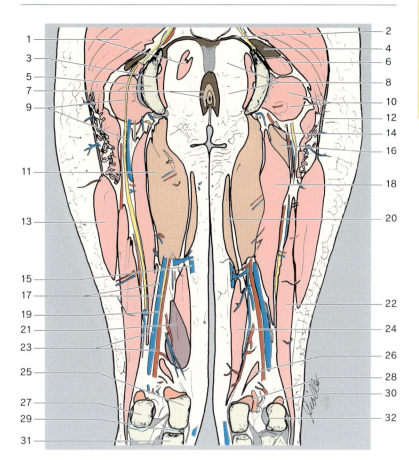

- 8 坐骨肛門窩 Ischioanal fossa
- 9 坐骨神経 Sciatic nerve
- 10 大腿方形筋 Quadratus femoris muscle
- 11 大内転筋 Adductor magnus muscle
- 12 腸脛靱帯 Iliotibial tract
- 13 外側広筋 Vastus lateralis muscle
- 14 小内転筋 Adductor minimus muscle
- 15 大伏在静脈 Great saphenous vein
- 16 短内転筋 Adductor brevis muscle
- 17 大腿動静脈 Femoral artery and vein
- 18 半腱様筋 Semitendinosus muscle
- 19 伏在神経 Saphenous nerve
- 20 薄筋 Gracilis muscle
- 21 内側広筋 Vastus medialis muscle
- 22 大腿二頭筋(長頭) Biceps femoris muscle (long head)
- 23 膝窩動静脈 Popliteal artery and vein
- 24 縫工筋 Sartorius muscle
- 25 大腿骨内側顆 Medial femoral condyle
- 26 半膜様筋 Semimembranosus muscle
- 27 大腿骨外側顆 Lateral femoral condyle
- 28 腓腹筋(内側頭,付着部) Gastrocnemius muscle(medial head, attachment)
- 29 膝関節 Knee joint
- 30 腓腹筋(外側頭,付着部) Gastrocnemius muscle(lateral head, attachment)
- 31 脛骨(頭) Tibia(head)
- 32 前十字靱帯 Anterior cruciate ligament

290 下肢

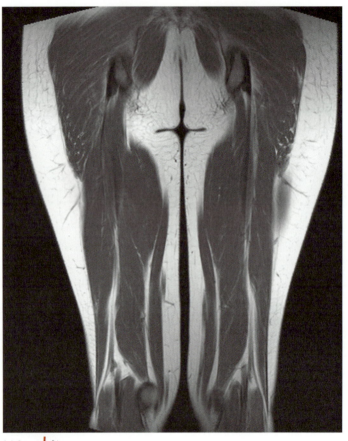

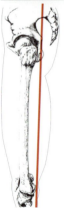

頭側

遠位

大腿，冠状断 **291**

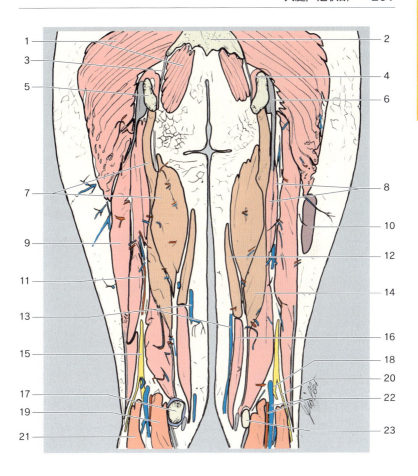

1 大殿筋 Gluteus maximus muscle
2 仙骨 Sacrum
3 仙結節靱帯 Sacrotuberous ligament
4 内閉鎖筋 Obturator internus muscle
5 坐骨 Ischium
6 半腱様筋 Semitendinosus muscle, 大腿二頭筋 Biceps femoris muscle 共通腱付着部
7 大内転筋 Adductor magnus muscle
8 半腱様筋 Semitendinosus muscle
9 大腿二頭筋(長頭) Biceps femoris muscle (long head)
10 外側広筋 Vastus lateralis muscle
11 貫通動脈 Perforating artery
12 薄筋 Gracilis muscle
13 大伏在静脈 Great saphenous vein
14 半膜様筋 Semimembranosus muscle
15 坐骨神経 Sciatic nerve
16 縫工筋 Sartorius muscle
17 大腿骨内側顆 Medial femoral condyle
18 脛骨神経 Tibial nerve
19 腓腹筋(内側頭) Gastrocnemius muscle (medial head)
20 総腓骨神経 Common fibular nerve
21 腓腹筋(外側頭) Gastrocnemius muscle (lateral head)
22 膝窩動静脈 Popliteal artery and vein
23 関節包 Joint capsule, 半膜様筋の滑液包 Semimembranosus bursa

292 下 肢

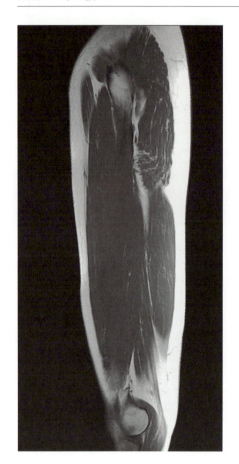

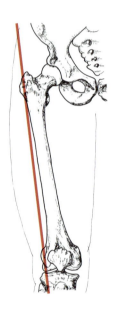

大腿，矢状断 293

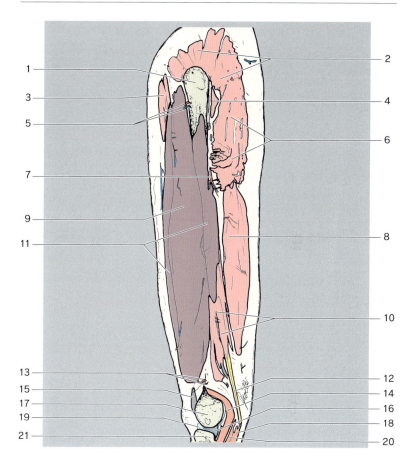

1 大転子 Greater trochanter
2 中殿筋 Gluteus medius muscle
3 大腿筋膜張筋 Tensor fasciae latae muscle
4 大腿方形筋 Quadratus femoris muscle
5 外側大腿回旋動静脈 Lateral circumflex femoral artery and vein
6 大殿筋 Gluteus maximus muscle
7 貫通動脈 Perforating arteries
8 大腿二頭筋（長頭） Biceps femoris muscle (long head)
9 中間広筋 Vastus intermedius muscle
10 大腿二頭筋（短頭） Biceps femoris muscle (short head)
11 外側広筋 Vastus lateralis muscle
12 総腓骨神経 Common fibular nerve
13 外側上膝動静脈 Superior lateral genicular artery and vein
14 腓腹筋（外側頭） Gastrocnemius muscle (lateral head)
15 大腿四頭筋腱 Quadriceps tendon
16 外側半月板 Lateral meniscus
17 大腿骨外側顆 Lateral femoral condyle
18 ヒラメ筋 Soleus muscle
19 膝関節 Knee joint
20 足底筋 Plantaris muscle
21 脛骨外側顆 Lateral tibial condyle

294 下　肢

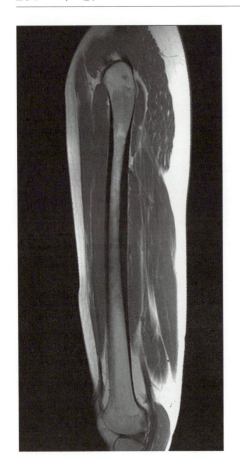
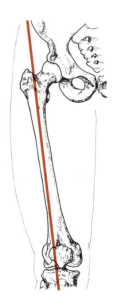

頭側
腹側　　背側
遠位

大腿, 矢状断 295

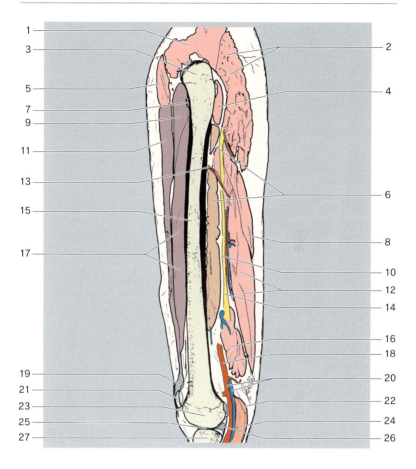

1 中殿筋 Gluteus medius muscle
2 大殿筋 Gluteus maximus muscle
3 大転子 Greater trochanter
4 大腿方形筋 Quadratus femoris muscle
5 大腿筋膜張筋 Tensor fasciae latae muscle
6 大内転筋 Adductor magnus muscle
7 外側大腿回旋動静脈 Lateral circumflex femoral artery and vein
8 大腿二頭筋(長頭) Biceps femoris muscle (long head)
9 外側広筋 Vastus lateralis muscle
10 坐骨神経 Sciatic nerve
11 大腿直筋 Rectus femoris muscle
12 半腱様筋 Semitendinosus muscle
13 貫通動脈 Perforating arteries
14 脛骨神経 Tibial nerve, 総腓骨神経 Common fibular nerve
15 大腿骨(体) Femur(shaft)
16 半膜様筋 Semimembranosus muscle
17 中間広筋 Vastus intermedius muscle
18 大腿動静脈 Femoral artery and vein
19 大腿四頭筋腱 Quadriceps tendon
20 膝窩動静脈 Popliteal artery and vein
21 膝蓋骨 Patella
22 腓腹筋(外側頭) Gastrocnemius muscle (lateral head)
23 大腿骨外側顆 Lateral femoral condyle
24 ヒラメ筋 Soleus muscle
25 膝関節 Knee joint
26 外側半月板 Lateral meniscus, posterior horn
27 脛骨外側顆 Lateral tibial condyle

296 下 肢

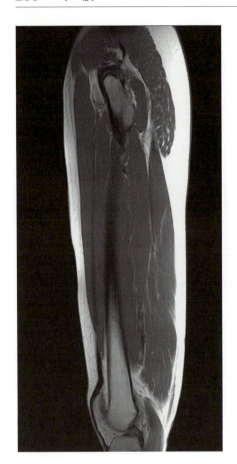

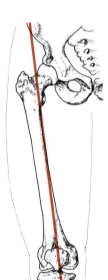

1 **中殿筋** Gluteus medius muscle
2 **大殿筋** Gluteus maximus muscle
3 **大腿筋膜張筋** Tensor fasciae latae muscle
4 **大腿方形筋** Quadratus femoris muscle
5 **腸骨大腿靱帯** Iliofemoral ligament
6 **小転子** Lesser trochanter

大腿，矢状断

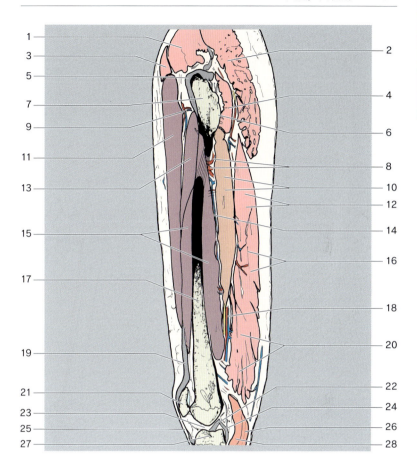

7 大腿骨(頸) Femur (neck)
8 貫通動脈 Perforating arteries
9 外側大腿回旋動静脈 Lateral circumflex femoral artery and vein
10 大内転筋 Adductor magnus muscle
11 大腿直筋 Rectus femoris muscle
12 大腿二頭筋(長頭) Biceps femoris muscle (long head)
13 内側広筋 Vastus medialis muscle
14 大腿深動静脈 Deep artery and vein of thigh
15 中間広筋 Vastus intermedius muscle
16 半腱様筋 Semitendinosus muscle
17 大腿骨(体) Femur (shaft)
18 大腿動静脈 Femoral artery and vein
19 大腿直筋(腱) Rectus femoris muscle (tendon)
20 半膜様筋 Semimembranosus muscle
21 膝蓋骨 Patella
22 前十字靱帯 Anterior cruciate ligament
23 膝関節 Knee joint
24 後十字靱帯 Posterior cruciate ligament
25 膝蓋靱帯 Patellar ligament
26 腓腹筋(外側頭) Gastrocnemius muscle (lateral head)
27 脛骨(頭) Tibia (head)
28 ヒラメ筋 Soleus muscle

298 下肢

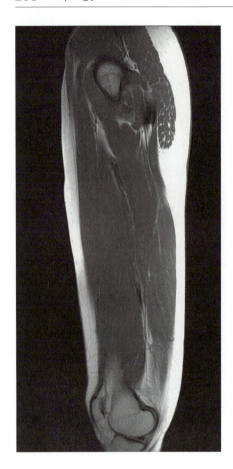

頭側
腹側 □ 背側
遠位

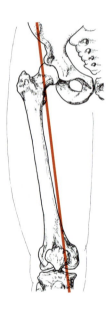

1 中殿筋 Gluteus medius muscle
2 大殿筋 Gluteus maximus muscle
3 大腿筋膜張筋 Tensor fasciae latae muscle
4 梨状筋 Piriformis muscle
5 縫工筋 Sartorius muscle
6 内閉鎖筋 Obturator internus muscle, 双子筋 Gemellus muscles
7 大腿骨(頭) Femur(head)
8 坐骨 Ischium
9 外閉鎖筋 Obturator externus muscle
10 大腿方形筋 Quadratus femoris muscle

大腿，矢状断

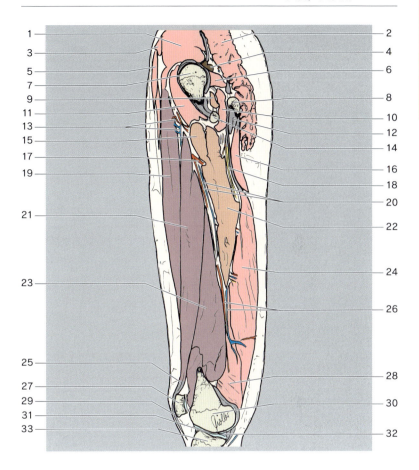

11 腸腰筋 Iliopsoas muscle
12 半膜様筋 Semimembranosus muscle, 半腱様筋 Semitendinosus muscle 腱付着部
13 外側大腿回旋動静脈 Lateral circumflex femoral artery and vein
14 小転子 Lesser trochanter
15 恥骨筋 Pectineus muscle
16 大腿二頭筋（長頭）Biceps femoris muscle (long head)
17 貫通動脈 Perforating arteries
18 坐骨神経 Sciatic nerve
19 大腿直筋 Rectus femoris muscle
20 大腿深動静脈 Deep femoral artery and vein
21 中間広筋 Vastus intermedius muscle
22 大内転筋 Adductor magnus muscle
23 内側広筋 Vastus medialis muscle
24 半腱様筋 Semitendinosus muscle
25 大腿四頭筋腱 Quadriceps tendon
26 大腿動静脈 Femoral artery and vein
27 膝蓋骨 Patella
28 半膜様筋 Semimembranosus muscle
29 膝蓋靱帯 Patellar ligament
30 大腿骨内側顆 Medial femoral condyle
31 膝関節 Knee joint
32 内側半月板（後角）Medial meniscus (posterior horn)
33 脛骨内側顆 Medial tibial condyle

300 下肢

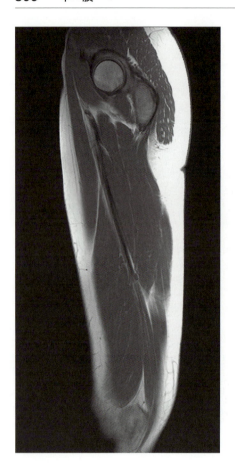

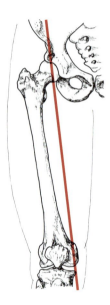

1 中殿筋 Gluteus medius muscle
2 小殿筋 Gluteus minimus muscle
3 腸骨 Ilium
4 大殿筋 Gluteus maximus muscle
5 腸腰筋 Iliopsoas muscle

大腿，矢状断　**301**

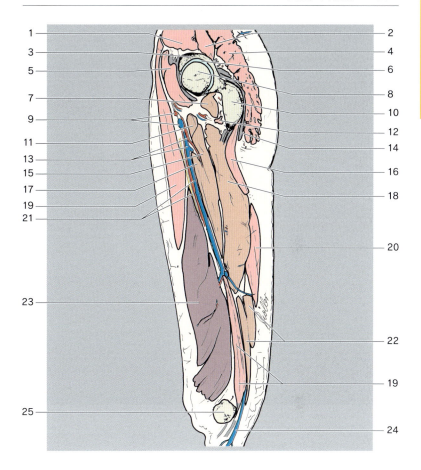

- 6 股関節 Hip joint
- 7 外閉鎖筋 Obturator externus muscle
- 8 大腿骨(頭) Femur (head)
- 9 外側大腿回旋動静脈 Lateral circumflex femoral artery and vein
- 10 坐骨 Ischium
- 11 恥骨筋 Pectineus muscle
- 12 大腿方形筋 Quadratus femoris muscle
- 13 大腿深動脈 Deep artery of thigh
- 14 大腿二頭筋(長頭,付着部部) Biceps femoris muscle (long head, attachment)
- 15 短内転筋 Adductor brevis muscle
- 16 半腱様筋 Semitendinosus muscle
- 17 長内転筋 Adductor longus muscle
- 18 大内転筋 Adductor magnus muscle
- 19 縫工筋 Sartorius muscle
- 20 半膜様筋 Semimembranosus muscle
- 21 大腿動静脈, 伏在神経 Femoral artery and vein, Saphenous nerve
- 22 薄筋 Gracilis muscle
- 23 内側広筋 Vastus medialis muscle
- 24 大伏在静脈 Great saphenous vein
- 25 大腿骨内側顆 Medial femoral condyle

302　下 肢

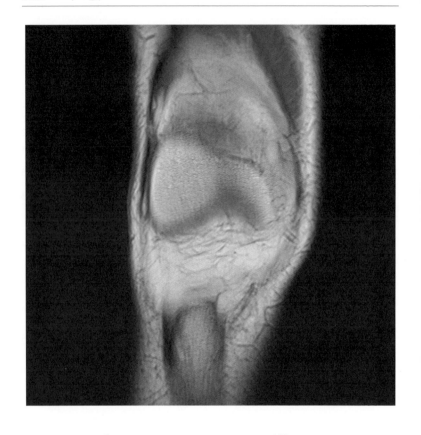

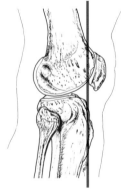

近位

外側　　　内側

遠位

膝，冠状断

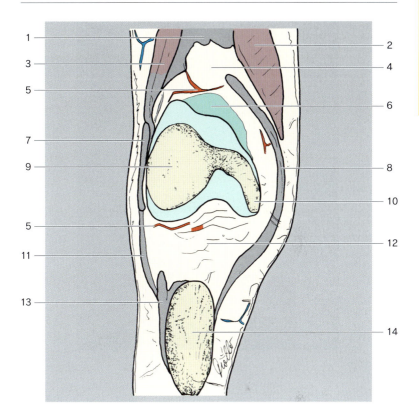

1 大腿四頭筋腱 Quadriceps tendon
2 内側広筋 Vastus medialis muscle
3 外側広筋 Vastus lateralis muscle
4 膝蓋上脂肪体 Suprapatellar fat pad
5 膝関節動脈網 Genicular anastomosis
6 膝蓋上包 Suprapatellar bursa
7 腸脛靱帯 Iliotibial tract
8 内側膝蓋支帯 Medial patellar retinaculum
9 大腿骨外側顆 Lateral femoral condyle
10 大腿骨内側顆 Medial femoral condyle
11 外側膝蓋支帯 Lateral patellar retinaculum
12 膝蓋下脂肪体 Infrapatellar fat pad
13 膝蓋靱帯 Patellar ligament
14 脛骨粗面 Tibial tuberosity

304 下 肢

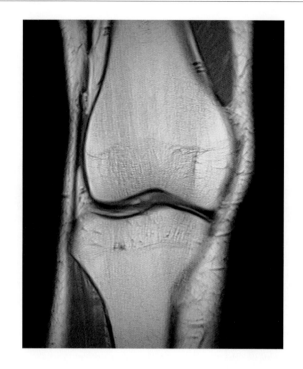

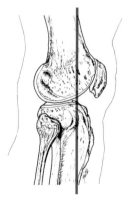

近位

外側 ☐ 内側

遠位

膝，冠状断　**305**

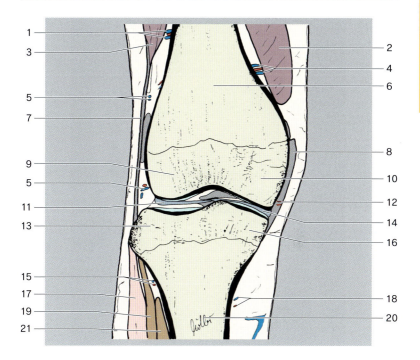

1 外側上膝動静脈 Superior lateral genicular artery artery and vein
2 内側広筋 Vastus medialis muscle
3 外側広筋 Vastus lateralis muscle
4 内側上膝動静脈 Superior medial genicular artery and vein
5 膝関節動脈網 Genicular anastomosis
6 大腿骨(体) Femur (shaft)
7 腸脛靱帯 Iliotibial tract
8 内側側副靱帯 Medial collateral ligament
9 大腿骨外側顆 Lateral femoral condyle
10 大腿骨内側顆 Medial femoral condyle
11 外側半月板(前角) Lateral meniscus (anterior horn)
12 下行膝動脈(関節枝) Descending genicular vein (articular branches)
13 脛骨外側顆 Lateral tibial condyle
14 内側半月板(前角) Medial meniscus (anterior horn)
15 外側下膝動脈 Inferior lateral genicular artery
16 脛骨内側顆 Medial tibial condyle
17 長腓骨筋 Peroneus (fibularis) longus muscle
18 内側下膝動脈 Inferior medial genicular artery
19 長趾伸筋 Extensor digitorum longus muscle
20 脛骨(体) Tibia (shaft)
21 前脛骨筋 Tibialis anterior muscle

306　下 肢

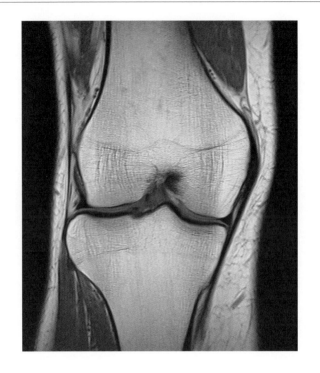

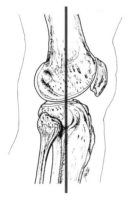

近位
外側　　内側
遠位

膝，冠状断　307

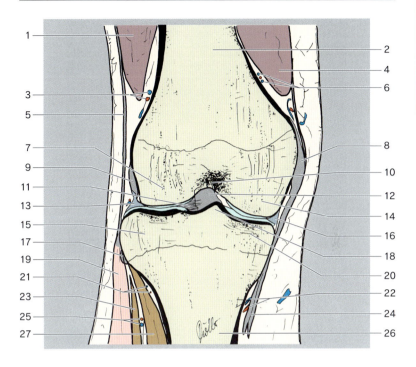

1 外側広筋　Vastus lateralis muscle
2 大腿骨(体)　Femur(shaft)
3 外側上膝動静脈　Superior lateral genicular artery and vein
4 内側広筋　Vastus medialis muscle
5 腸脛靱帯　Iliotibial tract
6 内側上膝動静脈　Superior medial genicular artery and vein
7 大腿骨外側顆　Lateral femoral condyle
8 内側側副靱帯　Medial collateral ligament
9 膝窩筋(腱)　Popliteus muscle(tendon)
10 顆間窩　Intercondylar fossa
11 膝横靱帯　Transverse ligament of knee
12 前十字靱帯　Anterior cruciate ligament
13 外側半月板(体部)　Lateral meniscus(body)
14 大腿骨内側顆　Medial femoral condyle
15 脛骨外側顆　Lateral tibial condyle
16 内側半月板(体部)　Medial meniscus(body)
17 前腓骨頭靱帯　Anterior ligament of fibular head
18 内側顆間結節　Medial intercondylar tubercle
19 長腓骨筋　Peroneus(fibularis)longus muscle
20 脛骨内側顆　Medial tibial condyle
21 外側下膝動静脈　Inferior lateral genicular artery and vein
22 内側下膝動静脈　Inferior medial genicular artery and vein
23 長趾伸筋　Extensor digitorum longus muscle
24 浅鵞足　Superficial pes anserinus
25 前脛骨反回動静脈　Anterior tibial recurrent artery and vein
26 脛骨(体)　Tibia(shaft)
27 前脛骨筋　Tibialis anterior muscle

308　下　肢

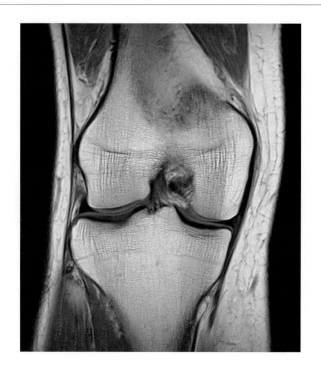

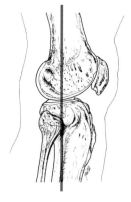

近位

外側　□　内側

遠位

膝，冠状断　　**309**

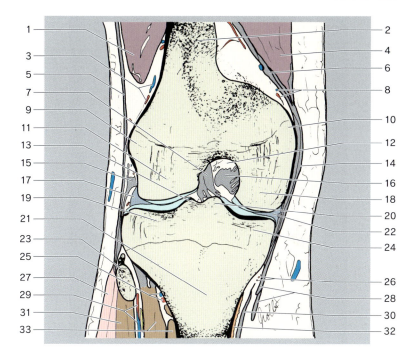

1 外側広筋 Vastus lateralis muscle
2 大腿骨(体) Femur(shaft)
3 外側上膝動静脈 Superior lateral genicular artery and vein
4 内側広筋 Vastus medialis muscle
5 腸脛靱帯 Iliotibial tract
6 大内転筋(腱) Adductor magnus muscle (tendon)
7 前十字靱帯 Anterior cruciate ligament
8 内側上膝動静脈 Superior medial genicular artery and vein
9 外側上顆 Lateral epicondyle
10 内側上顆 Medial epicondyle
11 大腿骨外側顆 Lateral femoral condyle
12 顆間窩 Intercondylar fossa
13 外側顆間結節 Lateral intercondylar tubercle
14 内側側副靱帯 Medial collateral ligament
15 膝窩筋(腱) Popliteus muscle(tendon)
16 後十字靱帯 Posterior cruciate ligament
17 外側半月板(体部) Lateral meniscus(body)
18 大腿骨内側顆 Medial femoral condyle
19 脛骨外側顆 Lateral tibial condyle
20 内側顆間結節 Medial intercondylar tubercle
21 脛骨(体) Tibia(shaft)
22 内側半月板(体部) Medial meniscus(body)
23 腓骨(頭) Fibula(head)
24 脛骨内側顆 Medial tibial condyle
25 外側下膝動静脈 Inferior lateral genicular artery and vein
26 内側下膝動静脈 Inferior medial genicular artery and vein
27 長腓骨筋 Peroneus(fibularis)longus muscle
28 浅鵞足 Superficial pes anserinus
29 前脛骨反回動静脈 Anterior tibial recurrent artery and vein
30 半膜様筋(脛骨付着部) Semimembranosus muscle (tibial attachment) 深鵞足 deep pes anserinus
31 長趾伸筋 Extensor digitorum longus muscle
32 膝窩筋(脛骨付着部) Popliteus muscle(tibial attachment)
33 前脛骨筋 Tibialis anterior muscle

310 下 肢

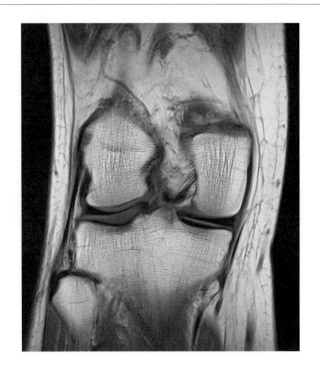

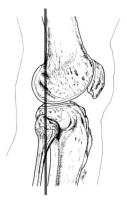

近位
外側　　　内側
遠位

膝，冠状断

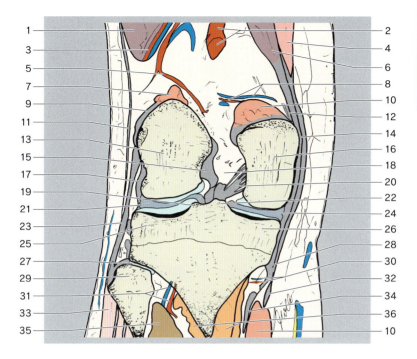

1 外側広筋 Vastus lateralis muscle
2 膝窩動脈 Popliteal artery
3 外側上膝動脈 Superior lateral genicular artery
4 縫工筋 Sartorius muscle
5 中膝動脈 Medial genicular artery
6 内側広筋 Vastus medialis muscle
7 腓腹筋(外側頭,大腿骨付着部) Gastrocnemius muscle(lateral head, femoral attachment)
8 内側上膝動静脈 Superior medial genicular artery and vein
9 足底筋(腱) Plantaris muscle(tendon)
10 腓腹筋(内側頭) Gastrocnemius muscle (medial head)
11 腸脛靱帯 Iliotibial tract
12 大内転筋(腱付着部) Adductor magnus muscle(tendon attachment)
13 大腿骨外側顆 Lateral femoral condyle
14 内側側副靱帯 Medial collateral ligament
15 前十字靱帯 Anterior cruciate ligament
16 大腿骨内側顆 Medial femoral condyle
17 膝筋(腱) Popliteus muscle(tendon)
18 顆間窩 Intercondylar fossa
19 外側顆間結節 Lateral intercondylar tubercle
20 後十字靱帯 Posterior cruciate ligament
21 外側半月板(後角) Lateral meniscus (posterior horn)
22 内側顆間結節 Medial intercondylar tubercle
23 外側側副靱帯 Fibular collateral ligament
24 内側半月板(後角) Medial meniscus (posterior horn)
25 脛骨外側顆 Lateral tibial condyle
26 脛骨内側顆 Medial tibial condyle
27 脛腓関節 Tibiofibular joint
28 浅鵞足 Superficial pes anserinus
29 腓骨(頭) Fibula(head)
30 内側下膝動静脈 Inferior medial genicular artery and vein
31 外側下膝動静脈 Inferior lateral genicular artery and vein
32 半腱様筋(腱) Semitendinosus muscle (tendon)
33 長腓骨筋 Peroneus(fibularis)longus muscle
34 半膜様筋(脛骨付着部) Semimembranosus muscle(tibial attachment) 深鵞足 deep pes anserinus
35 後脛骨筋 Tibialis posterior muscle
36 膝窩筋 Popliteus muscle

312　下 肢

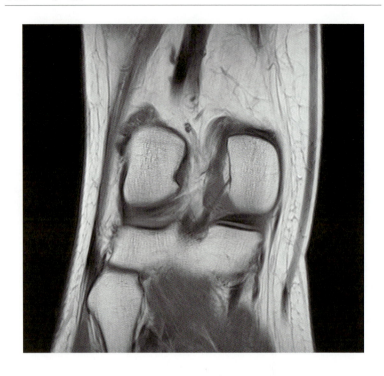

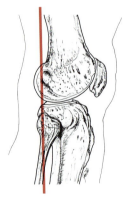

近位
外側 ☐ 内側
遠位

膝，冠状断　**313**

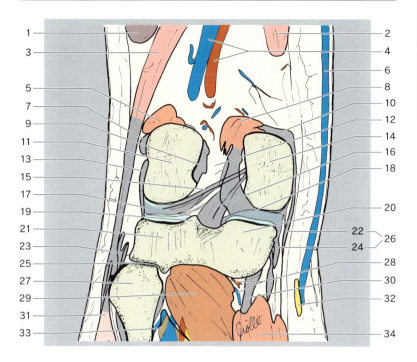

1 外側広筋 Vastus lateralis muscle
2 縫工筋 Sartorius muscle
3 大腿二頭筋 Biceps femoris muscle
4 膝窩動静脈 Popliteal artery and vein
5 腓腹筋(外側頭,大腿骨付着部) Gastrocnemius muscle(lateral head, femoral attachment)
6 大伏在静脈 Great saphenous vein
7 足底筋(腱付着部) Plantaris muscle(tendon attachment)
8 腓腹筋(内側頭,大腿骨付着部) Gastrocnemius muscle(medial head, femoral attachment)
9 前十字靱帯 Anterior cruciate ligament
10 関節包 Joint capsule
11 大腿骨外側顆 Lateral femoral condyle
12 顆間窩 Intercondylar fossa
13 膝窩筋(腱) Popliteus muscle(tendon)
14 大腿骨内側顆 Medial femoral condyle
15 後半月大腿靱帯(Wrisberg 靱帯) Posterior meniscofemoral ligament(Wrisberg ligament)
16 後十字靱帯 Posterior cruciate ligament
17 外側半月板(後角) Lateral meniscus(posterior horn)
18 内側半月板(後角) Medial meniscus(posterior horn)
19 外側顆間結節 Lateral intercondylar tubercle
20 脛骨内側顆 Medial tibial condyle
21 脛骨外側顆 Lateral tibial condyle
22 薄筋(腱) Gracilis muscle(tendon)
23 外側側副靱帯 Fibular collateral ligament
24 半腱様筋(腱) Semitendinosus muscle (tendon)
25 脛腓関節 Tibiofibular joint(proximal)
26 浅鵞足 Superficial pes anserinus
27 腓骨(頭) Fibula(head)
28 内側下膝動静脈 Inferior medial genicular artery and vein
29 膝窩筋 Popliteus muscle
30 半膜様筋(脛骨付着部) Semimembranosus muscle(tibial attachment) 深鵞足 deep pes anserinus
31 長腓骨筋 Peroneus(fibularis)longus muscle
32 伏在神経 Saphenous nerve
33 後脛骨筋 Tibialis posterior muscle
34 腓腹筋(内側頭) Gastrocnemius muscle (medial head)

314　下　肢

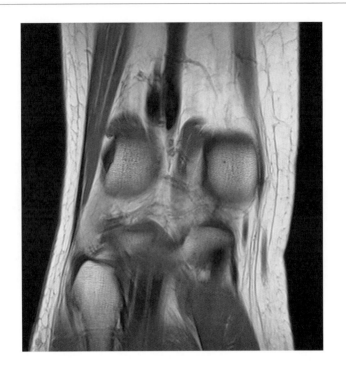

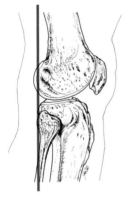

　　　　　　　近位

外側　□　内側

　　　　　　　遠位

膝, 冠状断 315

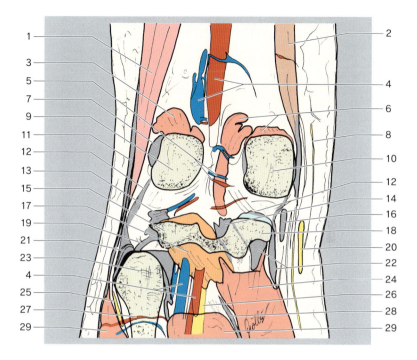

1 大腿二頭筋 Biceps femoris muscle
2 薄筋 Gracilis muscle
3 腓腹筋(外側頭) Gastrocnemius muscle (lateral head)
4 膝窩動静脈 Popliteal artery and vein
5 腓腹動静脈 Sural arteries and veins
6 腓腹筋(内側頭,大腿骨付着部) Gastrocnemius muscle (medial head, femoral attachment)
7 足底筋(腱) Plantaris muscle (tendon)
8 伏在神経(枝) Saphenous nerve (branch)
9 大腿骨外側顆 Lateral femoral condyle
10 大腿骨内側顆 Medial femoral condyle
11 腸脛靱帯 Iliotibial tract
12 関節包 Joint capsule
13 弓状膝窩靱帯 Arcuate popliteal ligament
14 斜膝窩靱帯 Oblique popliteal ligament
15 脛骨外側顆 Lateral tibial condyle
16 半腱様筋(腱) Semitendinosus muscle (tendon)
17 膝窩筋(腱) Popliteus muscle (tendon)
18 脛骨内側顆 Medial tibial condyle
19 外側側副靱帯 Fibular collateral ligament
20 伏在神経 Saphenous nerve
21 後腓骨頭靱帯 Posterior ligament of fibular head
22 半膜様筋(脛骨付着部) Semimembranosus muscle (tibial attachment) 深鵞足 deep pes anserinus
23 腓骨(頭) Fibula (head)
24 腓腹筋(内側頭) Gastrocnemius muscle (medial head)
25 総腓骨神経 Common fibular nerve
26 脛骨神経 Tibial nerve
27 後脛骨動脈(腓骨回旋枝) Posterior tibial artery (circumflex fibular branch)
28 足底筋(腱) Plantaris muscle (tendon)
29 ヒラメ筋 Soleus muscle

316　下 肢

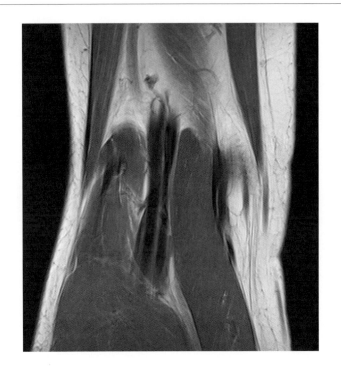

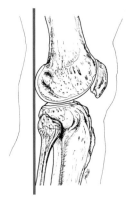

近位

外側　　　内側

遠位

膝, 冠状断　317

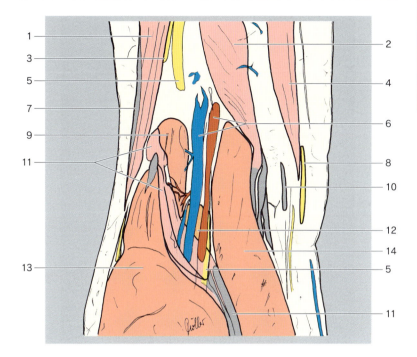

1　大腿二頭筋 Biceps femoris muscle
2　半膜様筋 Semimembranosus muscle
3　総腓骨神経 Common fibular nerve
4　薄筋 Gracilis muscle
5　脛骨神経 Tibial nerve
6　膝窩動静脈 Popliteal artery and vein
7　腸脛靱帯 Iliotibial tract
8　伏在神経 Saphenous nerve
9　腓腹筋(外側頭) Gastrocnemius muscle (lateral head)
10　半腱様筋(腱) Semitendinosus muscle (tendon)
11　足底筋(＋腱) Plantaris muscle(＋tendon)
12　膝窩筋 Popliteus muscle
13　ヒラメ筋 Soleus muscle
14　腓腹筋(内側頭) Gastrocnemius muscle (medial head)

318 下 肢

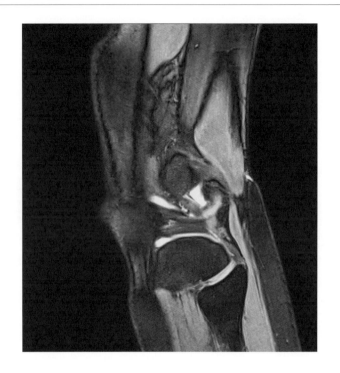

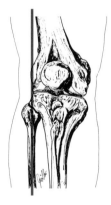

近位
腹側 □ 背側
遠位

膝，矢状断

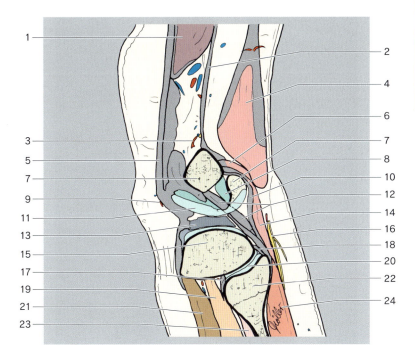

1 **外側広筋** Vastus lateralis muscle
2 **腸脛靱帯** Iliotibial tract
3 **膝関節動脈網へ向かう血管** Blood vessels to genicular anastomosis
4 **大腿二頭筋** Biceps femoris muscle
5 **外側膝蓋支帯** Lateral patellar retinaculum
6 **腓腹筋（外側頭）** Gastrocnemius muscle (lateral head)
7 **大腿骨外側顆** Lateral femoral condyle
8 **外側関節陥凹** Lateral joint recess
9 **外側下膝動脈** Inferior lateral genicular artery
10 **関節包** Joint capsule
11 **大腿骨（外側顆，関節軟骨）** Femur (lateral condyle, joint cartilage)
12 **膝窩筋（腱）** Popliteus muscle (tendon)
13 **外側半月板（体部）** Lateral meniscus (body)
14 **足底筋（＋腱付着部）** Plantaris muscle (+tendon attachment)
15 **脛骨外側顆** Lateral tibial condyle
16 **総腓骨神経** Common fibular nerve
17 **前腓骨頭靱帯** Anterior ligament of fibular head
18 **後腓骨頭靱帯** Posterior ligament of fibular head
19 **後脛骨筋** Tibialis posterior muscle
20 **脛腓関節** Tibiofibular joint
21 **前脛骨筋** Tibialis anterior muscle
22 **腓骨（頭）** Fibula (head)
23 **長腓骨筋** Peroneus (fibularis) longus muscle
24 **ヒラメ筋** Soleus muscle

320　下　肢

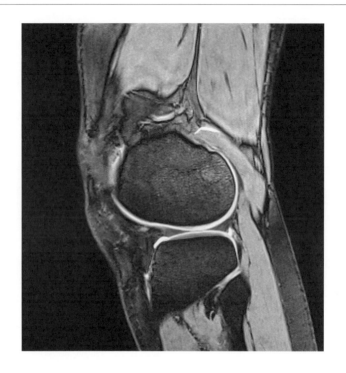

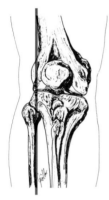

近位

腹側　□　背側

遠位

膝, 矢状断

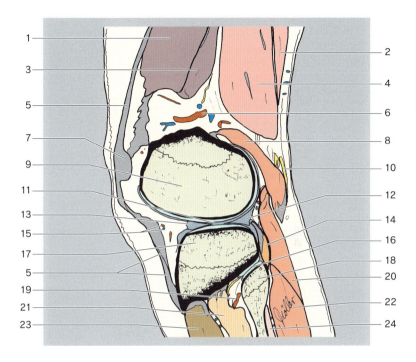

1 外側広筋 Vastus lateralis muscle
2 大腿二頭筋(長頭) Biceps femoris muscle (long head)
3 中間広筋 Vastus intermedius muscle
4 大腿二頭筋(短頭) Biceps femoris muscle (short head)
5 外側膝蓋支帯 Lateral patellar retinaculum (longitudinal)
6 外側上膝動静脈 Superior lateral genicular artery and vein
7 外側膝蓋支帯 Lateral patellar retinaculum
8 腓腹筋(外側頭) Gastrocnemius muscle (lateral head)
9 大腿骨外側顆 Lateral femoral condyle
10 総腓骨神経 Common fibular nerve
11 膝関節 Knee joint
12 外側半月板(後角) Lateral meniscus (posterior horn)
13 外側半月板(前角) Lateral meniscus (anterior horn)
14 膝窩筋(+腱) Popliteus muscle (+tendon)
15 外側下膝動静脈 Inferior lateral genicular artery and vein
16 (近位)脛腓関節 Tibiofibular joint (proximal)
17 脛骨外側顆 Lateral tibial condyle
18 腓骨(頭) Fibula (head)
19 前脛骨動脈 Anterior tibial artery
20 足底筋 Plantaris muscle
21 後脛骨筋 Tibialis posterior muscle
22 ヒラメ筋 Soleus muscle
23 前脛骨筋 Tibialis anterior muscle
24 長腓骨筋 Peroneus (fibularis) longus muscle

322 下肢

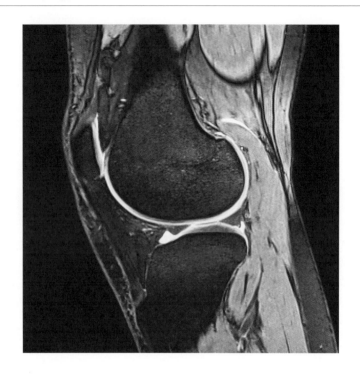

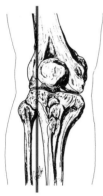

近位
腹側 　　 背側
遠位

膝，矢状断　**323**

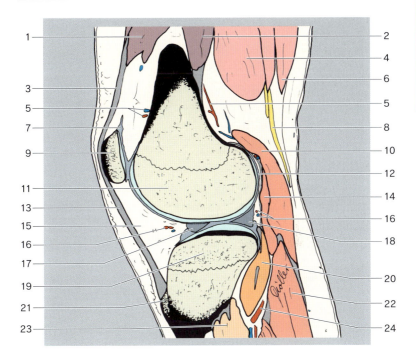

1 外側広筋 Vastus lateralis muscle
2 中間広筋 Vastus intermedius muscle
3 大腿四頭筋腱 Quadriceps tendon
4 大腿二頭筋(短頭) Biceps femoris muscle (short head)
5 外側上膝動静脈 Superior lateral genicular artery and vein
6 大腿二頭筋(長頭) Biceps femoris muscle (long head)
7 膝蓋上包 Suprapatellar bursa
8 総腓骨神経 Common fibular nerve
9 膝蓋骨 Patella
10 腓腹筋(外側頭) Gastrocnemius muscle (lateral head)
11 大腿骨外側顆 Lateral femoral condyle
12 関節包 Joint capsule
13 膝蓋靱帯 Patellar ligament
14 足底筋 Plantaris muscle
15 膝蓋下脂肪体 Infrapatellar fat pad
16 外側下膝動静脈 Inferior lateral genicular artery and vein
17 外側半月板(前角) Lateral meniscus (anterior horn)
18 外側半月板(後角) Lateral meniscus (posterior horn)
19 脛骨外側顆 Lateral tibial condyle
20 膝窩筋 Popliteus muscle
21 脛骨粗面 Tibial tuberosity
22 ヒラメ筋 Soleus muscle
23 後脛骨筋 Tibialis posterior muscle
24 前脛骨動脈 Anterior tibial artery

324　下 肢

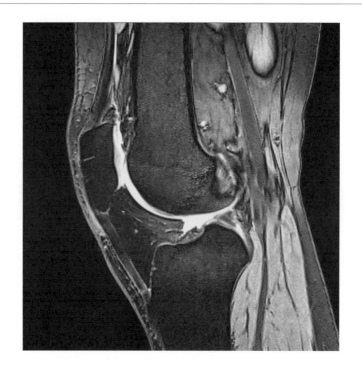

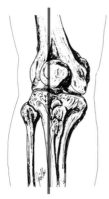

近位

腹側　　背側

遠位

膝，矢状断 325

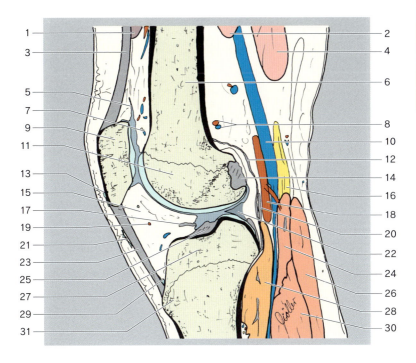

1 内側広筋 Vastus medialis muscle
2 大腿二頭筋 Biceps femoris muscle
3 大腿四頭筋腱 Quadriceps tendon
4 半膜様筋 Semimembranosus muscle
5 膝蓋上包 Suprapatellar bursa
6 大腿骨(体) Femur(shaft)
7 膝蓋動静脈網 Patellar anastomosis
8 外側上膝動静脈 Superior lateral genicular artery and vein
9 膝蓋骨 Patella
10 膝窩静脈 Popliteal vein
11 大腿骨外側顆 Lateral femoral condyle
12 関節包 Joint capsule
13 膝蓋前皮下包 Subcutaneous prepatellar bursa
14 前十字靱帯(大腿骨付着部) Anterior cruciate ligament(femoral attachment)
15 膝蓋下脂肪体 Infrapatellar fat pad
16 脛骨神経 Tibial nerve
17 膝横靱帯 Transverse ligament of knee
18 膝窩動脈 Popliteal artery
19 外側下膝動静脈 Inferior lateral genicular artery and vein
20 斜膝窩靱帯 Oblique popliteal ligament
21 膝蓋下皮下包 Subcutaneous infrapatellar bursa
22 外側半月板(後角,内付着部) Lateral meniscus (posterior horn, inner attachment)
23 膝蓋靱帯 Patellar ligament
24 足底筋 Plantaris muscle
25 前十字靱帯(脛骨起始部) Anterior cruciate ligament(tibial origin)
26 腓腹筋(外側頭) Gastrocnemius muscle (lateral head)
27 脛骨(頭) Tibia(head)
28 膝窩筋 Popliteus muscle
29 深膝蓋下包 Deep infrapatellar bursa
30 ヒラメ筋 Soleus muscle
31 脛骨粗面 Tibial tuberosity

326 下 肢

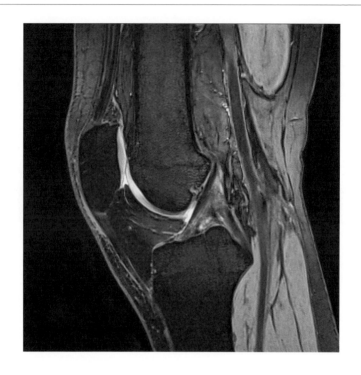

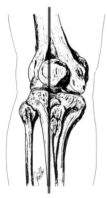

近位

腹側 ☐ 背側

遠位

膝，矢状断 327

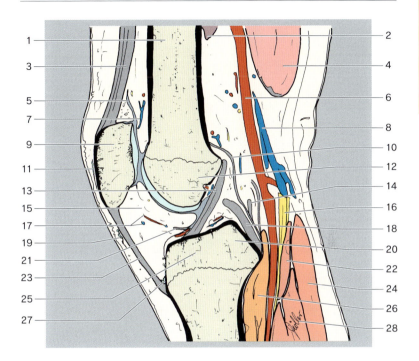

1 大腿骨(体) Femur(shaft)
2 内側広筋 Vastus medialis muscle
3 大腿四頭筋腱 Quadriceps tendon
4 半膜様筋 Semimembranosus muscle
5 膝蓋上包 Suprapatellar bursa
6 膝窩動脈 Popliteal artery
7 膝蓋動静脈網 Patellar anastomosis
8 膝窩静脈 Popliteal vein
9 膝蓋骨 Patella
10 関節包 Joint capsule
11 膝蓋前皮下包 Subcutaneous prepatellar bursa
12 大腿骨(顆間部) Femur(intercondylar part)
13 前十字靱帯 Anterior cruciate ligament
14 斜膝窩靱帯 Oblique popliteal ligament
15 膝蓋下脂肪体 Infrapatellar fat pad
16 脛骨神経 Tibial nerve
17 外側下膝動静脈 Inferior lateral genicular artery and vein
18 後十字靱帯 Posterior cruciate ligament
19 膝蓋下皮下包 Subcutaneous infrapatellar bursa
20 内側顆間結節 Medial intercondylar tubercle
21 膝横靱帯 Transverse ligament of knee
22 足底筋 Plantaris muscle
23 膝蓋靱帯 Patellar ligament
24 腓腹筋(外側頭) Gastrocnemius muscle (lateral head)
25 脛骨(頭) Tibia(head)
26 膝窩筋 Popliteus muscle
27 深膝蓋下包 Deep infrapatellar bursa
28 ヒラメ筋 Soleus muscle

328 下　肢

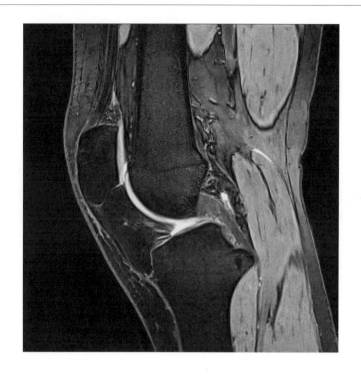

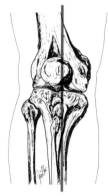

近位

腹側　　背側

遠位

膝，矢状断 329

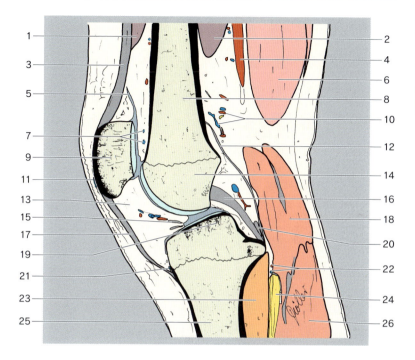

1 大腿直筋 Rectus femoris muscle
2 内側広筋 Vastus medialis muscle
3 大腿四頭筋腱 Quadriceps tendon
4 大腿動脈 Femoral artery
5 膝蓋上包 Suprapatellar bursa
6 半膜様筋 Semimembranosus muscle
7 膝蓋動脈網 Patellar anastomosis
8 大腿骨(体) Femur(shaft)
9 膝蓋骨 Patella
10 内側上膝動静脈 Superior medial genicular artery and vein
11 膝蓋前皮下包 Subcutaneous prepatellar bursa
12 関節包 Joint capsule
13 膝蓋下脂肪体 Infrapatellar fat pad
14 大腿骨内側顆 Medial femoral condyle
15 膝横靱帯 Transverse ligament of knee
16 後十字靱帯 Posterior cruciate ligament
17 膝蓋靱帯 Patellar ligament
18 腓腹筋(内側頭) Gastrocnemius muscle (medial head)
19 脛骨内側顆間結節 Medial intercondylar tubercle of tibial condyle
20 後半月大腿靱帯(Wrisberg 靱帯) Posterior meniscofemoral ligament (Wrisberg ligament)
21 深膝蓋下包 Deep infrapatellar bursa
22 内側下膝動静脈 Inferior medial genicular artery and vein
23 膝窩筋 Popliteus muscle
24 脛骨神経 Tibial nerve
25 脛骨(体) Tibia(shaft)
26 腓腹筋(外側頭) Gastrocnemius muscle (lateral head)

330　下　肢

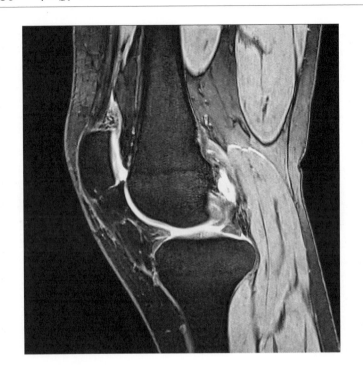

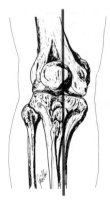

近位　腹側　背側　遠位

膝，矢状断　**331**

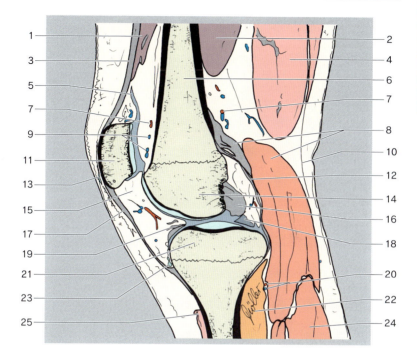

1 大腿直筋　Rectus femoris muscle
2 内側広筋　Vastus medialis muscle
3 大腿四頭筋腱　Quadriceps tendon
4 半膜様筋　Semimembranosus muscle
5 膝蓋上包　Suprapatellar bursa
6 大腿骨(体)　Femur(shaft)
7 内側上膝動静脈　Superior medial genicular artery and vein
8 腓腹筋(内側頭, 筋付着部)　Gastrocnemius muscle(medial head, muscle attachment)
9 膝蓋動静脈網　Patellar anastomosis
10 深下腿筋膜　Deep fascia of leg
11 膝蓋骨　Patella
12 関節包　Joint capsule
13 膝蓋前皮下包　Subcutaneous prepatellar bursa
14 大腿骨内側顆　Medial femoral condyle
15 膝蓋下脂肪体　Infrapatellar fat pad
16 後十字靱帯(付着部)　Posterior cruciate ligament(attachment)
17 膝蓋靱帯　Patellar ligament
18 内側半月板(後角, 関節内付着部)　Medial meniscus(posterior horn, inner attachment)
19 膝横靱帯　Transverse ligament of knee
20 内側下膝動静脈　Inferior medial genicular artery and vein
21 脛骨内側顆　Medial tibial condyle
22 膝窩筋　Popliteus muscle
23 深膝蓋下包　Deep infrapatellar bursa
24 腓腹筋(外側頭)　Gastrocnemius muscle (lateral head)
25 縫工筋(付着部)　Sartorius muscle(attachment)
浅鵞足　Superficial pes anserinus の一部

332　下　肢

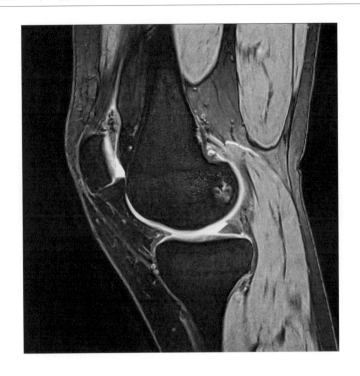

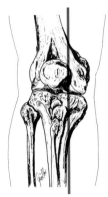

近位

腹側　□　背側

遠位

膝，矢状断 **333**

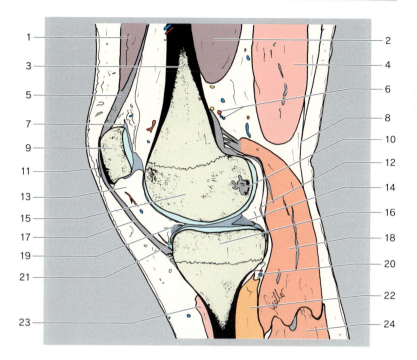

1 大腿直筋 Rectus femoris muscle
2 内側広筋 Vastus medialis muscle
3 大腿骨(体) Femur(shaft)
4 半膜様筋 Semimembranosus muscle
5 大腿四頭筋腱 Quadriceps tendon
6 内側上膝動静脈 Superior medial genicular artery and vein
7 膝蓋上包 Suprapatellar bursa
8 深下腿筋膜 Deep fascia of leg
9 膝蓋骨 Patella
10 後十字靱帯(付着部) Posterior cruciate ligament(attachment)
11 膝蓋前皮下包 Subcutaneous prepatellar bursa
12 関節包 Joint capsule
13 膝蓋下脂肪体 Infrapatellar fat pad
14 内側半月板(後角) Medial meniscus(posterior horn)
15 大腿骨内側顆 Medial femoral condyle
16 脛骨内側顆 Medial tibial condyle
17 膝蓋靱帯 Patellar ligament
18 腓腹筋(内側頭) Gastrocnemius muscle(medial head)
19 膝横靱帯 Transverse ligament of knee
20 内側下膝動静脈 Inferior medial genicular artery and vein
21 深膝蓋下包 Deep infrapatellar bursa
22 膝窩筋 Popliteus muscle
23 縫工筋(付着部) Sartorius muscle(attachment) 浅鵞足 Superficial pes anserinus の一部
24 腓腹筋(外側頭) Gastrocnemius muscle(lateral head)

334　下 肢

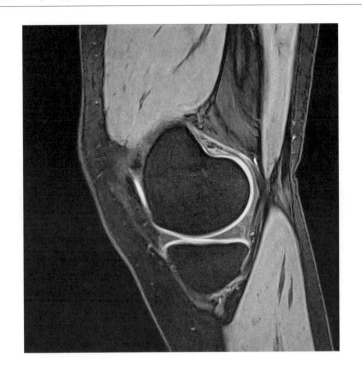

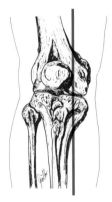

　　　　近位

腹側　☐　背側

　　　　遠位

膝，矢状断 **335**

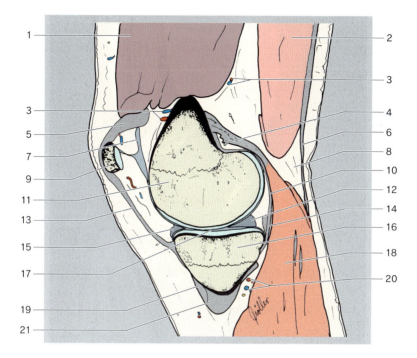

1 内側広筋 Vastus medialis muscle
2 半膜様筋 Semimembranosus muscle
3 内側上膝動静脈 Superior medial genicular artery and vein
4 腓腹筋の内側腱下包 Medial subtendinous bursa of gastrocnemius
5 内側膝蓋支帯 Medial patellar retinaculum
6 深下腿筋膜 Deep fascia of leg
7 膝蓋上包 Suprapatellar bursa
8 膝窩 Popliteal fossa
9 膝蓋骨 Patella
10 関節包 Joint capsule
11 大腿骨内側顆 Medial femoral condyle
12 内側半月板(後角) Medial meniscus (posterior horn)
13 内側膝蓋支帯 Medial patellar retinaculum
14 斜膝窩靱帯 Oblique popliteal ligament
15 内側半月板(前角) Medial meniscus (anterior horn)
16 脛骨内側顆 Medial tibial condyle
17 膝関節 Knee joint
18 腓腹筋(内側頭) Gastrocnemius muscle (medial head)
19 縫工筋(付着部) Sartorius muscle (attachment) 浅鵞足 Superficial pes anserinus の一部
20 内側下膝動静脈 Inferior medial genicular artery and vein
21 浅鵞足 Superficial pes anserinus

336　下　肢

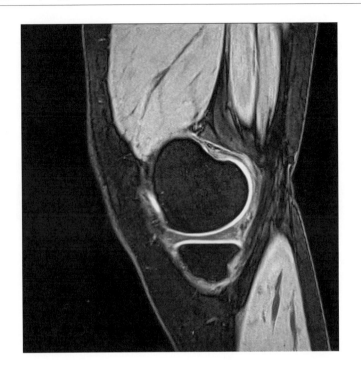

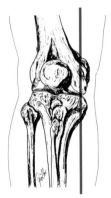

近位

腹側　□　背側

遠位

膝，矢状断   *337*

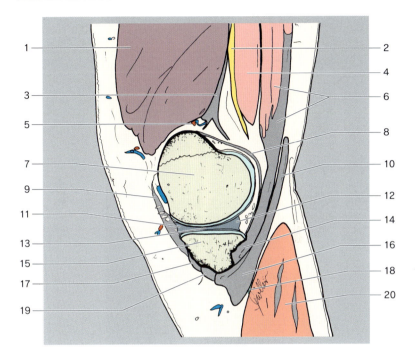

1 内側広筋 Vastus medialis muscle
2 伏在神経 Saphenous nerve
3 大内転筋(腱) Adductor magnus muscle (tendon)
4 縫工筋 Sartorius muscle
5 内側上膝動静脈 Superior medial genicular artery and vein
6 半膜様筋(＋腱) Semimembranosus muscle (+tendon)
7 大腿骨内側顆 Medial femoral condyle
8 関節包 Joint capsule
9 内側膝蓋支帯 Medial patellar retinaculum
10 半腱様筋(腱) Semitendinosus muscle (tendon)
11 内側半月板(前角) Medial meniscus (anterior horn)
12 内側半月板(後角) Medial meniscus (posterior horn)
13 内側半月板(体部) Medial meniscus (body)
14 深鵞足 Deep pes anserinus
15 脛骨内側顆 Medial tibial condyle
16 浅鵞足 Superficial pes anserinus
17 縫工筋(付着部) Sartorius muscle (attachment) 浅鵞足 Superficial pes anserinus の一部
18 鵞足包 Anserine bursa
19 薄筋(付着部) Gracilis muscle (attachment) 浅鵞足 Superficial pes anserinus の一部
20 腓腹筋(内側頭) Gastrocnemius muscle (medial head)

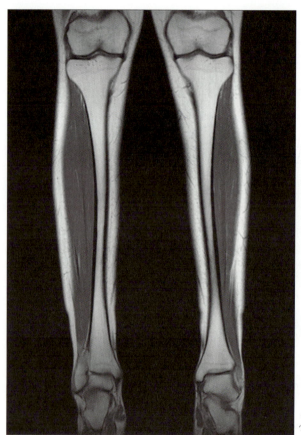
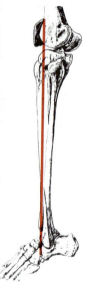

1 腓腹筋(内側頭,大腿骨付着部) Gastrocnemius muscle(medial head, femoral attachment)
2 腓腹筋(外側頭,大腿骨付着部) Gastrocnemius muscle(lateral head, femoral attachment)
3 足底筋(腱) Plantaris muscle(tendon)
4 内側側副靱帯 Medial collateral ligament
5 外側側副靱帯 Fibular collateral ligament
6 大腿骨内側顆 Medial femoral condyle
7 膝窩筋(腱) Popliteus muscle(tendon)
8 大腿骨外側顆 Lateral femoral condyle
9 外側半月板(体部) Lateral meniscus(body)
10 腸脛靱帯 Iliotibial tract

下腿，冠状断 **339**

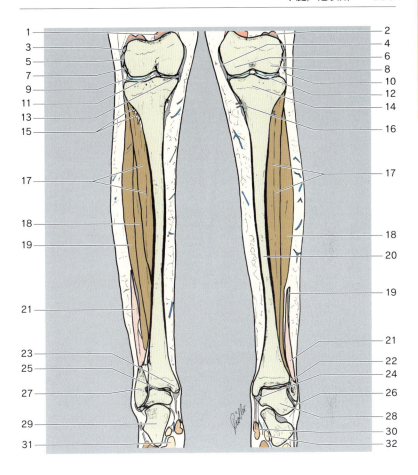

11 前十字靱帯 Anterior cruciate ligament
12 膝関節 Knee joint
13 内側半月板(体部) Medial meniscus (body)
14 脛骨(頭) Tibia (head)
15 外側下膝動静脈 Inferior lateral genicular artery and vein
16 内側下膝動静脈 Inferior medial genicular artery and vein
17 前脛骨筋 Tibialis anterior muscle
18 長趾伸筋 Extensor digitorum longus muscle
19 長母趾伸筋(腱) Extensor hallucis longus muscle (tendon)
20 脛骨(体) Tibia (shaft)

21 短腓骨筋 Peroneus (fibularis) brevis muscle
22 距腓関節 Talofibular joint
23 内果 Medial malleolus
24 三角靱帯 Deltoid ligament
25 足関節 Ankle joint (距腿関節 Talocrural joint)
26 前距腓靱帯 Anterior talofibular ligament
27 腓骨 Fibula
28 距骨 Talus
29 踵骨 Calcaneus
30 母趾外転筋 Abductor hallucis muscle
31 短趾屈筋 Flexor digitorum brevis muscle
32 足底方形筋 Quadratus plantae muscle

340　下　肢

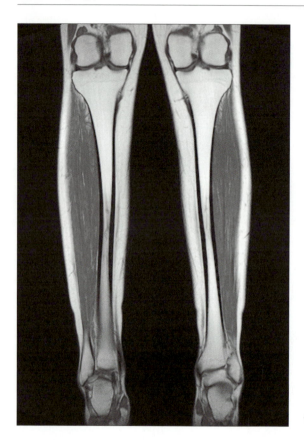

頭側

遠位

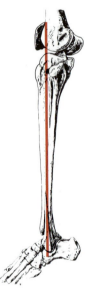

1　大腿二頭筋　Biceps femoris muscle
2　内側側副靱帯　Medial collateral ligament
3　腓腹筋（外側頭，大腿骨付着部）Gastrocnemius muscle (lateral head, femoral attachment)
4　大腿骨内側顆　Medial femoral condyle
5　腓腹筋（内側頭，大腿骨付着部）Gastrocnemius muscle (medial head, femoral attachment)
6　顆間窩　Intercondylar fossa
7　膝窩筋（腱）Popliteus muscle (tendon)
8　大腿骨外側顆　Lateral femoral condyle
9　外側半月板（体部）Lateral meniscus (body)
10　腸脛靱帯　Iliotibial tract
11　後十字靱帯　Posterior cruciate ligament
12　膝関節　Knee joint
13　前十字靱帯　Anterior cruciate ligament
14　脛骨外側顆　Lateral tibial condyle
15　内側半月板（体部）Medial meniscus (body)
16　顆間結節　Intercondylar tubercle
17　膝窩筋（脛骨付着部）Popliteus muscle (tibial attachment)
18　脛骨内側顆　Medial tibial condyle
19　前脛骨動静脈　Anterior tibial artery and vein, 深腓骨神経　Deep fibular nerve
20　浅鵞足　Superficial pes anserinus
21　長腓骨筋　Peroneus (fibularis) longus muscle
22　長趾伸筋　Extensor digitorum longus muscle

下腿，冠状断

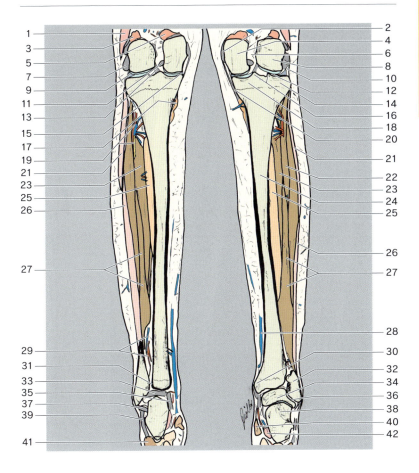

23 前脛骨筋 Tibialis anterior muscle
24 脛骨(体) Tibia (shaft)
25 後脛骨筋 Tibialis posterior muscle
26 短腓骨筋 Peroneus (fibularis) brevis muscle
27 長母趾伸筋 Extensor hallucis longus muscle
28 大伏在静脈 Great saphenous vein
29 腓骨動静脈 Fibular artery and vein
30 内果 Medial malleolus
31 下脛腓関節(靱帯結合) Inferior tibiofibular joint (syndesmosis)
32 外果 Lateral malleolus
33 後距腓靱帯 Posterior talofibular ligament
34 距骨 Talus
35 長趾屈筋 Flexor digitorum longus muscle (tendon)
36 距腓関節 Talofibular joint
37 踵腓靱帯 Calcaneofibular ligament
38 踵骨 Calcaneus
39 長腓骨筋(腱) Peroneus (fibularis) longus muscle (tendon), 短腓骨筋(腱) Peroneus (fibularis) brevis muscle (tendon)
40 母趾外転筋 Abductor hallucis muscle
41 小趾外転筋 Abductor digiti minimi muscle
42 足底方形筋 Quadratus plantae muscle

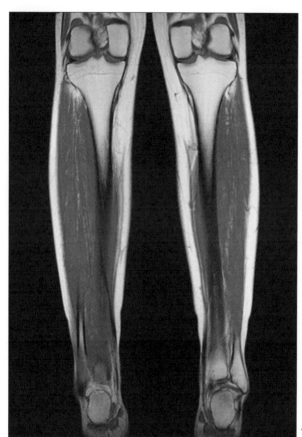

頭側

遠位
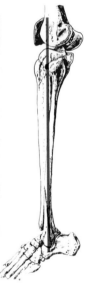

1 大腿二頭筋 Biceps femoris muscle
2 縫工筋(腱) Sartorius muscle (tendon), 薄筋(腱) Gracilis muscle (tendon)
3 大腿骨内側顆 Medial femoral condyle
4 腓腹筋(外側頭,大腿骨付着部) Gastrocnemius muscle (lateral head, femoral attachment)
5 大腿骨外側顆 Lateral femoral condyle
6 腓腹筋(内側頭,大腿骨付着部) Gastrocnemius muscle (medial head, femoral attachment)
7 足底筋(腱) Plantaris muscle (tendon)
8 外側側副靱帯 Lateral collateral ligament
9 後十字靱帯 Posterior cruciate ligament
10 内側半月板(体部) Medial meniscus (body)
11 膝窩筋(腱) Popliteus muscle (tendon)
12 膝窩筋(脛骨付着部) Popliteus muscle (tibial attachment)
13 外側半月板(体部) Lateral meniscus (body)
14 長腓骨筋 Peroneus (fibularis) longus muscle
15 前十字靱帯 Anterior cruciate ligament
16 前脛骨筋 Tibialis anterior muscle
17 脛骨(頭) Tibia (head)
18 ヒラメ筋 Soleus muscle
19 内側側副靱帯 Medial collateral ligament
20 脛骨(体) Tibia (shaft)

下腿，冠状断 343

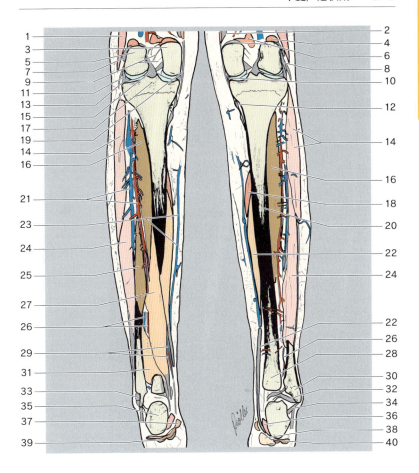

21 前脛骨動静脈 Anterior tibial artery and vein, 深腓骨神経 Deep fibular nerve
22 長趾屈筋 Flexor digitorum longus muscle
23 大伏在静脈 Great saphenous vein
24 短腓骨筋 Peroneus (fibularis) brevis muscle
25 長母趾伸筋 Extensor hallucis longus muscle
26 腓骨動静脈 Fibular artery and vein
27 後脛骨筋 Tibialis posterior muscle
28 脛骨 Tibia
29 後脛骨動静脈 Posterior tibial artery and vein
30 腓骨 Fibula
31 長母趾屈筋 Flexor hallucis longus muscle
32 後距腓靱帯 Posterior talofibular ligament
33 長腓骨筋（腱） Peroneus (fibularis) longus muscle (tendon), 短腓骨筋（腱） Peroneus (fibularis) brevis muscle (tendon)
34 踵腓靱帯 Calcaneofibular ligament
35 踵骨 Calcaneus
36 足底方形筋 Quadratus plantae muscle
37 母趾外転筋 Abductor hallucis muscle
38 短趾屈筋 Flexor digitorum brevis muscle
39 短趾屈筋 Flexor digitorum brevis muscle, 足底腱膜 Plantar aponeurosis
40 小趾外転筋 Abductor digiti minimi muscle

344 下肢

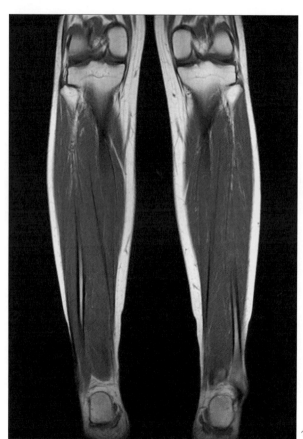
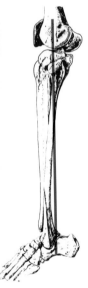

頭側

遠位

1 大腿二頭筋 Biceps femoris muscle
2 縫工筋(腱) Sartorius muscle(tendon), 薄筋(腱) Gracilis muscle(tendon)
3 大腿骨内側顆 Medial femoral condyle
4 腓腹筋(外側頭,大腿骨付着部) Gastrocnemius muscle(lateral head, femoral attachment)
5 大腿骨外側顆 Lateral femoral condyle
6 腓腹筋(内側頭,大腿骨付着部) Gastrocnemius muscle(medial head, femoral attachment)
7 前十字靱帯 Anterior cruciate ligament
8 後十字靱帯 Posterior cruciate ligament
9 脛骨(頭) Tibia(head)
10 外側半月板(体部) Lateral meniscus(body)
11 外側側副靱帯 Fibular collateral ligament
12 内側半月板(体部) Medial meniscus(body)
13 脛腓関節 Tibiofibular joint
14 腓骨(頭) Fibula(head)
15 膝窩筋(脛骨付着部) Popliteus muscle (tibial attachment)
16 脛骨(体) Tibia(shaft)
17 前脛骨動静脈 Anterior tibial artery and vein, 深腓骨神経 Deep fibular nerve

下腿，冠状断

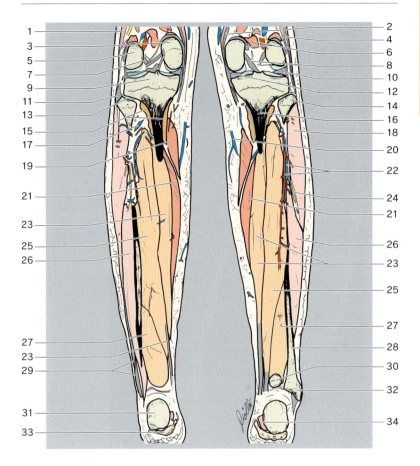

18 **長腓骨筋** Peroneus (fibularis) longus muscle
19 **腓腹筋(内側頭)** Gastrocnemius muscle (medial head)
20 **大伏在静脈** Great saphenous vein
21 **ヒラメ筋** Soleus muscle
22 **腓骨動静脈** Fibular artery and vein
23 **長趾屈筋** Flexor digitorum longus muscle
24 **浅腓骨神経** Superficial fibular nerve
25 **後脛骨筋** Tibialis posterior muscle
26 **短腓骨筋** Peroneus (fibularis) brevis muscle
27 **長母趾屈筋** Flexor hallucis longus muscle
28 **腓骨(体)** Fibula (shaft)
29 **長腓骨筋(腱)** Peroneus (fibularis) longus muscle (tendon), **短腓骨筋(腱)** Peroneus (fibularis) brevis muscle (tendon)
30 **脛骨** Tibia
31 **踵骨** Calcaneus
32 **外果** Lateral malleolus
33 **短趾屈筋** Flexor digitorum brevis muscle
34 **足底方形筋** Quadratus plantae muscle

346 下　肢

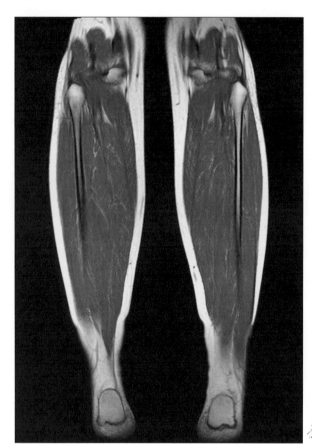

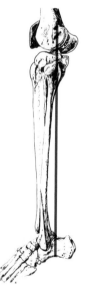

頭側

遠位

1 薄筋(腱)　Gracilis muscle (tendon)
2 腓腹筋(内側頭)　Gastrocnemius muscle (medial head)
3 縫工筋(腱)　Sartorius muscle (tendon)
4 膝窩動静脈　Popliteal artery and vein
5 半膜様筋(腱)　Semimembranosus muscle (tendon)

下腿，冠状断 347

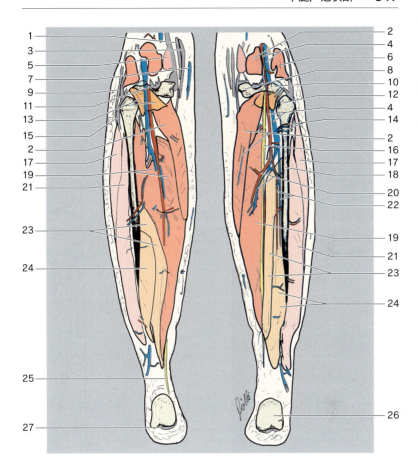

- 6 腓腹筋(外側頭) Gastrocnemius muscle (lateral head)
- 7 大伏在静脈 Great saphenous vein
- 8 脛骨内側顆 Medial tibial condyle
- 9 腸脛靱帯 Iliotibial tract
- 10 脛骨外側顆 Lateral tibial condyle
- 11 前十字靱帯 Anterior cruciate ligament
- 12 腓骨(頭) Fibula(head)
- 13 膝窩筋 Popliteus muscle
- 14 後脛骨反回動静脈 Posterior tibial recurrent artery and vein
- 15 外側側副靱帯 Fibular collateral ligament
- 16 後脛骨神経 Posterior tibial nerve
- 17 長腓骨筋 Peroneus(fibularis)longus muscle
- 18 腓骨(体) Fibula(shaft)
- 19 ヒラメ筋 Soleus muscle
- 20 後脛骨動静脈 Posterior tibial artery and vein
- 21 短腓骨筋 Peroneus(fibularis)brevis muscle
- 22 腓骨動静脈 Fibular artery and vein
- 23 後脛骨筋 Tibialis posterior muscle
- 24 長母趾屈筋 Flexor hallucis longus muscle
- 25 脛骨神経 Tibial nerve
- 26 踵骨 Calcaneus
- 27 足底腱膜 Plantar aponeurosis

348 下 肢

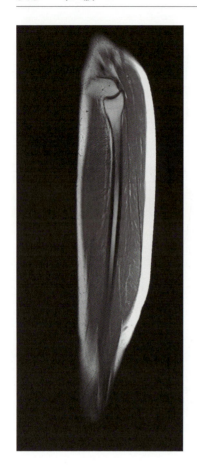

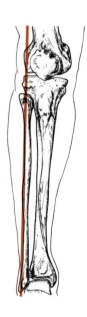

下腿，矢状断　　**349**

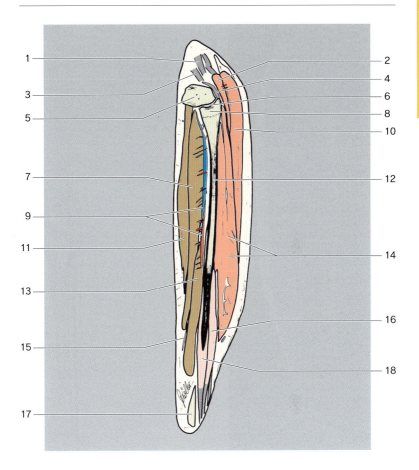

1　腸脛靱帯　Iliotibial tract
2　足底筋(+腱)　Plantaris muscle(+tendon)
3　外側膝蓋支帯　Lateral patellar retinaculum
4　膝窩筋　Popliteus muscle,
　　弓状膝窩靱帯　Arcuate popliteal ligament
5　脛骨(頭)　Tibia(head)
6　脛腓関節(上脛腓関節)　Tibiofibular joint (superior tibiofibular joint)
7　長趾伸筋　Extensor digitorum longus muscle
8　腓骨(頭)　Fibula(head)
9　前脛骨動静脈　Anterior tibial artery and vein
10　腓腹筋(外側頭)　Gastrocnemius muscle (lateral head)
11　前脛骨筋　Tibialis anterior muscle
12　腓骨(体)　Fibula(shaft)
13　長母趾伸筋　Extensor hallucis longus muscle
14　ヒラメ筋　Soleus muscle
15　浅腓骨神経　Superficial fibular nerve
16　長腓骨筋　Peroneus(fibularis)longus muscle
17　腓骨(外果)　Fibula(lateral malleolus)
18　短腓骨筋　Peroneus(fibularis)brevis muscle

350 下 肢

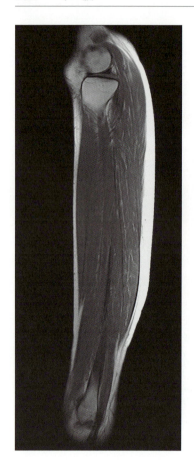

頭側
腹側 □ 背側
遠位

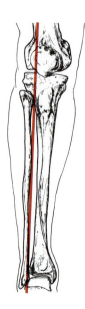

1 腸脛靱帯 Iliotibial tract
2 大腿二頭筋(腱) Biceps femoris muscle (tendon)
3 外側膝蓋支帯 Lateral patellar retinaculum
4 腓腹筋(外側頭,付着部) Gastrocnemius muscle (lateral head, attachment)
5 膝関節 Knee joint

下腿，矢状断 **351**

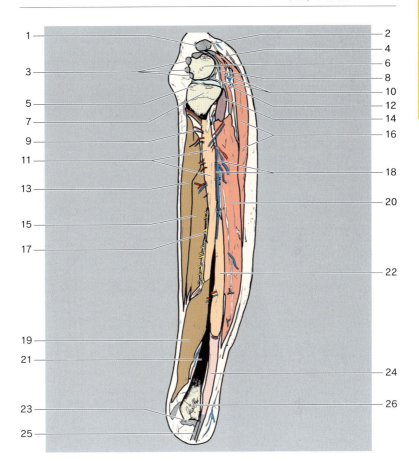

- 6 大腿骨外側顆 Lateral femoral condyle
- 7 脛骨（頭）Tibia (head)
- 8 関節包 Joint capsule of knee
- 9 前脛骨動静脈 Anterior tibial artery and vein
- 10 足底筋（+腱）Plantaris muscle (+tendon)
- 11 後脛骨筋 Tibialis posterior muscle
- 12 外側半月板（後角）Lateral meniscus (posterior horn)
- 13 前脛骨筋 Tibialis anterior muscle
- 14 膝窩筋 Popliteus muscle
- 15 長趾伸筋 Extensor digitorum longus muscle
- 16 腓腹筋（外側頭）Gastrocnemius muscle (lateral head)
- 17 浅腓骨神経 Superficial fibular nerve
- 18 腓骨動静脈 Fibular artery and vein
- 19 長母趾伸筋 Extensor hallucis longus muscle
- 20 ヒラメ筋 Soleus muscle
- 21 腓骨（体）Fibula (shaft)
- 22 長母趾屈筋 Flexor hallucis longus muscle
- 23 踵腓靱帯 Calcaneofibular ligament
- 24 長腓骨筋 Peroneus (fibularis) longus muscle
- 25 短腓骨筋（腱）Peroneus (fibularis) brevis muscle (tendon)
- 26 腓骨（外果）Fibula (lateral malleolus)

352 下 肢

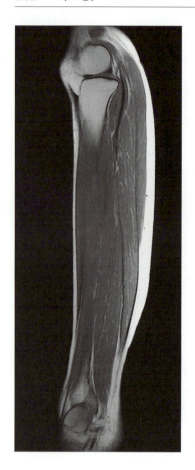

頭側
腹側 ☐ 背側
遠位

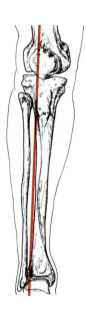

1 **腸脛靭帯** Iliotibial tract
2 **大腿二頭筋(腱)** Biceps femoris muscle (tendon)
3 **外側膝蓋支帯** Lateral patellar retinaculum
4 **腓腹筋(外側頭,付着部)** Gastrocnemius muscle (lateral head, attachment)

下腿, 矢状断 353

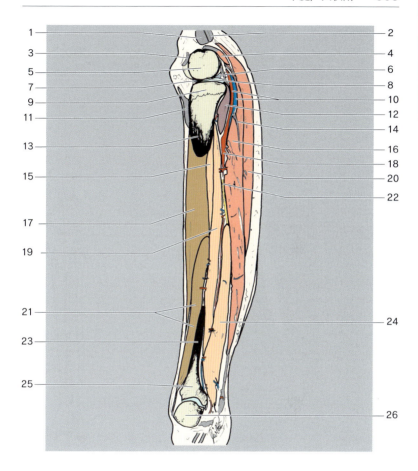

5 大腿骨外側顆 Lateral femoral condyle
6 外側半月板(後角) Lateral meniscus(posterior horn)
7 外側半月板(前角) Lateral meniscus(anterior horn)
8 膝関節 Knee joint
9 脛骨(頭) Tibia(head)
10 膝窩動静脈 Popliteal artery and vein
11 膝蓋靱帯 Patellar ligament
12 膝窩筋 Popliteus muscle
13 脛骨(体) Tibia(shaft)
14 足底筋(＋腱) Plantaris muscle(＋tendon)
15 長趾屈筋 Flexor digitorum longus muscle
16 ヒラメ筋 Soleus muscle
17 前脛骨筋 Tibialis anterior muscle
18 脛腓動脈幹 Tibiofibular trunk
19 後脛骨筋 Tibialis posterior muscle
20 腓腹筋(外側頭) Gastrocnemius muscle (lateral head)
21 長母趾伸筋 Extensor hallucis longus muscle
22 脛骨神経 Tibial nerve
23 脛骨(体) Tibia(shaft)
24 長母趾屈筋 Flexor hallucis longus muscle
25 脛骨 Tibia
26 距骨 Talus

354　下 肢

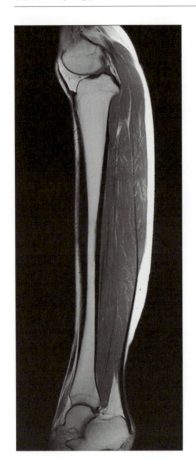

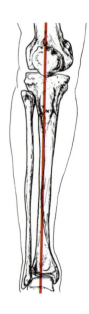

1 **外側上膝動静脈** Superior lateral genicular artery and vein
2 **脛骨神経** Tibial nerve
3 **大腿骨** Femur
4 **膝窩動静脈** Popliteal artery and vein
5 **膝蓋下(Hoffa)脂肪体** Infrapatellar(Hoffa)fat pad
6 **腓腹筋(外側頭)** Gastrocnemius muscle(lateral head)
7 **膝蓋靱帯** Patellar ligament
8 **後十字靱帯** Posterior cruciate ligament
9 **脛骨粗面** Tibial tuberosity
10 **前十字靱帯** Anterior cruciate ligament
11 **脛骨(体)** Tibia(shaft)
12 **脛骨(頭)** Tibia(head)

下腿，矢状断　355

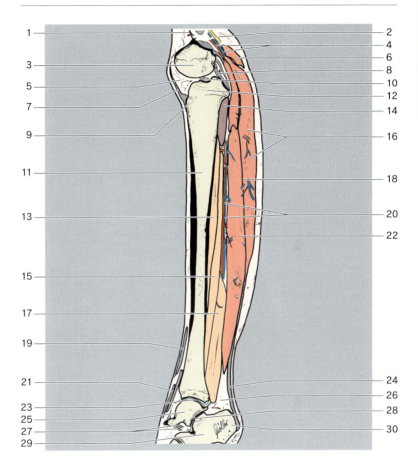

13 長趾屈筋 Flexor digitorum longus muscle
14 膝窩筋 Popliteus muscle
15 後脛骨筋 Tibialis posterior muscle
16 腓腹筋(内側頭) Gastrocnemius muscle (medial head)
17 長母趾屈筋 Flexor hallucis longus muscle
18 足底筋(腱) Plantaris muscle (tendon)
19 前脛骨筋(腱) Tibialis anterior muscle (tendon)
20 後脛骨動静脈 Posterior tibial artery and vein, 脛骨神経 Tibial nerve
21 長趾伸筋(腱) Extensor digitorum longus muscle (tendon),
   長母趾伸筋(腱) Extensor hallucis longus muscle (tendon)
22 ヒラメ筋 Soleus muscle
23 足関節 Ankle joint (距腿関節 Talocrural joint)
24 アキレス腱(踵骨腱) Achilles tendon (calcaneal tendon)
25 距骨 Talus
26 アキレス腱前脂肪体 Pre-Achilles fat body
27 骨間距踵靱帯 Talocalcaneal interosseous ligament
28 距骨下関節 Subtalar joint
29 踵骨 Calcaneus
30 踵骨結節 Calcaneal tuberosity

356 下　肢

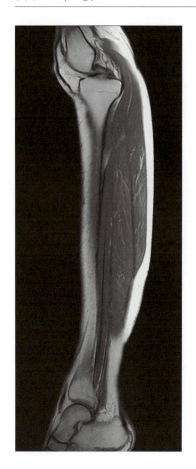

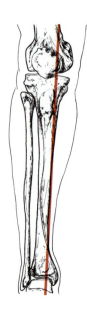

頭側
腹側 □ 背側
遠位

1　大腿四頭筋腱　Quadriceps tendon
2　膝窩動静脈　Popliteal artery and vein
3　膝蓋骨　Patella
4　腓腹筋(外側頭)　Gastrocnemius muscle (lateral head)
5　大腿骨　Femur
6　後十字靱帯　Posterior cruciate ligament
7　膝蓋下(Hoffa)脂肪体　Infrapatellar (Hoffa) fat pad
8　内側半月板(後角)　Medial meniscus (posterior horn)
9　膝蓋靱帯　Patellar ligament
10　前十字靱帯　Anterior cruciate ligament

下腿，矢状断 *357*

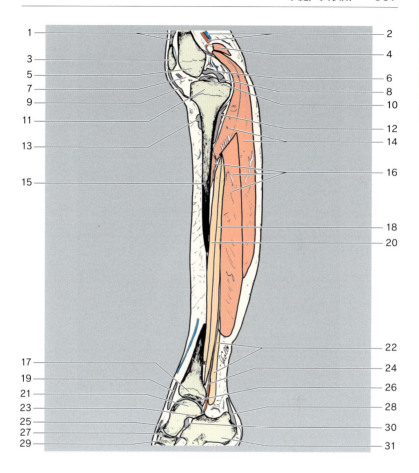

11 脛骨(頭) Tibia(head)
12 膝窩筋 Popliteus muscle
13 鵞足腱 Pes anserinus tendon
14 腓腹筋(内側頭) Gastrocnemius muscle (medial head)
15 脛骨(体) Tibia(shaft)
16 ヒラメ筋 Soleus muscle
17 脛骨 Tibia
18 後脛骨筋 Tibialis posterior muscle
19 前脛骨筋(腱) Tibialis anterior muscle (tendon)
20 長趾屈筋 Flexor digitorum longus muscle
21 距骨 Talus
22 長母趾屈筋 Flexor hallucis longus muscle
23 距骨下関節 Subtalar joint
24 後脛骨動静脈 Posterior tibial artery and vein, 脛骨神経 Tibial nerve
25 長趾伸筋(腱) Extensor digitorum longus muscle(tendon)
26 足関節 Ankle joint (距腿関節 Talocrural joint)
27 距舟関節 Talonavicular joint
28 アキレス腱(踵骨腱) Achilles tendon (calcaneal tendon)
29 舟状骨 Navicular
30 骨間距踵靱帯 Talocalcaneal interosseous ligament
31 踵骨 Calcaneus

358 下 肢

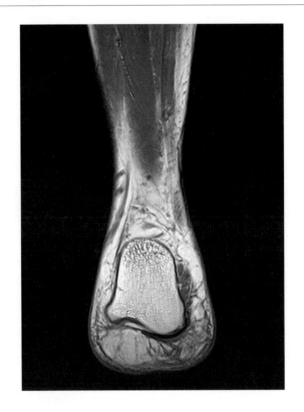

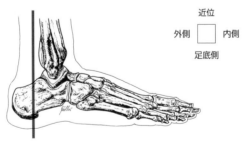

近位
外側 内側
足底側

足，冠状断

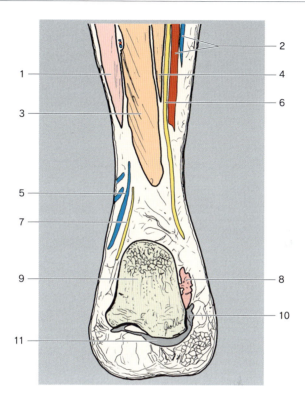

1 短腓骨筋 Peroneus (fibularis) brevis muscle
2 後脛骨動静脈 Posterior tibial artery and vein
3 長母趾屈筋 Flexor hallucis longus muscle
4 長趾屈筋 Flexor digitorum longus muscle
5 小伏在静脈 Small saphenous vein
6 脛骨神経 Tibial nerve
7 腓腹神経 Sural nerve
8 足底方形筋 Quadratus plantae muscle
9 踵骨 Calcaneus
10 母趾外転筋(腱) Abductor hallucis muscle (tendon)
11 足底腱膜 Plantar aponeurosis

360 下肢

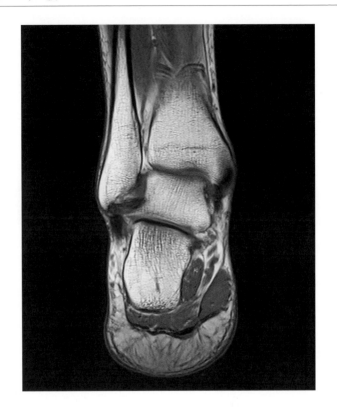

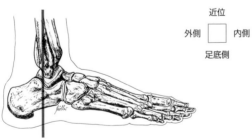

近位
外側 　　 内側
足底側

足, 冠状断

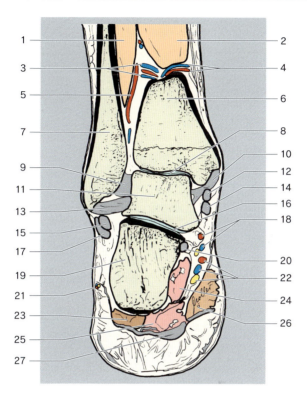

1 長母趾屈筋 Flexor hallucis longus muscle
2 後脛骨筋 Tibialis posterior muscle
3 腓骨動静脈(交通枝) Fibular artery and vein (communicating branch)
4 後脛骨動静脈(交通枝) Posterior tibial artery and vein (communicating branch)
5 腓骨動脈 Fibular artery
6 脛骨 Tibia
7 腓骨 Fibula
8 足関節 Ankle joint (距腿関節 Talocrural joint)
9 関節包の背側部 Dorsal capsule
10 三角靱帯 Deltoid ligament
11 距骨 Talus
12 後脛骨筋(腱) Tibialis posterior muscle (tendon)
13 後距腓靱帯 Posterior talofibular ligament
14 長趾屈筋(腱) Flexor digitorum longus muscle (tendon)
15 短腓骨筋(腱) Peroneus (fibularis) brevis muscle (tendon)
16 距骨下関節 Subtalar joint
17 長腓骨筋(腱) Peroneus (fibularis) longus muscle (tendon)
18 内側足底動静脈, 神経 Medial plantar artery, vein and nerve
19 踵骨 Calcaneus
20 長母趾屈筋(腱) Flexor hallucis longus muscle (tendon)
21 腓腹神経 Sural nerve および伴行血管
22 外側足底動静脈, 神経 Lateral plantar artery, vein and nerve
23 小趾外転筋 Abductor digiti minimi muscle
24 足底方形筋 Quadratus plantae muscle
25 短趾屈筋 Flexor digitorum brevis muscle
26 母趾外転筋 Abductor hallucis muscle
27 足底腱膜 Plantar aponeurosis

362　下　肢

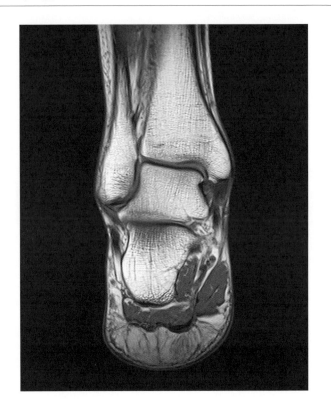

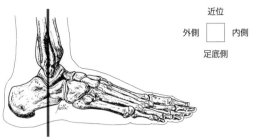

近位

外側　□　内側

足底側

足，冠状断

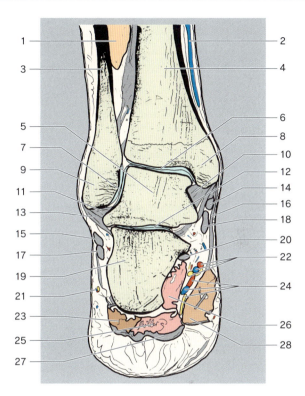

1 長母趾屈筋 Flexor hallucis longus muscle
2 大伏在静脈 Great saphenous vein
3 腓骨 Fibula
4 脛骨 Tibia
5 距骨 Talus
6 足関節 Ankle joint（距腿関節 Talocrural joint）
7 距腓関節 Talofibular joint
8 内果 Medial malleolus
9 外果 Lateral malleolus
10 三角靱帯（後距部）Deltoid ligament (posterior tibiotalar part)
11 後距腓靱帯 Posterior talofibular ligament
12 距骨下関節 Subtalar joint
13 踵腓靱帯 Calcaneofibular ligament
14 後脛骨筋（腱）Tibialis posterior muscle (tendon)
15 短腓骨筋（腱）Peroneus (fibularis) brevis muscle (tendon)
16 屈筋支帯 Flexor retinaculum
17 長腓骨筋（腱）Peroneus (fibularis) longus muscle (tendon)
18 長趾屈筋（腱）Flexor digitorum longus muscle (tendon)
19 踵骨 Calcaneus
20 長母趾屈筋（腱）Flexor hallucis longus muscle (tendon)
21 腓腹神経 Sural nerve および伴行血管
22 内側足底動静脈，神経 Medial plantar artery, vein and nerve
23 小趾外転筋 Abductor digiti minimi muscle
24 外側足底動静脈，神経 Lateral plantar artery, vein and nerve
25 短趾屈筋 Flexor digitorum brevis muscle
26 足底方形筋 Quadratus plantae muscle
27 足底腱膜 Plantar aponeurosis
28 母趾外転筋 Abductor hallucis muscle

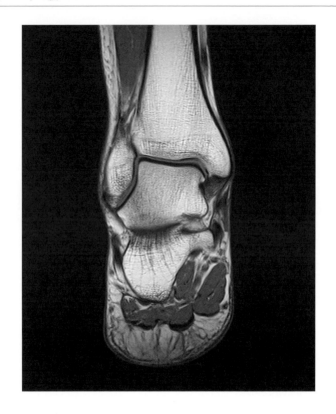

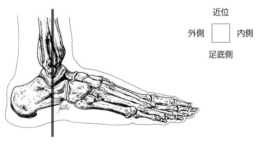

足，冠状断　　*365*

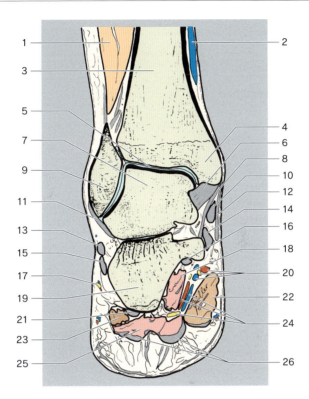

1 長趾伸筋 Extensor digitorum longus muscle
2 大伏在静脈 Great saphenous vein
3 脛骨 Tibia
4 内果 Medial malleolus
5 足関節 Ankle joint（距腿関節 Talocrural joint）
6 三角靱帯（後脛距部）Deltoid ligament (posterior tibiotalar part)
7 距骨 Talus
8 三角靱帯（脛踵部）Deltoid ligament (tibiocalcaneal part)
9 腓骨（外果）Fibula (lateral malleolus)
10 後脛骨筋（腱）Tibialis posterior muscle (tendon)
11 踵腓靱帯 Calcaneofibular ligament
12 屈筋支帯 Flexor retinaculum
13 短腓骨筋（腱）Peroneus (fibularis) brevis muscle (tendon)
14 長趾屈筋（腱）Flexor digitorum longus muscle (tendon)
15 長腓骨筋（腱）Peroneus (fibularis) longus muscle (tendon)
16 長母趾屈筋（腱）Flexor hallucis longus muscle (tendon)
17 腓腹神経 Sural nerve および伴行血管
18 足底方形筋 Quadratus plantae muscle
19 踵骨 Calcaneus
20 内側足底動静脈，神経 Medial plantar artery, vein and nerve
21 長足底靱帯 Long plantar ligament
22 母趾外転筋 Abductor hallucis muscle
23 小趾外転筋 Abductor digiti minimi muscle
24 外側足底動静脈，神経 Lateral plantar artery, vein, and nerve
25 短趾屈筋 Flexor digitorum brevis muscle
26 足底腱膜 Plantar aponeurosis

366　下　肢

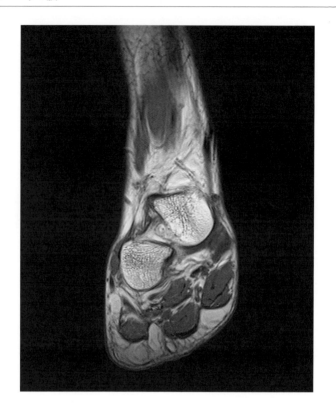

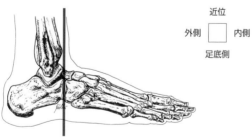

近位
外側 　　内側
足底側

足，冠状断   367

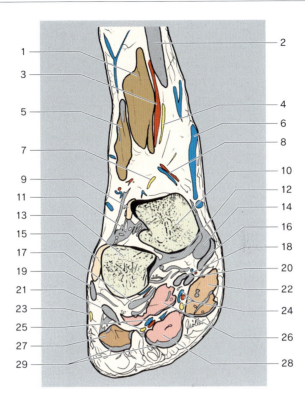

1 長母趾伸筋 Extensor hallucis longus muscle
2 前脛骨筋(腱) Tibialis anterior muscle (tendon)
3 前脛骨動脈 Anterior tibial artery
4 深腓骨神経 Deep fibular nerve
5 長趾伸筋 Extensor digitorum longus muscle
6 大伏在静脈 Great saphenous vein
7 深腓骨神経(皮枝) Deep fibular nerve (cutaneous branch)
8 内側足根動脈 Medial tarsal artery
9 短母趾伸筋(腱) Extensor hallucis brevis muscle (tendon)
10 距骨 Talus
11 骨間距踵靱帯 Talocalcaneal interosseous ligament
12 底側踵舟靱帯 Plantar calcaneonavicular ligament
13 踵骨 Calcaneus
14 三角靱帯(脛舟部) Deltoid ligament (tibionavicular part)
15 短趾伸筋 Extensor digitorum brevis muscle
16 後脛骨筋(腱) Tibialis posterior muscle (tendon)
17 長足底靱帯 Long plantar ligament
18 長母趾屈筋(腱) Flexor hallucis longus muscle (tendon)
19 短腓骨筋 Peroneus (fibularis) brevis muscle
20 長趾屈筋(腱) Flexor digitorum longus muscle (tendon)
21 長腓骨筋(腱) Peroneus (fibularis) longus muscle (tendon)
22 母趾外転筋 Abductor hallucis muscle
23 外側足背皮神経 Lateral dorsal cutaneous nerve
24 内側足底動静脈，神経 Medial plantar artery, vein, and nerve
25 外側足底動静脈，神経 Lateral plantar artery, vein, and nerve
26 足底方形筋 Quadratus plantae muscle
27 小趾外転筋 Abductor digiti minimi muscle
28 短趾屈筋 Flexor digitorum brevis muscle
29 足底腱膜 Plantar aponeurosis

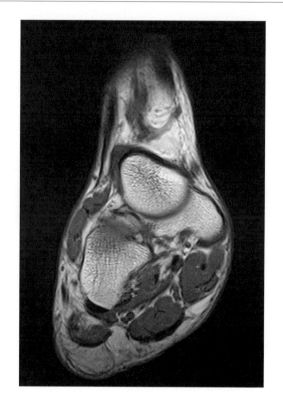

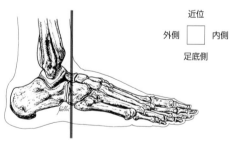

近位

外側 　　　 内側

足底側

1 **長母趾伸筋(腱)** Extensor hallucis longus muscle(tendon)
2 **前脛骨筋(腱)** Tibialis anterior muscle (tendon)
3 **長趾伸筋(腱)** Extensor digitorum longus muscle(tendon)
4 **前脛骨動脈** Anterior tibial artery

足，冠状断　369

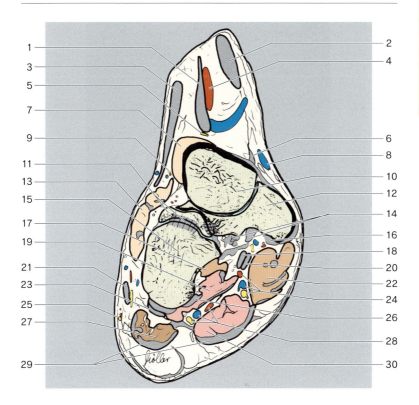

- 5 深腓骨神経(内側枝) Deep fibular nerve (medial branch)
- 6 三角靱帯(前脛距部) Deltoid ligament (anterior tibiotalar part)
- 7 短母趾伸筋 Extensor hallucis brevis muscle
- 8 大伏在静脈 Great saphenous vein
- 9 深腓骨神経(外側枝) Deep fibular nerve (lateral branch)
- 10 距骨 Talus
- 11 踵骨 Calcaneus, 二分靱帯 Bifurcate ligament
- 12 舟状骨 Navicular
- 13 短趾伸筋 Extensor digitorum brevis muscle
- 14 底側踵舟靱帯 Plantar calcaneonavicular ligament
- 15 立方骨 Cuboid
- 16 後脛骨筋(腱) Tibialis posterior muscle (tendon)
- 17 母趾内転筋(斜頭) Adductor hallucis muscle (oblique head)
- 18 長母趾屈筋(腱) Flexor hallucis longus muscle (tendon)
- 19 足底方形筋 Quadratus plantae muscle
- 20 長趾屈筋(腱) Flexor digitorum longus muscle (tendon)
- 21 短腓骨筋(腱) Peroneus (fibularis) brevis muscle (tendon)
- 22 母趾外転筋 Abductor hallucis muscle
- 23 長腓骨筋(腱) Peroneus (fibularis) longus muscle (tendon)
- 24 内側足底動静脈, 神経 Medial plantar artery, vein, and nerve
- 25 外側足背皮神経 Lateral dorsal cutaneous nerve
- 26 長足底靱帯 Long plantar ligament
- 27 小趾外転筋 Abductor digiti minimi muscle
- 28 外側足底動静脈, 神経 Lateral plantar artery, vein, and nerve
- 29 足底腱膜 Plantar aponeurosis
- 30 短趾屈筋 Flexor digitorum brevis muscle

370 下肢

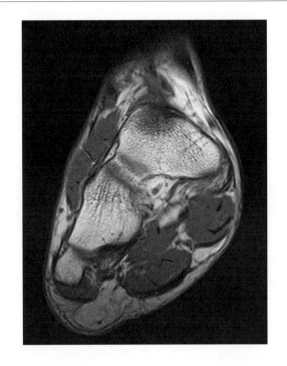

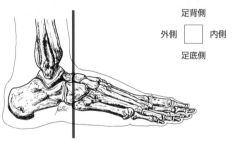

足背側
外側　　　内側
足底側

足，冠状断 *371*

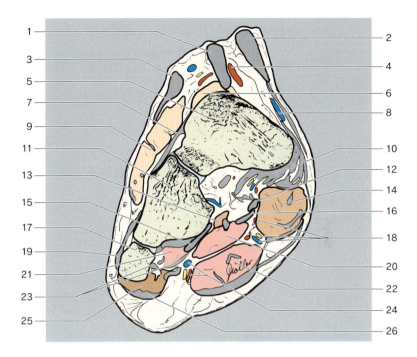

1 長母趾伸筋（腱） Extensor hallucis longus muscle (tendon)
2 前脛骨筋（腱） Tibialis anterior muscle (tendon)
3 長趾伸筋（腱） Extensor digitorum longus muscle (tendon)
4 前脛骨動脈 Anterior tibial artery
5 舟状骨 Navicular
6 短母趾伸筋 Extensor hallucis brevis muscle
7 背側足根靱帯 Dorsal tarsal ligaments
8 大伏在静脈 Great saphenous vein
9 短趾伸筋 Extensor digitorum brevis muscle
10 後脛骨筋（腱） Tibialis posterior muscle (tendon)
11 立方骨 Cuboid
12 長母趾屈筋（腱） Flexor hallucis longus muscle (tendon)
13 母趾内転筋（斜頭） Adductor hallucis muscle (oblique head)
14 母趾外転筋 Abductor hallucis muscle
15 長腓骨筋（腱） Peroneus (fibularis) longus muscle (tendon)
16 長趾屈筋（腱） Flexor digitorum longus muscle (tendon)
17 第5中足骨（底） MetatarsalV (base)
18 内側足底動静脈，神経 Medial plantar artery, vein, and nerve
19 短腓骨筋（腱） Peroneus (fibularis) brevis muscle (tendon)
20 足底方形筋 Quadratus plantae muscle
21 骨間筋 Interosseous muscles
22 短趾屈筋 Flexor digitorum brevis muscle
23 長足底靱帯 Long plantar ligament
24 外側足底動静脈，神経 Lateral plantar artery, vein, and nerve
25 小趾外転筋 Abductor digiti minimi muscle
26 足底腱膜 Plantar aponeurosis

372 下 肢

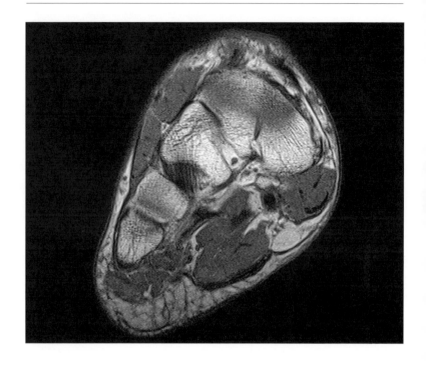

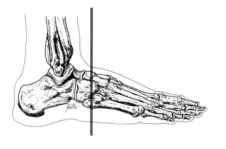

足背側

外側　内側

足底側

足，冠状断　**373**

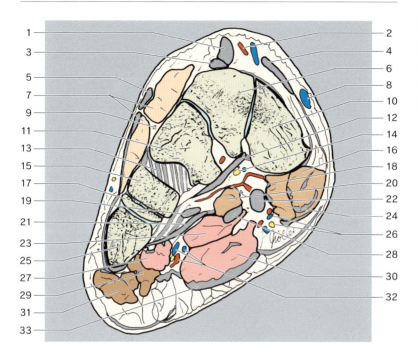

1 長母趾伸筋(腱) Extensor hallucis longus muscle(tendon)
2 前脛骨動脈 Anterior tibial artery
3 短母趾伸筋(腱) Extensor hallucis brevis muscle(tendon)
4 前脛骨筋(腱) Tibialis anterior muscle (tendon)
5 長趾伸筋(腱) Extensor digitorum longus muscle(tendon)
6 中間楔状骨 Intermediate cuneiform
7 短趾伸筋 Extensor digitorum brevis muscle
8 大伏在静脈 Great saphenous vein
9 深腓骨神経(外側枝) Deep fibular nerve (lateral branch)
10 内側楔状骨 Medial cuneiform
11 外側楔状骨 Lateral cuneiform
12 後脛骨筋(腱付着部) Tibialis posterior muscle (tendon attachment)
13 背側足根靱帯 Dorsal tarsal ligaments
14 外側足底神経(深枝) Lateral plantar nerve (deep branch)
15 立方骨 Cuboid
16 母趾外転筋 Abductor hallucis muscle
17 第4中足骨(底) MetatarsalⅣ(base)
18 足底の内側筋間中隔 Medial plantar septum
19 長腓骨筋(腱) Peroneus(fibularis)longus muscle(tendon)
20 母趾内転筋(斜頭) Adductor hallucis muscle (oblique head), 深足底動脈弓 Deep plantar arch
21 長足底靱帯 Long plantar ligament
22 長母趾屈筋(腱) Flexor hallucis longus muscle(tendon)
23 足底方形筋 Quadratus plantae muscle
24 短母趾屈筋 Flexor hallucis brevis muscle
25 第5中足骨(底) MetatarsalⅤ(base)
26 内側足底動静脈，神経 Medial plantar artery, vein, and nerve
27 骨間筋 Interosseous muscles
28 長趾屈筋(腱) Flexor digitorum longus muscle(tendon)
29 短小趾屈筋 Flexor digiti minimi brevis muscle
30 短趾屈筋 Flexor digitorum brevis muscle
31 小趾外転筋 Abductor digiti minimi muscle
32 外側足底動静脈，神経 Lateral plantar artery, vein, and nerve
33 足底腱膜 Plantar aponeurosis

374　下肢

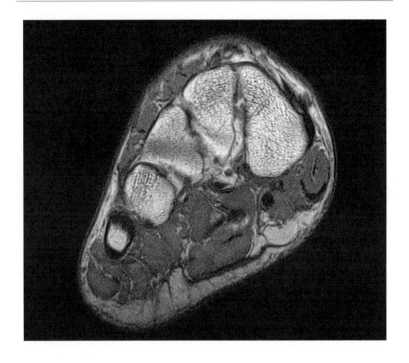

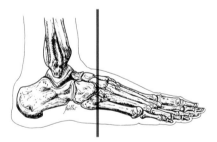

足背側

外側　　内側

足底側

1 **短母趾伸筋(腱)** Extensor hallucis brevis muscle (tendon)
2 **長母趾伸筋(腱)** Extensor hallucis longus muscle (tendon)
3 **短趾伸筋** Extensor digitorum brevis muscle
4 **前脛骨動脈** Anterior tibial artery
5 **長趾伸筋(腱)** Extensor digitorum longus muscle (tendons)

足，冠状断　375

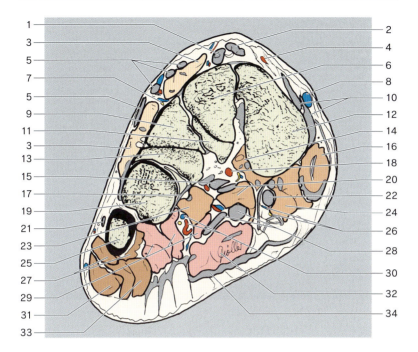

- 6 中間楔状骨 Intermediate cuneiform
- 7 深腓骨神経（外側枝）Deep fibular nerve (lateral branch)
- 8 大伏在静脈 Great saphenous vein
- 9 外側楔状骨 Lateral cuneiform
- 10 前脛骨筋（腱）Tibialis anterior muscle (tendon)
- 11 第2中足骨(底) Metatarsal II (base)
- 12 内側楔状骨 Medial cuneiform
- 13 第3中足骨(底) Metatarsal III (base)
- 14 短母趾屈筋（外側頭）Flexor hallucis brevis muscle (lateral head)
- 15 長腓骨筋（腱）Peroneus (fibularis) longus muscle (tendon)
- 16 母趾外転筋 Abductor hallucis muscle
- 17 長足底靱帯 Long plantar ligament
- 18 深足底動脈弓 Deep plantar arch
- 19 第4中足骨(底) Metatarsal IV (base)
- 20 母趾内転筋（斜頭＋腱）Adductor hallucis muscle (oblique head + tendon)
- 21 短小趾伸筋（腱）Extensor digiti minimi brevis muscle (tendon)
- 22 長母趾屈筋（腱）Flexor hallucis longus muscle (tendon)
- 23 短母趾屈筋（外側頭）Flexor hallucis brevis muscle (lateral head)
- 24 短母趾屈筋（内側頭）Flexor hallucis brevis muscle (medial head)
- 25 第5中足骨(底) Metatarsal V (base)
- 26 内側足底動脈静脈，神経 Medial plantar artery, vein, and nerve (superficial branch)
- 27 小趾対立筋 Opponens digiti minimi muscle
- 28 長趾屈筋（腱）Flexor digitorum longus muscle (tendon)
- 29 骨間筋 Interosseous muscles
- 30 外側足底動脈静脈，神経 Lateral plantar artery, vein, and nerve
- 31 小趾外転筋 Abductor digiti minimi muscle
- 32 短趾屈筋 Flexor digitorum brevis muscle
- 33 短小趾屈筋 Flexor digiti minimi brevis muscle
- 34 足底腱膜 Plantar aponeurosis

376 下 肢

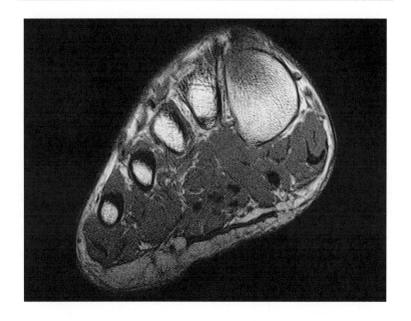

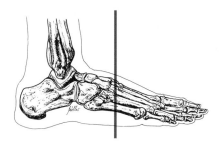

足背側

外側 　　 内側

足底側

足，冠状断　*377*

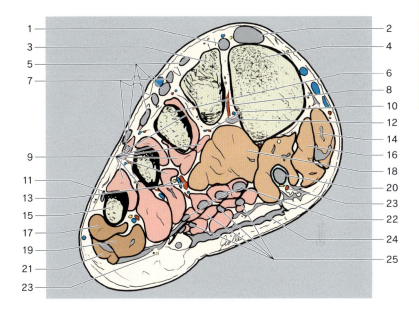

1 短母趾伸筋(腱) Extensor hallucis brevis muscle(tendon)
2 長母趾伸筋(腱) Extensor hallucis longus muscle(tendon)
3 第2中足骨(底) MetatarsalⅡ(base)
4 第1中足骨(底) MetatarsalⅠ(base)
5 長趾伸筋(腱) Extensor digitorum longus muscle(tendons)
6 第3中足骨(底) MetatarsalⅢ(base)
7 短趾伸筋 Extensor digitorum brevis muscle
8 底側中足動脈 Plantar metatarsal arteries
9 骨間筋 Interosseous muscles
10 (第1背側骨間筋の)貫通静脈 Perforating veins(of first dorsal interosseous muscle)
11 短小趾伸筋(腱) Extensor digiti minimi brevis muscle(tendon)
12 長腓骨筋(付着部) Peroneus(fibularis)longus muscle(attachment)
13 外側足底神経(深枝) Lateral plantar nerve (deep branch), 底側中足動脈 Plantar metatarsal arteries
14 母趾外転筋 Abductor hallucis muscle
15 第5中足骨 MetatarsalⅤ
16 短母趾屈筋(外側頭) Flexor hallucis brevis muscle(lateral head)
17 小趾対立筋 Opponens digiti minimi muscle
18 母趾内転筋(斜頭) Adductor hallucis muscle (oblique head)
19 短小趾屈筋 Flexor digiti minimi brevis muscle
20 長母趾屈筋(腱) Flexor hallucis longus muscle(tendon)
21 小趾外転筋 Abductor digiti minimi muscle
22 長趾屈筋(＋腱) Flexor digitorum longus muscle(+tendon)
23 固有底側趾動脈 Proper plantar digital artery
24 足底腱膜 Plantar aponeurosis
25 短趾屈筋(＋腱) Flexor digitorum brevis muscle(+tendon)

378 下 肢

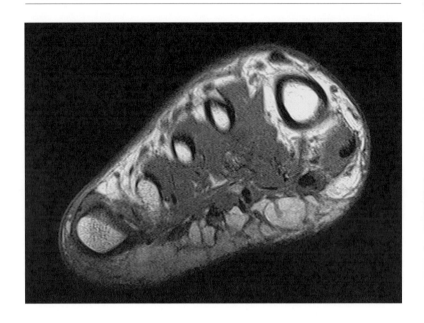

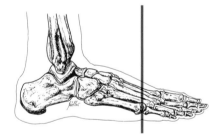

足背側
外側　　内側
足底側

足，冠状断　*379*

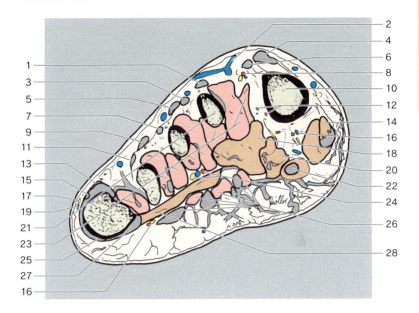

1 第2趾の長趾伸筋（腱）Extensor digitorum longus II muscle (tendon)
2 足背静脈弓 Dorsal venous arch of foot
3 第2趾の短趾伸筋（腱）Extensor digitorum brevis II muscle (tendon)
4 長母趾伸筋（腱）Extensor hallucis longus muscle (tendon)
5 第3趾の長趾伸筋（腱）Extensor digitorum longus III muscle (tendon)
6 短母趾伸筋（腱）Extensor hallucis brevis muscle (tendon)
7 第3趾の短趾伸筋（腱）Extensor digitorum brevis III muscle (tendon)
8 背側中足動静脈 Dorsal metatarsal arteries and veins
9 第4趾の短趾伸筋（腱）Extensor digitorum brevis IV muscle (tendon)
10 第1中足骨 Metatarsal I
11 第4趾の短趾伸筋（腱）Extensor digitorum brevis IV muscle (tendon)
12 底側中足動静脈（第1骨間筋への貫通枝）Plantar metatarsal artery and vein (perforating branch of first dorsal interosseous muscle)
13 第5趾の長趾伸筋（腱）Extensor digitorum longus V muscle (tendons)
14 母趾外転筋 Abductor hallucis muscle
15 第5趾の短趾伸筋（腱）Extensor digitorum brevis V muscle (tendon)
16 固有底側趾動静脈，神経 Proper plantar digital arteries, veins, and nerve
17 足背趾皮神経 Dorsal digital cutaneous nerve of foot
18 母趾内転筋（斜頭）Adductor hallucis muscle (oblique head)
19 小伏在静脈 Small saphenous vein
20 短母趾屈筋（外側頭）Flexor hallucis brevis muscle (lateral head)
21 中足骨 Metatarsals
22 長母趾屈筋（腱）Flexor hallucis longus muscle (tendon)
23 底側骨間筋 Plantar interosseous muscles, 背側骨間筋 Dorsal interosseous muscle
24 外側足底神経（深枝）Lateral plantar nerve (deep branch), 底側中足動脈 Plantar metatarsal arteries
25 小趾外転筋（付着部）Abductor digiti minimi muscle (attachment)
26 長趾屈筋（腱）Flexor digitorum longus muscle (tendon), 短趾屈筋（腱）Flexor digitorum brevis muscle (tendon)
27 短小趾伸筋（腱）Extensor digiti minimi brevis muscle (tendon)
28 母趾内転筋（横頭）Adductor hallucis muscle (transverse head)

380　下　肢

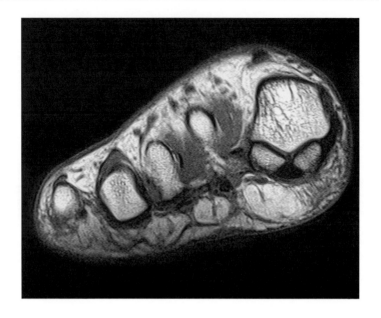

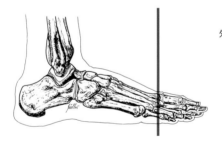

足背側

外側　　内側

足底側

足，冠状断 *381*

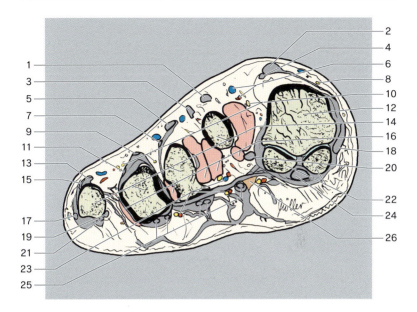

1 第2趾の長趾伸筋(腱) Extensor digitorum longus II muscle (tendon)
2 長母趾伸筋(腱) Extensor hallucis longus muscle (tendon)
3 第2趾の短趾伸筋(腱) Extensor digitorum brevis II muscle (tendon)
4 短母趾伸筋(腱) Extensor hallucis brevis muscle (tendon)
5 第3趾の長趾伸筋(腱) Extensor digitorum longus III muscle (tendon)
6 背側中足動静脈 Dorsal metatarsal arteries and veins
7 第3趾の短趾伸筋(腱) Extensor digitorum brevis III muscle (tendon)
8 第1趾の内側背側皮神経 Medial dorsal cutaneous nerve I
9 第4趾の長趾伸筋(腱) Extensor digitorum longus IV muscle (tendon)
10 背側趾神経 Dorsal digital nerves of foot
11 第4趾の短趾伸筋(腱) Extensor digitorum brevis IV muscle (tendon)
12 第1中足骨(頭) Metatarsal I (head)
13 第5趾の長趾伸筋(腱) Extensor digiti minimi longus muscle (tendon)
14 第2-5中足骨 Metatarsals II-V
15 短小趾伸筋(腱) Extensor digiti minimi brevis muscle (tendon)
16 背側骨間筋 Dorsal interosseous muscle, 底側骨間筋 Plantar interosseous muscle
17 小趾外転筋(腱付着部) Abductor digiti minimi muscle (tendon attachment)
18 母趾外転筋(腱) Abductor hallucis muscle (tendon)
19 第5趾の長趾屈筋(腱) Flexor digiti minimi longus muscle (tendon)
20 母趾内転筋(腱) Adductor hallucis muscle (tendon)
21 短小趾屈筋(腱) Flexor digiti minimi brevis muscle (tendon)
22 種子骨 Sesamoid bones
23 固有底側趾動静脈 Plantar digital artery and vein proper, 固有底側趾神経 Proper plantar digital nerve
24 長母趾屈筋(腱) Flexor hallucis longus muscle (tendon)
25 長趾屈筋(腱) Flexor digitorum longus muscle (tendon), 短趾屈筋(腱) Flexor digitorum brevis muscle (tendon)
26 母趾内転筋(横頭) Adductor hallucis muscle (transverse head)

382　下 肢

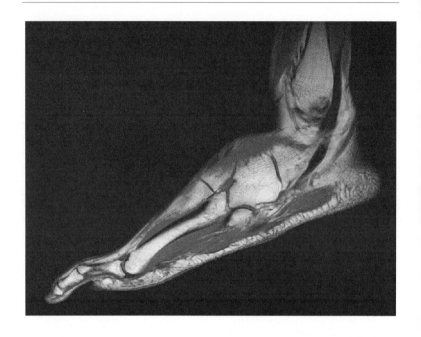

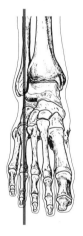

近位
足背側
前　　　後
遠位
足底側

足, 矢状断　*383*

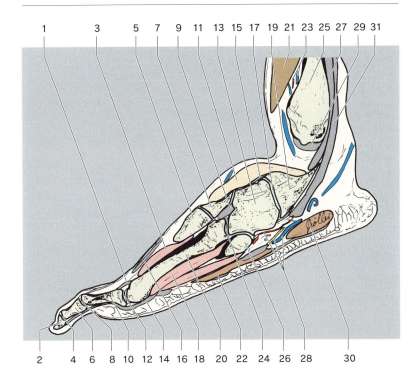

1 背側中足靱帯 Dorsal metatarsal ligaments
2 第4末節骨 Distal phalanx Ⅳ
3 背側骨間筋 Dorsal interosseous muscle
4 第4遠位趾節間関節 Distal interphalangeal joint Ⅳ
5 中足骨 Metatarsal Ⅲ (base)
6 第4中節骨 Middle phalanx Ⅳ
7 外側楔状骨 Lateral cuneiform
8 第4近位趾節間関節 Proximal interphalangeal joint Ⅳ
9 骨間楔立方靱帯 Cuneocuboid interosseous ligament
10 第4基節骨 Proximal phalanx Ⅳ
11 短趾伸筋 Extensor digitorum brevis muscle
12 第4中足趾節関節 Metatarsophalangeal joint Ⅳ
13 立方骨 Cuboid
14 長趾屈筋(腱) Flexor digitorum longus muscle (tendon)
15 二分靱帯 Bifurcate ligament
16 趾伸筋(腱) Extensor digitorum muscle (tendon)
17 踵立方関節 Calcaneocuboid joint
18 底側骨間筋 Plantar interosseous muscle
19 踵骨 Calcaneus
20 第4中足骨 Metatarsal Ⅳ
21 長趾伸筋 Extensor digitorum longus muscle
22 短小趾屈筋 Flexor digiti minimi brevis muscle
23 前外果動脈 Anterior lateral malleolar artery
24 第4足根中足関節 Tarsometatarsal joint Ⅳ
25 腓骨 Fibula
26 第5中足骨(底) Metatarsal Ⅴ (base)
27 短腓骨筋(腱) Peroneus (fibularis) brevis muscle (tendon)
28 外側足底動静脈, 神経 Lateral plantar artery, vein, and nerve
29 踵腓靱帯 Calcaneofibular ligament
30 小趾外転筋 Abductor digiti minimi muscle
31 長腓骨筋(腱) Peroneus (fibularis) longus muscle (tendon)

384　下　肢

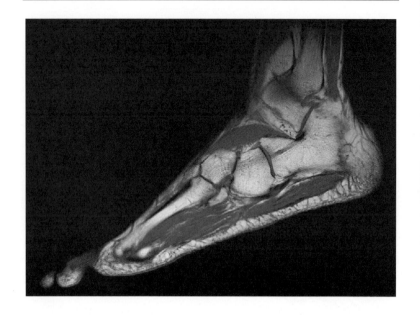

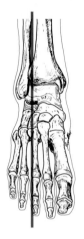

近位

足背側

前　後

遠位

足底側

足,矢状断

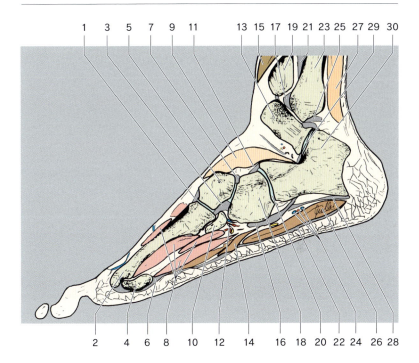

1 背側中足靱帯 Dorsal metatarsal ligaments
2 第3中足骨 MetatarsalⅢ
3 骨間楔立方靱帯 Cuneocuboid interosseous ligament
4 第4中足骨(頭) MetatarsalⅣ(head)
5 外側楔状骨 Lateral cuneiform
6 長趾屈筋(腱) Flexor digitorum longus muscle(tendon)
7 背側足根靱帯 Dorsal tarsal ligaments
8 背側骨間筋 Dorsal interosseous muscle, 底側骨間筋 Plantar interosseous muscles
9 短趾伸筋 Extensor digitorum brevis muscle
10 第4中足骨(底) MetatarsalⅣ(base)
11 二分靱帯 Bifurcate ligament
12 深足底動脈弓 Deep plantar arch
13 距骨 Talus
14 短小趾屈筋 Flexor digiti minimi brevis muscle
15 長趾伸筋 Extensor digitorum longus muscle
16 長腓骨筋(腱) Peroneus(fibularis)longus muscle(tendon)
17 前距腓靱帯 Anterior talofibular ligament
18 立方骨 Cuboid
19 脛骨 Tibia
20 踵立方関節 Calcaneocuboid joint
21 脛腓靱帯結合 Tibiofibular syndesmosis (前脛腓靱帯 Anterior tibiofibular ligament)
22 足底腱膜 Plantar aponeurosis
23 腓骨 Fibula
24 外側足底動静脈,神経 Lateral plantar artery, vein, and nerve
25 後距腓靱帯 Posterior talofibular ligament
26 小趾外転筋 Abductor digiti minimi muscle
27 短腓骨筋 Peroneus(fibularis)brevis muscle
28 長足底靱帯 Long plantar ligament
29 距骨下関節 Subtalar joint
30 踵骨 Calcaneus

386　下 肢

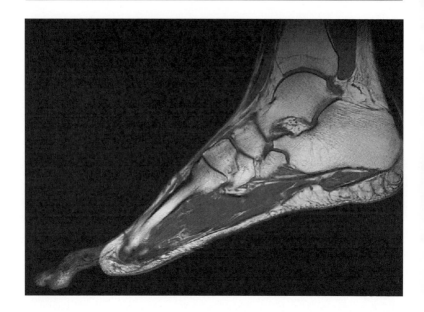

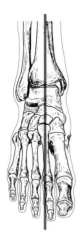

近位
足背側

前　　　後

遠位
足底側

足，矢状断　　*387*

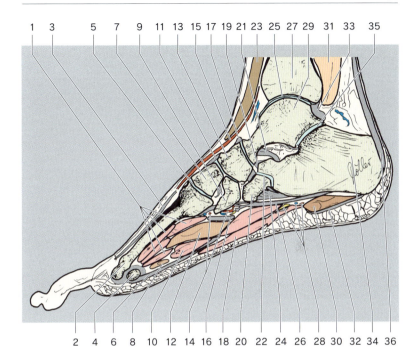

1 骨間筋 Interosseous muscles
2 第2中足骨 Metatarsal II
3 第2趾の趾伸筋(腱) Extensor digitorum II muscle (tendon)
4 第2中足骨(頭) Metatarsal II (head)
5 足根中足関節 Tarsometatarsal joint II
6 長趾屈筋(腱) Flexor digitorum longus muscle (tendon)
7 中間楔状骨 Intermediate cuneiform
8 母趾内転筋(横頭) Adductor hallucis muscle (transverse head)
9 外側楔状骨 Lateral cuneiform
10 虫様筋 Lumbrical muscle
11 背側足根靱帯 Dorsal tarsal ligaments
12 母趾内転筋(斜頭) Adductor hallucis muscle (oblique head)
13 舟状骨 Navicular
14 深足底動脈弓 Deep plantar arch
15 足背動脈 Dorsalis pedis artery
16 長腓骨筋(腱) Peroneus (fibularis) longus muscle (tendon)
17 背側距舟靱帯 Dorsal talonavicular ligament
18 短趾屈筋 Flexor digitorum brevis muscle
19 二分靱帯 Bifurcate ligament
20 立方骨 Cuboid
21 骨間距踵靱帯 Talocalcaneal interosseous ligament
22 踵立方関節 Calcaneocuboid joint
23 長趾伸筋 Extensor digitorum longus muscle
24 ばね靱帯(底側踵舟靱帯) Spring ligament (plantar calcaneonavicular ligament)
25 足関節 Ankle joint (距腿関節 Talocrural joint)
26 長足底靱帯 Long plantar ligament
27 脛骨 Tibia
28 外側足底動静脈，神経 Lateral plantar artery, vein, and nerve
29 距骨 Talus
30 小趾外転筋 Abductor digiti minimi muscle
31 長母趾屈筋 Flexor hallucis longus muscle
32 足底腱膜 Plantar aponeurosis
33 後距腓靱帯 Posterior talofibular ligament
34 踵骨 Calcaneus
35 距骨下関節 Subtalar joint
36 アキレス腱(踵骨腱) Achilles tendon (calcaneal tendon)

388　下　肢

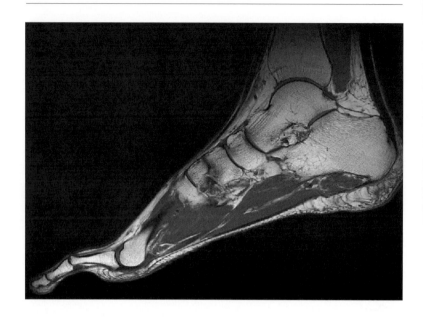

近位
足背側
前　　　後
遠位
足底側

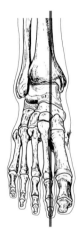

足，矢状断　389

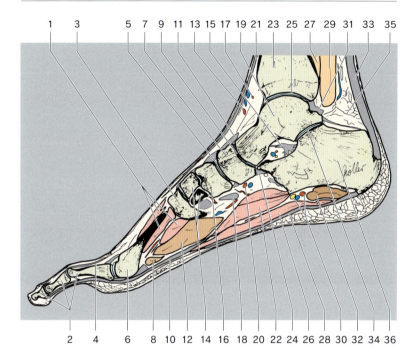

1 骨間筋 Interosseous muscle
2 第2基節骨, 中節骨, 末節骨 Proximal, middle, and distal phalanx II
3 第1中足骨(底) Metatarsal I (base)
4 趾伸筋(腱) Extensor digitorum muscle (tendon)
5 楔舟関節 Cuneonavicular joint
6 第2中足骨(頭) Metatarsal II (head)
7 舟状骨 Navicular
8 母趾内転筋(横頭) Adductor hallucis muscle (transverse head)
9 距舟関節 Talonavicular joint
10 長趾屈筋(腱) Flexor digitorum longus muscle (tendon)
11 距舟靱帯 Talonavicular ligament
12 母趾内転筋(斜頭) Adductor hallucis muscle (oblique head)
13 内側足根動脈 Medial tarsal artery
14 内側楔状骨 Medial cuneiform
15 骨間距踵靱帯 Talocalcaneal interosseous ligament
16 中間楔状骨 Intermediate cuneiform
17 前内果動脈 Anterior medial malleolar artery
18 長腓骨筋(腱) Peroneus (fibularis) longus muscle (tendon)
19 距骨 Talus
20 深足底動脈弓 Deep plantar arch
21 長母趾伸筋(腱) Extensor hallucis longus muscle (tendon)
22 足底方形筋 Quadratus plantae muscle
23 脛骨 Tibia
24 底側踵舟靱帯 Plantar calcaneonavicular ligament
25 足関節 Ankle joint (距腿関節 Talocrural joint)
26 短趾屈筋 Flexor digitorum brevis muscle
27 後脛骨筋 Tibialis posterior muscle
28 足底腱膜 Plantar aponeurosis
29 長母趾屈筋 Flexor hallucis longus muscle
30 外側足底動静脈, 神経 Lateral plantar artery, vein, and nerve
31 後距腓靱帯 Posterior talofibular ligament
32 小趾外転筋 Abductor digiti minimi muscle
33 アキレス腱(踵骨腱) Achilles tendon (calcaneal tendon)
34 距骨下関節 Subtalar joint
35 アキレス腱前脂肪体 Pre-Achilles fat body
36 踵骨 Calcaneus

390　下 肢

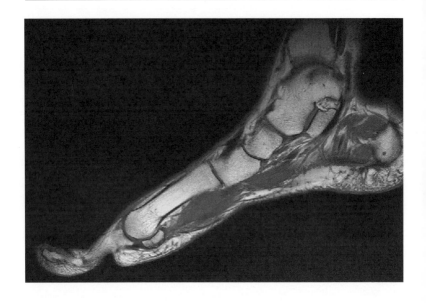

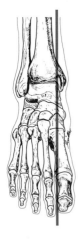

近位
足背側
前　　　後
遠位
足底側

足，矢状断   391

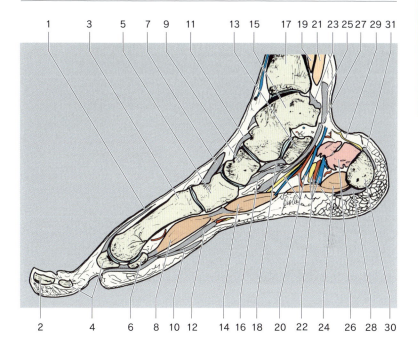

1 長母趾伸筋 Extensor hallucis longus muscle
2 第1末節骨 Distal phalanx I
3 第1中足骨 Metatarsal I
4 第1基節骨 Proximal phalanx I
5 内側楔状骨 Medial cuneiform
6 種子骨 Sesamoid bone
7 前脛骨筋 Tibialis anterior muscle
8 短母趾屈筋(外側頭) Flexor hallucis brevis muscle (lateral head)
9 舟状骨 Navicular
10 足底腱膜 Plantar aponeurosis
11 距舟靱帯 Talonavicular ligament
12 長母趾屈筋(腱) Flexor hallucis longus muscle (tendon)
13 踵骨 Calcaneus
14 短母趾屈筋(内側頭) Flexor hallucis brevis muscle (medial head)
15 距骨 Talus
16 後脛骨筋(腱) Tibialis posterior muscle (tendon)
17 脛骨 Tibia
18 ばね靱帯(底側踵舟靱帯) Spring ligament (plantar calcaneonavicular ligament)
19 後脛骨筋 Tibialis posterior muscle
20 内側足底動静脈,神経 Medial plantar artery, vein, and nerve
21 長趾屈筋(腱) Flexor digitorum longus muscle (tendon)
22 外側足底動静脈,神経 Lateral plantar artery, vein, and nerve
23 三角靱帯(後脛部) Deltoid ligament (posterior tibiotalar part)
24 母趾外転筋 Abductor hallucis muscle
25 長母趾屈筋(腱) Flexor hallucis longus muscle (tendon)
26 足底方形筋 Quadratus plantae muscle
27 長趾屈筋(腱) Flexor digitorum longus muscle (tendon)
28 足底腱膜 Plantar aponeurosis
29 踵骨動脈網 Calcaneal anastomosis
30 踵骨(踵骨隆起) Calcaneus (tuber)
31 アキレス腱(踵骨腱) Achilles tendon (calcaneal tendon)

392　下　肢

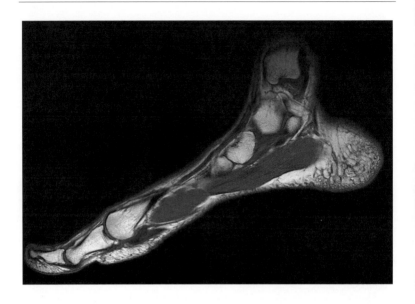

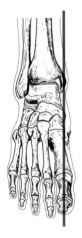

近位
足背側

前　　　後

遠位
足底側

足, 矢状断 393

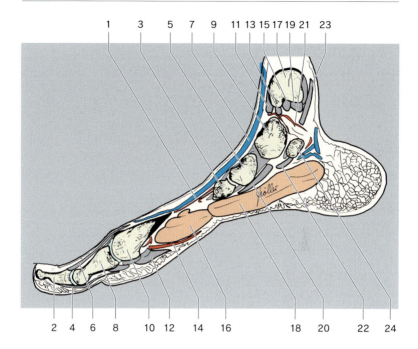

1 内側足根動脈 Medial tarsal arteries
2 第1末節骨 Distal phalanx I
3 内側楔状骨 Medial cuneiform
4 長母趾屈筋(腱) Flexor hallucis longus muscle (tendon)
5 舟状骨 Navicular
6 長母趾伸筋 Extensor hallucis longus muscle
7 足背静脈 Dorsalis pedis vein 大伏在静脈へ
8 第1基節骨 Proximal phalanx I
9 距骨 Talus
10 第1中足骨(頭) Metatarsal I (head)
11 三角靱帯(前脛距部) Deltoid ligament (anterior tibiotalar part)
12 足底腱膜 Plantar aponeurosis
13 三角靱帯(脛舟部) Deltoid ligament (tibionavicular part)
14 内側足底動脈・神経(浅枝) Medial plantar artery and nerve (superficial branch)
15 三角靱帯(脛踵部) Deltoid ligament (tibiocalcaneal part)
16 短母趾屈筋 Flexor hallucis brevis muscle
17 脛骨(内果) Tibia (medial malleolus)
18 母趾外転筋 Abductor hallucis muscle
19 三角靱帯(後脛距部) Deltoid ligament (posterior tibiotalar part)
20 後脛骨筋(腱) Tibialis posterior muscle (tendon)
21 後脛骨動脈 Posterior tibial artery (medial malleolar branches)
22 長母趾屈筋(腱) Flexor hallucis longus muscle (tendon)
23 長趾屈筋(腱) Flexor digitorum longus muscle (tendon)
24 踵骨 Calcaneus

色分けコード：脊椎　　*395*

- 動脈
- 神経
- 静脈
- 骨
- 脂肪組織
- 軟骨
- 腱
- 関節円板, 椎間板
- 液体, 脳脊髄液
- リンパ節
- 食道
- 肝臓, 腺
- 空気

脊柱起立筋（外側筋列）：
　腸肋筋
　最長筋
　頭板状筋, 頸板状筋
　横突間筋
　肋骨挙筋

脊柱起立筋（内側筋列）：
　棘筋系：
　　棘間筋
　　胸棘筋, 頸棘筋, 頭棘筋
　横突棘筋系：
　　長回旋筋, 短回旋筋
　　多裂筋
　　胸半棘筋, 頸半棘筋, 頭半棘筋

短い項筋：
　大後頭直筋, 後頭直筋
　上頭斜筋, 頭斜筋

頸部の椎前筋：
　頭長筋, 頸長筋
　外側頭直筋, 前頭直筋

胸郭の筋：
　外肋間筋, 内肋間筋, 最内肋間筋
　胸横筋
　肋下筋
　前斜角筋, 中斜角筋, 下斜角筋

体幹～上肢帯の筋：
　大菱形筋, 小菱形筋
　胸鎖乳突筋
　肩甲挙筋
　前鋸筋
　大胸筋, 小胸筋
　僧帽筋
　広背筋

体幹～下肢帯の筋：
　腰筋
　腰方形筋
　梨状筋
　中殿筋

顔面筋と前頸筋：
　顎二腹筋
　茎突舌骨筋
　胸骨舌骨筋

396 脊 椎

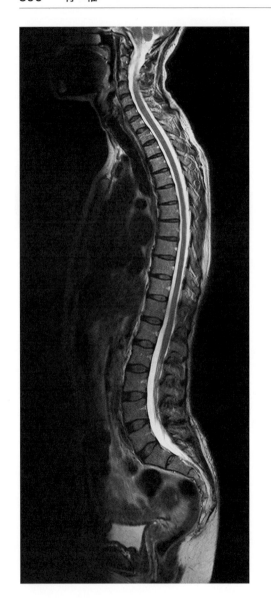

頭側
腹側 背側
尾側

脊椎，矢状断 397

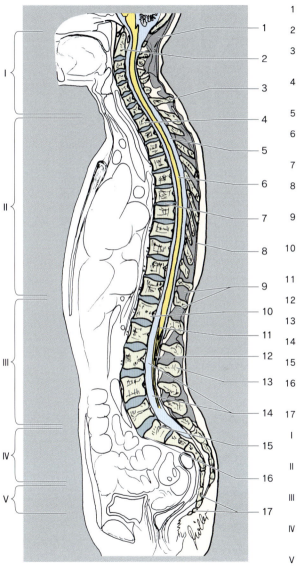

1 項靱帯 Nuchal ligament
2 軸椎歯突起, C2 Dens axis, C2
3 隆椎, C7 Vertebra prominens, C7
4 Th1椎体 Body of thoracic vertebra T1
5 脊柱管 Vertebral canal
6 胸髄 Thoracic spinal cord
7 椎間板 Intervertebral disk
8 棘上靱帯 Supraspinous ligament
9 棘間靱帯 Interspinous ligaments
10 L1椎体 Body of lumbar vertebra L1
11 脊髄円錐 Conus medullaris
12 馬尾 Cauda equina
13 棘突起 Spinous process
14 硬膜嚢 Thecal sac
15 仙骨(S1) Sacrum(S1)
16 仙骨の岬角 Promontory of sacrum
17 尾骨 Coccyx

I 頸椎(C1-7) Cervical vertebrae C1-7
II 胸椎(Th1-12) Thoracic vertebrae T1-12
III 腰椎(L1-5) Lumbar vertebrae L1-5
IV 仙骨(S1-5) Sacrum(sacral vertebrae 1-5)
V 尾骨(第1～3あるいは第1～4尾椎) Coccyx(coccygeal vertebrae 1-3 or 1-4)

398 脊 椎

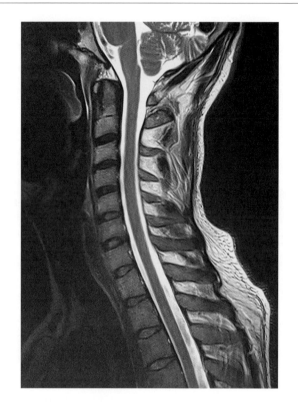

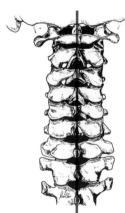

1 **大(後頭)孔** Foramen magnum
2 **僧帽筋(下行部)** Trapezius muscle (descending part)
3 **蓋膜** Tectorial membrane
4 **後頭骨(内後頭隆起)** Occipital bone (internal occipital protuberance)
5 **前環椎後頭膜** Anterior atlanto-occipital membrane
6 **頭半棘筋** Semispinalis capitis muscle
7 **歯尖靱帯** Apical ligament of dens

頸椎，矢状断

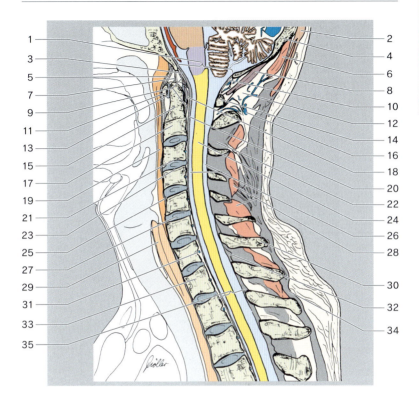

- 8 **小後頭直筋** Rectus capitis posterior minor muscle
- 9 **縦束** Longitudinal fasciculi
- 10 **後環椎後頭膜** Posterior atlanto-occipital membrane
- 11 **環椎(前弓)** Atlas (anterior arch)
- 12 **後頭下脂肪織** Suboccipital fatty tissue
- 13 **正中環軸関節** Median atlanto-axial joint
- 14 **環椎(後弓)** Atlas (posterior arch)
- 15 **軸椎(歯突起)** Axis (dens)
- 16 **深頸静脈** Deep cervical veins
- 17 **軸椎(椎体)** Axis (vertebral body)
- 18 **環椎横靱帯** Transverse ligament of atlas
- 19 **頭長筋** Longus capitis muscle
- 20 **後縦靱帯** Posterior longitudinal ligament
- 21 **C3椎体下面の終板** Inferior vertebral endplate C3
- 22 **棘間靱帯** Interspinous ligament
- 23 **C4椎体上面の終板** Superior vertebral endplate C4
- 24 **頸髄** Cervical spinal cord
- 25 **前縦靱帯** Anterior longitudinal ligament
- 26 **脊髄前方および後方のクモ膜下腔** Premedullary and postmedullary subarachnoid space
- 27 **椎間板** Intervertebral disk
- 28 **棘間筋** Interspinales muscles
- 29 **食道** Esophagus
- 30 **C7棘突起** Spinous process C7
- 31 **椎体静脈** Basivertebral veins
- 32 **黄色靱帯** Ligamentum flavum
- 33 **Th1椎体** Thoracic vertebral body T1
- 34 **棘上靱帯** Supraspinous ligament
- 35 **骨性脊柱管** Bony vertebral canal

400 脊 椎

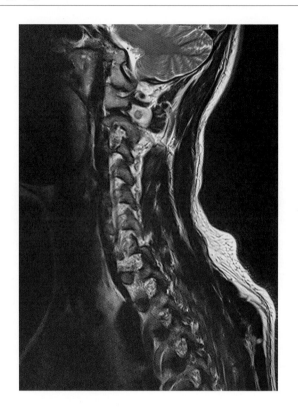

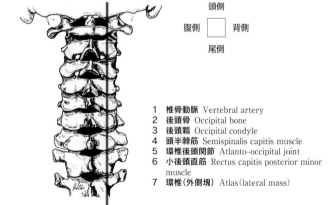

頭側

腹側 □ 背側

尾側

1 **椎骨動脈** Vertebral artery
2 **後頭骨** Occipital bone
3 **後頭顆** Occipital condyle
4 **頭半棘筋** Semispinalis capitis muscle
5 **環椎後頭関節** Atlanto–occipital joint
6 **小後頭直筋** Rectus capitis posterior minor muscle
7 **環椎(外側塊)** Atlas (lateral mass)

頸椎，矢状断　　401

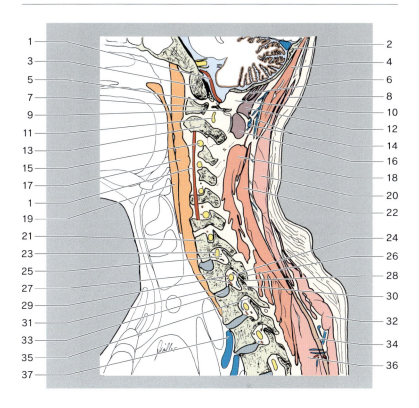

8	僧帽筋（下行部）Trapezius muscle (descending part)
9	環椎（後弓）Atlas (posterior arch)
10	後頭下脂肪織 Suboccipital fatty tissue
11	第2頸神経 Spinal nerve C2
12	大後頭直筋 Rectus capitis posterior major muscle
13	軸椎（椎体）Axis (body)
14	深頸静脈 Deep cervical veins
15	第3頸神経の脊髄神経節 Spinal ganglion C3
16	下頭斜筋 Obliquus capitis inferior muscle
17	頭長筋 Longus capitis muscle
18	頸棘筋 Spinalis cervicis muscle, 多裂筋 Multifidus muscle
19	口蓋咽頭筋 Palatopharyngeus muscle
20	頭板状筋 Splenius capitis muscle
21	C7椎体 Body of cervical vertebra C7
22	頸半棘筋 Semispinalis cervicis muscle
23	第8頸神経の脊髄神経節 Spinal ganglion C8
24	第1胸神経の脊髄神経節 Spinal ganglion T1
25	椎間孔 Intervertebral foramen
26	下関節突起 Inferior articular process
27	Th1椎体 First thoracic vertebral body
28	椎間関節 Zygapophyseal joint
29	肋間動脈（背枝の脊髄枝, 根枝）Posterior intercostal artery (spinal and radicular branches of dorsal branch)
30	上関節突起 Superior articular process
31	頸長筋 Longus colli muscle
32	僧帽筋（横行部）Trapezius muscle (transverse part)
33	椎間板 Intervertebral disk
34	菱形筋 Rhomboid muscle
35	黄色靱帯 Ligamentum flavum
36	頸板状筋 Splenius cervicis muscle
37	肋間静脈 Posterior intercostal vein

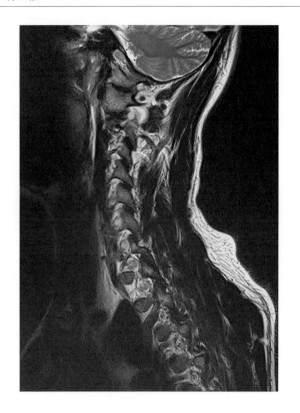

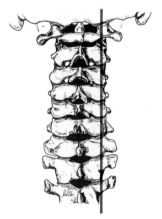

頭側

腹側 □ 背側

尾側

頸椎，矢状断　　403

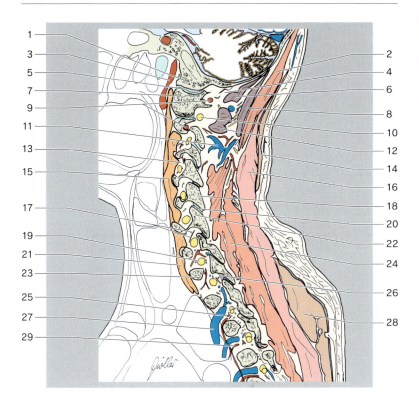

1　後頭顆　Occipital condyle
2　頭半棘筋　Semispinalis capitis muscle
3　内頸動脈　Internal carotid artery
4　後頭下脂肪織　Suboccipital fatty tissue
5　環椎後頭関節　Atlanto-occipital joint
6　小後頭直筋　Rectus capitis posterior minor muscle
7　環椎（外側塊）　Atlas (lateral mass)
8　大後頭直筋　Rectus capitis posterior major muscle
9　椎骨動脈　Vertebral artery
10　第2頸神経　Spinal nerve C2
11　深頸静脈　Deep cervical veins
12　下頭斜筋　Obliquus capitis inferior muscle
13　椎間孔　Intervertebral foramen
14　僧帽筋（下行部）　Trapezius muscle (descending part)
15　頭長筋　Longus capitis muscle
16　頭板状筋　Splenius capitis muscle
17　椎骨動脈（脊髄枝，根枝）　Vertebral artery (spinal and radicular branches)
18　下関節突起　Inferior articular process
19　第8頸神経の脊髄神経節　Spinal ganglion C8
20　椎間関節　Zygapophyseal joint
21　頸長筋　Longus colli muscle
22　上関節突起　Superior articular process
23　Th1椎体　First thoracic vertebral body
24　頸棘筋　Spinalis cervicis muscle, 多裂筋　Multifidus muscle
25　肋間動脈（背枝の脊髄枝，根枝）　Posterior intercostal artery (spinal and radicular branches of dorsal branch)
26　黄色靱帯　Ligamentum flavum
27　肋間静脈　Posterior intercostal vein
28　僧帽筋（横行部）　Trapezius muscle (transverse part)
29　肋間動脈（背枝）　Posterior intercostal artery (dorsal branch)

404　脊椎

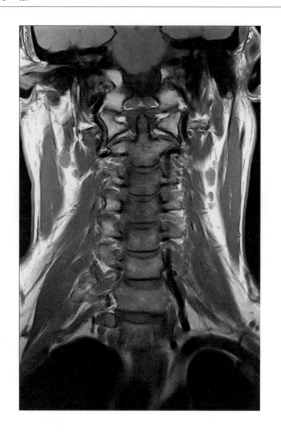

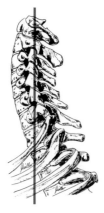

頭側
右　□　左
尾側

1　**外耳道** External auditory canal
2　**茎乳突孔** Stylomastoid foramen
3　**椎骨静脈** Vertebral vein
4　**内頸静脈** Internal jugular vein
5　**後頭顆** Occipital condyle
6　**乳様突起** Mastoid process
7　**耳下腺** Parotid gland

頸椎，冠状断

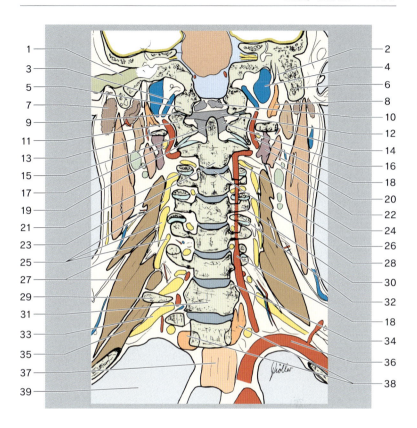

8	外側頭直筋 Rectus capitis lateralis muscle	24	第3頸神経の脊髄神経節 Spinal ganglion C3
9	環椎後頭関節 Atlanto-occipital joint	25	頸神経叢 Cervical plexus
10	蓋膜 Tectorial membrane	26	胸鎖乳突筋 Sternocleidomastoid muscle
11	環椎（外側塊）Atlas (lateral mass)	27	中斜角筋 Scalenus medius muscle
12	横靱帯 Transverse ligament	28	C2/3椎間板 Intervertebral disk (C2/C3)
13	環椎（横突起）Atlas (transverse process)	29	C7横突起 Transverse process C7
14	顎二腹筋（後腹）Digastric muscle (posterior belly)	30	C4上関節突起 Superior articular process C4
15	軸椎（歯突起）Axis (dens)	31	C7椎体 cervical vertebral body C7
16	翼状靱帯 Alar ligaments	32	下関節突起 Inferior articular process
17	第2頸神経 Spinal nerve C2	33	第8頸神経 Spinal nerve C8
18	椎骨動脈 Vertebral artery	34	C7鈎状突起 Uncinate process C7
19	外側環軸関節 Lateral atlantoaxial joint	35	後斜角筋 Scalenus posterior muscle
20	下頭斜筋 Obliquus capitis inferior muscle	36	鎖骨下動脈 Subclavian artery
21	椎間関節 Zygapophyseal joint	37	食道 Esophagus
22	肩甲挙筋 Levator scapulae muscle	38	頸長筋 Longus colli muscle
23	軸椎（椎体）Axis (vertebral body)	39	肺 Lung

406 脊椎

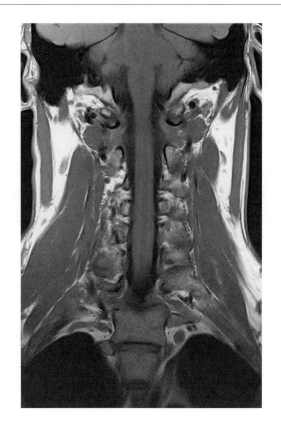

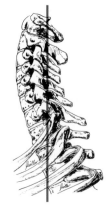

頭側
右 □ 左
尾側

1 延髄 Medulla oblongata
2 S状静脈洞 Sigmoid sinus
3 乳様突起 Mastoid process
4 大(後頭)孔 Foramen magnum
5 椎骨動脈 Vertebral artery
6 頭板状筋 Splenius capitis muscle

頸椎, 冠状断

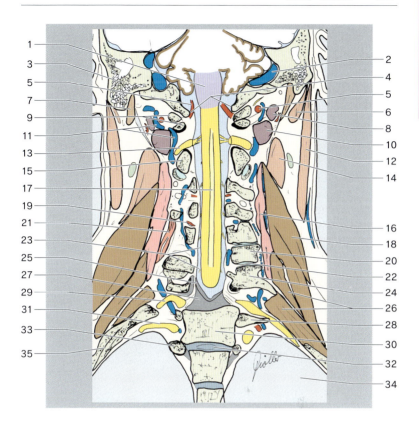

- 7 顎二腹筋（後腹）Digastric muscle (posterior belly)
- 8 上頭斜筋 Obliquus capitis superior muscle
- 9 環椎（後弓）Atlas (posterior arch)
- 10 下頭斜筋 Obliquus capitis inferior muscle
- 11 椎骨動脈 Vertebral artery
- 12 胸鎖乳突筋 Sternocleidomastoid muscle
- 13 第2頸神経の脊髄神経節 Spinal ganglion C2
- 14 肩甲挙筋 Levator scapulae muscle
- 15 軸椎（椎弓）Axis (vertebral arch)
- 16 頭板状筋 Splenius cervicis muscle
- 17 脊髄（中心管を伴う頸髄）Spinal cord (cervical pulp with central canal)
- 18 中斜角筋 Scalenus medius muscle
- 19 椎骨動脈（脊髄枝,根枝）Vertebral artery (spinal and radicular branches)
- 20 C6下関節突起 Inferior articular process C6
- 21 頸半棘筋 Semispinalis cervicis muscle
- 22 椎間関節 Zygapophyseal joint
- 23 脊柱管内の脳脊髄液 Cerebrospinal fluid in spinal canal
- 24 C7上関節突起 Superior articular process C7
- 25 脊髄硬膜 Spinal dura mater
- 26 後斜角筋 Scalenus posterior muscle
- 27 後縦靱帯 Posterior longitudinal ligament
- 28 第1肋骨（頸）First rib (neck)
- 29 第8頸神経 Spinal nerve C8
- 30 Th1椎体 Thoracic vertebral body T1
- 31 第1胸神経 Spinal nerve T1
- 32 椎間板 Intervertebral disk
- 33 第2肋骨（頭）Second rib (head)
- 34 左肺 Left lung
- 35 第1肋骨（体）First rib (body)

408　脊 椎

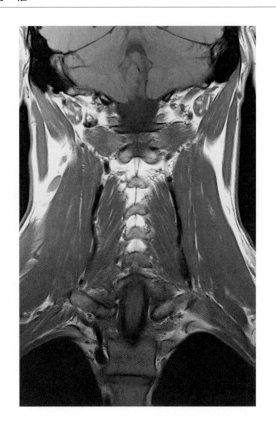

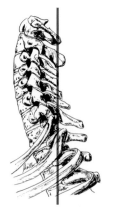

頭側
右　□　左
尾側

頸椎，冠状断

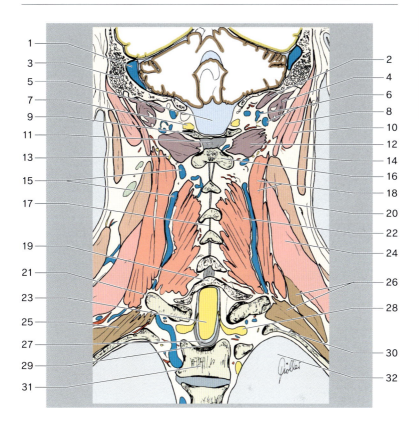

1. S状静脈洞 Sigmoid sinus
2. 大後頭直筋 Rectus capitis posterior major muscle
3. 乳様突起 Mastoid process
4. 上頭斜筋 Obliquus capitis superior muscle
5. 大槽 Cisterna magna
6. 後頭下静脈叢 Suboccipital venous plexus
7. 後頭下神経 Suboccipital nerve
8. 頭最長筋 Longissimus capitis muscle
9. 環椎(後弓) Atlas (posterior arch)
10. 頭板状筋 Splenius capitis muscle
11. 項靱帯 Nuchal ligament
12. 下頭斜筋 Obliquus capitis inferior muscle
13. 大後頭神経 Major occipital nerve
14. 胸鎖乳突筋 Sternocleidomastoid muscle
15. 深頸静脈 Deep cervical vein
16. C2棘突起 Spinous process C2
17. 棘間靱帯 Interspinous ligament
18. 頸半棘筋 Semispinalis cervicis muscle
19. C7椎弓 Vertebral arch C7
20. 肩甲挙筋 Levator scapulae muscle
21. 第1肋骨(頭,結節) First rib (neck and tubercle)
22. 頸棘筋 Spinalis cervicis muscle, 多裂筋 Multifidus muscle
23. 胸髄 Thoracic spinal cord
24. 頸板状筋 Splenius cervicis muscle
25. 肋間筋 Intercostal muscles
26. 後斜角筋 Scalenus posterior muscle
27. 脊柱管内の脳脊髄液 Cerebrospinal fluid in vertebral canal
28. 第1胸神経の脊髄神経節 Spinal ganglion T1
29. 脊髄硬膜 Spinal dura mater, 後縦靱帯 Posterior longitudinal ligament
30. 第2肋骨 Second rib
31. Th2椎体 Second thoracic vertebral body
32. 左肺 Left lung

410　脊　椎

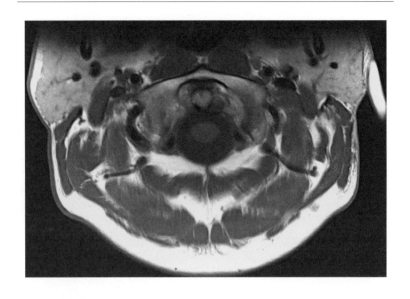

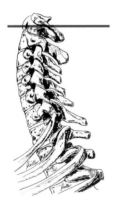

腹側

右　□　左

背側

頸椎，軸位断　　411

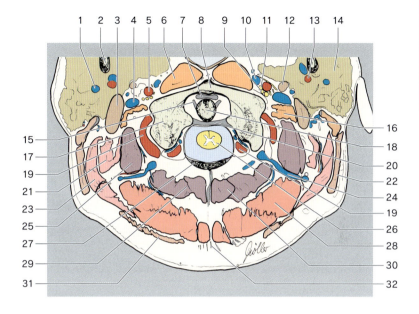

1 下顎後静脈 Retromandibular vein
2 下顎骨 Mandible
3 顎二腹筋（後腹）Digastric muscle (posterior belly)
4 内頸静脈 Internal jugular vein
5 内頸動脈 Internal carotid artery
6 頭長筋 Longus capitis muscle
7 正中環軸関節 Median atlantoaxial joint
8 環椎（前弓）Atlas (anterior arch)
9 舌下神経（第XII脳神経）Hypoglossal nerve (XII)
10 翼突筋静脈叢 Pterygoid venous plexus
11 迷走神経（第X脳神経）Vagus nerve (X)
12 茎突舌骨筋 Stylohyoid muscle
13 顎動脈（下顎部）Maxillary artery (mandibular part)
14 耳下腺 Parotid gland
15 翼状靱帯 Alar ligaments
16 外側頭直筋 Rectus capitis lateralis muscle
17 環椎（外側塊）Atlas (lateral mass)
18 軸椎（歯突起）Axis (dens)
19 椎骨動脈 Vertebral artery
20 環椎十字靱帯（縦束中央部）Cruciate ligament of atlas (longitudinal bands [=central part]), 環椎横靱帯（縦束外側部）transverse ligament of atlas [=lateral part]
21 頭最長筋 Longissimus capitis muscle
22 胸鎖乳突筋 Sternocleidomastoid muscle
23 頭板状筋 Splenius capitis muscle
24 深頸静脈 Deep cervical vein
25 上頭斜筋 Obliquus capitis superior muscle
26 脊髄 Spinal cord
27 環椎（後弓）Atlas (posterior arch)
28 頭半棘筋 Semispinalis capitis muscle
29 大後頭直筋 Rectus capitis posterior major muscle
30 小後頭直筋 Rectus capitis posterior minor muscle
31 僧帽筋 Trapezius muscle
32 項靱帯 Nuchal ligament

412 脊 椎

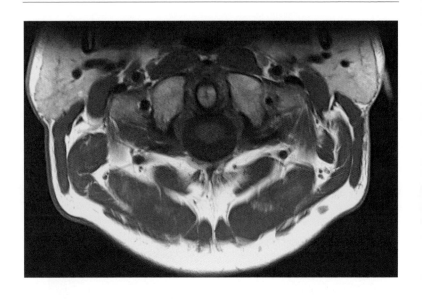

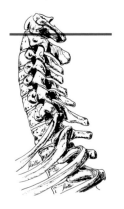

腹側
右 □ 左
背側

頸椎，軸位断

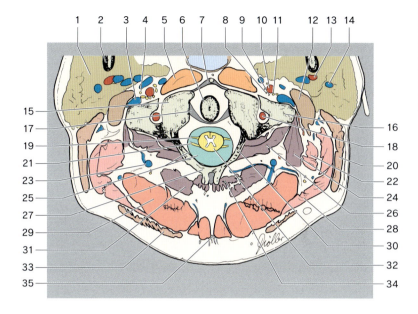

1 耳下腺 Parotid gland
2 下顎骨（下顎枝）Mandible(ramus)
3 内頸静脈 Internal jugular vein
4 舌咽神経（第Ⅸ脳神経）Glossopharyngeal nerve(Ⅸ)
5 頭長筋 Longus capitis muscle
6 軸椎（歯突起）Axis(dens)
7 前縦靭帯 Anterior longitudinal ligament
8 迷走神経（第Ⅹ脳神経）Vagus nerve(Ⅹ)
9 舌下神経（第Ⅻ脳神経）Hypoglossal nerve (Ⅻ)
10 内頸動脈 Internal carotid artery
11 副神経（第Ⅺ脳神経）Accessory nerve(Ⅺ)
12 顎二腹筋（後腹）Digastric muscle(posterior belly)
13 顎動脈（下顎部）Maxillary artery(mandibular part)
14 下顎後静脈 Retromandibular vein
15 環椎（外側塊）Atlas(lateral mass)
16 環椎（横突起）Atlas(transverse process)
17 環椎横靭帯 Transverse ligament of atlas
18 椎骨動脈 Vertebral artery
19 前根 Ventral root
20 胸鎖乳突筋 Sternocleidomastoid muscle
21 後根 Dorsal root
22 頭最長筋 Longissimus capitis muscle
23 深頸静脈 Deep cervical vein
24 上頭斜筋 Obliquus capitis superior muscle
25 硬膜 Dura mater, 脳脊髄液（クモ膜下腔）Cerebrospinal fluid (subarachnoid space)
26 下頭斜筋 Obliquus capitis inferior muscle
27 棘突起 Spinous process
28 頭板状筋 Splenius capitis muscle
29 頭半棘筋 Semispinalis capitis muscle
30 軸椎（後弓）Axis(posterior arch)
31 大後頭直筋 Rectus capitis posterior major muscle
32 脊髄 Spinal cord
33 僧帽筋 Trapezius muscle
34 小後頭直筋 Rectus capitis posterior minor muscle
35 項靭帯 Nuchal ligament

414 脊 椎

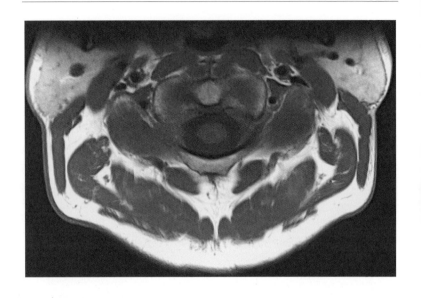

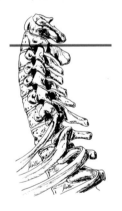

腹側
右 □ 左
背側

頸椎，軸位断

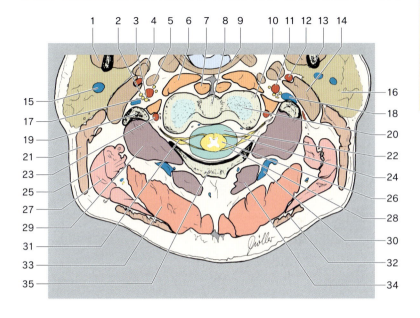

1 内側翼突筋 Medial pterygoid muscle
2 迷走神経（第X脳神経）Vagus nerve(X)
3 副神経（第XI脳神経）Accessory nerve(XI)
4 茎突舌骨筋 Styloglossus muscle
5 茎突咽頭筋 Stylopharyngeus muscle
6 頭長筋 Longus capitis muscle
7 頸長筋 Longus colli muscle
8 軸椎（椎体）Axis(body)
9 上咽頭収縮筋 Superior constrictor muscle of pharynx
10 環椎（関節突起）Atlas(articular process)
11 内頸動脈 Internal carotid artery
12 外頸動脈 External carotid artery
13 下顎骨（下顎枝）Mandible(ramus)
14 顎二腹筋（後腹）Digastric muscle(posterior belly)
15 下顎後静脈 Retromandibular vein
16 耳下腺 Parotid gland
17 舌下神経（第XII脳神経）Hypoglossal nerve(XII)
18 内頸静脈 Internal jugular vein
19 環椎（横突起）Atlas(transverse process)
20 軸椎（椎体）Axis(body)
21 胸鎖乳突筋 Sternocleidomastoid muscle
22 脊髄前方のクモ膜下腔 Premedullary subarachnoid space
23 椎骨動脈 Vertebral artery
24 第2頸神経の前根 Ventral root C2
25 頭最長筋 Longissimus capitis muscle
26 脊髄 Spinal cord
27 頭板状筋 Splenius capitis muscle
28 第2頸神経の後根 Dorsal root C2
29 下頭斜筋 Obliquus capitis inferior muscle
30 深頸静脈 Deep cervical vein
31 脊髄神経節（神経根）Spinal ganglion(nerve root)
32 僧帽筋 Trapezius muscle
33 頭半棘筋 Semispinalis capitis muscle
34 大後頭直筋 Rectus capitis posterior major muscle
35 軸椎（後弓）Axis(posterior arch)

416 脊 椎

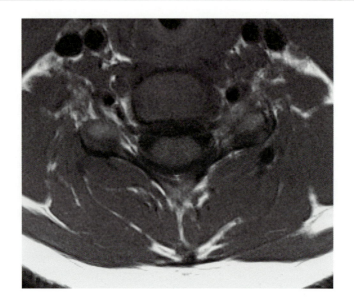

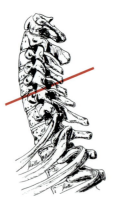

腹側
右 □ 左
背側

頸椎，軸位断

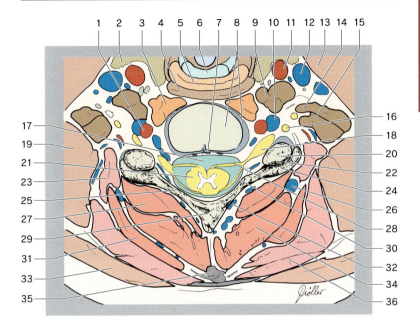

1 椎骨動脈 Vertebral artery
2 甲状腺 Thyroid gland
3 頸長筋 Longus colli muscle
4 上咽頭収縮筋 Superior constrictor muscle of pharynx
5 食道 Esophagus
6 輪状軟骨 Cricoid cartilage
7 椎体静脈 Basivertebral veins
8 C5椎体 Cervical vertebral body C5, C5/6椎間板 intervertebral space C5/C6
9 前斜角筋 Scalenus anterior muscle
10 椎骨静脈 Vertebral vein
11 総頸動脈 Common carotid artery
12 内頸静脈 Internal jugular vein
13 胸鎖乳突筋 Sternocleidomastoid muscle
14 中斜角筋 Scalenus medius muscle
15 後斜角筋 Scalenus posterior muscle
16 第5頸神経 Spinal nerve C5
17 脊髄前方のクモ膜下腔 Premedullary subarachnoid space
18 脊髄神経節(神経根) Spinal ganglion (nerve root)
19 肩甲挙筋 Levator scapulae muscle
20 上関節突起 Superior articular process
21 脊髄 Spinal cord
22 椎間関節 Zygapophyseal joint
23 頸最長筋 Longissimus cervicis muscle
24 下関節突起 Inferior articular process
25 C5椎弓(椎弓板) Vertebral arch C5 (lamina)
26 深頸静脈 Deep cervical vein
27 頸棘筋 Spinalis cervicis muscle, 多裂筋 Multifidus muscle
28 第6頸神経の前根 Ventral root C6
29 棘突起 Spinous process
30 第6頸神経の後根 Dorsal root C6
31 頭半棘筋 Semispinalis capitis muscle
32 後外椎骨静脈叢 Posterior external vertebral venous plexus
33 僧帽筋 Trapezius muscle
34 頸半棘筋 Semispinalis cervicis muscle
35 項靱帯 Nuchal ligament
36 頭板状筋 Splenius capitis muscle

418　脊椎

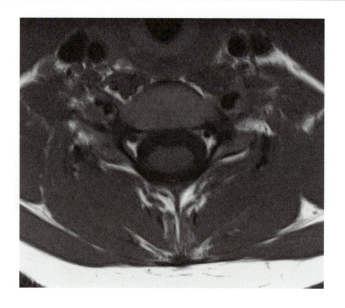

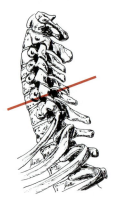

腹側
右 □ 左
背側

頸椎，軸位断

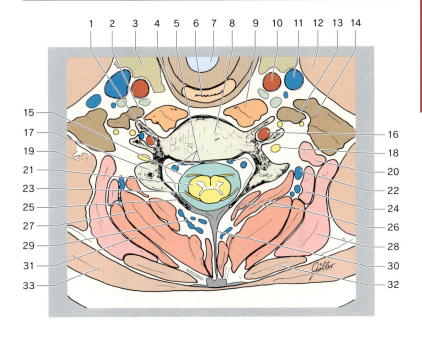

1 横突起 Transverse process
2 椎弓根 Pedicle of vertebral arch
3 甲状腺 Thyroid gland
4 上咽頭収縮筋 Superior constrictor muscle of pharynx
5 前内椎骨静脈叢 Anterior internal vertebral venous plexus
6 食道 Esophagus
7 喉頭 Larynx
8 C6椎体 Cervical vertebral body C6
9 頸長筋 Longus colli muscle
10 総頸動脈 Common carotid artery
11 内頸静脈 Internal jugular vein
12 胸鎖乳突筋 Sternocleidomastoid muscle
13 前斜角筋 Scalenus anterior muscle
14 中斜角筋 Scalenus medius muscle
15 第7頸神経の前根 Ventral root C7
16 椎骨動脈 Vertebral artery
17 関節突起 Articular process
18 第6頸神経 Spinal nerve C6
19 肩甲挙筋 Levator scapulae muscle
20 頭最長筋 Longissimus capitis muscle
21 脊髄 Spinal cord
22 深頸静脈 Deep cervical vein
23 第7頸神経の後根 Dorsal root C7
24 頸最長筋 Longissimus cervicis muscle
25 C6椎弓（椎弓板） Vertebral arch C6 (lamina)
26 頸棘筋 Spinalis cervicis muscle, 多裂筋 Multifidus muscle
27 頸半棘筋 Semispinalis cervicis muscle
28 頸板状筋 Splenius cervicis muscle
29 後外椎骨静脈叢 Posterior external vertebral venous plexus
30 項靱帯 Nuchal ligament
31 頭板状筋 Splenius capitis muscle
32 小菱形筋 Rhomboid minor muscle
33 僧帽筋 Trapezius muscle

420　脊 椎

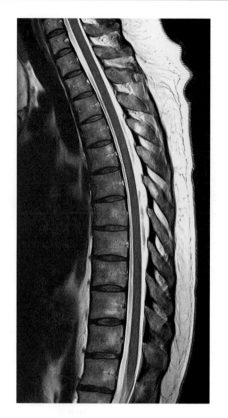

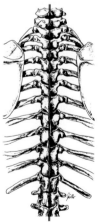

頭側
腹側　□　背側
尾側

胸椎, 矢状断 421

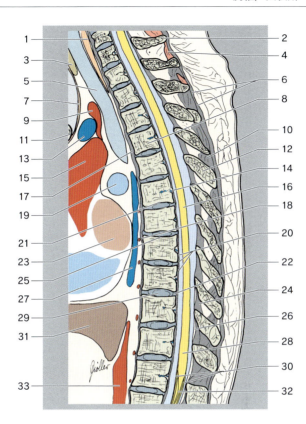

1. 食道 Esophagus
2. 隆椎 C7 Vertebra prominens C7
3. 甲状腺 Thyroid gland
4. 頸棘間筋 Interspinales cervicis muscles
5. 気管 Trachea
6. 棘上靱帯 Supraspinous ligament
7. 胸骨舌骨筋 Sternohyoid muscle
8. Th4椎体 Thoracic vertebral body T4
9. 腕頭動脈 Brachiocephalic trunk
10. 棘間靱帯 Interspinous ligament
11. 胸骨(柄) Sternum(manubrium)
12. 棘突起 Spinous process
13. 左腕頭静脈 Left brachiocephalic vein
14. 椎体静脈 Basivertebral vein
15. 上行大動脈 Ascending aorta
16. 胸髄 Thoracic spinal cord
17. 前縦靱帯 Anterior longitudinal ligament
18. 肋間動脈 Posterior intercostal artery
19. 肺動脈 Pulmonary artery
20. 後縦靱帯 Posterior longitudinal ligament
21. 第6胸椎下縁の終板 Inferior vertebral endplate T6
22. Th9/10椎間板(線維輪) Intervertebral disk T9-10 (anulus fibrosus)
23. 左心房 Left atrium
24. 黄色靱帯 Ligamentum flavum
25. 第7胸椎上縁の終板 Superior vertebral endplate T7
26. 硬膜外脂肪織 Epidural fatty tissue (retrospinal fat)
27. 奇静脈 Azygos vein
28. 脊髄円錐 Conus medullaris
29. Th9/10椎間板(髄核) Intervertebral disk T9-10 (nucleus pulposus)
30. 馬尾 Cauda equina
31. 肝臓 Liver
32. 終糸 Filum terminale
33. 下行大動脈 Descending aorta

422 脊椎

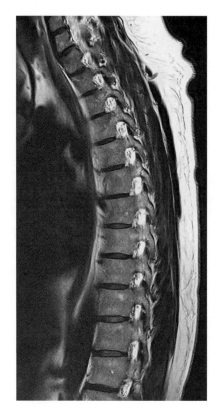

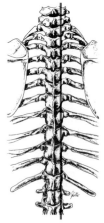

頭側

腹側 □ 背側

尾側

1 気管 Trachea
2 頸板状筋 Splenius cervicis muscle
3 甲状腺 Thyroid gland
4 頭半棘筋 Semispinalis capitis muscle
5 胸骨舌骨筋 Sternohyoid muscle
6 上後鋸筋 Serratus posterior superior muscle
7 食道 Esophagus
8 大菱形筋 Rhomboid major muscle

胸椎，矢状断

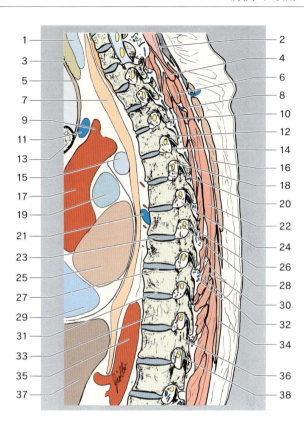

- 9 腕頭動脈 Brachiocephalic trunk
- 10 Th3/4椎間関節 Zygapophyseal joint T3-4
- 11 左腕頭静脈 Left brachiocephalic vein
- 12 Th4下関節突起 Inferior articular process T4
- 13 胸骨（柄）Sternum (manubrium)
- 14 Th5上関節突起 Superior articular process T5
- 15 左主気管支 Left main bronchus
- 16 僧帽筋 Trapezius muscle
- 17 上行大動脈 Ascending aorta
- 18 肋間動脈（脊髄枝）Posterior intercostal artery (spinal branch)
- 19 肺動脈 Pulmonary artery
- 20 椎間静脈 Intervertebral vein
- 21 半奇静脈 Hemiazygos vein
- 22 脊柱起立筋 Erector spinae muscle
- 23 Th7/8椎間板 Intervertebral disk T7-8
- 24 椎間孔 Intervertebral foramen
- 25 左心房 Left atrium
- 26 脊髄神経節（後根）Spinal ganglion (dorsal root)
- 27 Th9椎体上面の終板 Superior vertebral endplate T9
- 28 脊髄神経節（前根）Spinal ganglion (ventral root)
- 29 右心室 Right atrium
- 30 多裂筋 Multifidus muscle, 胸半棘筋 Semispinalis thoracis muscle
- 31 Th9椎体下面の終板 Inferior vertebral endplate T9
- 32 後外椎骨静脈叢 Posterior external vertebral venous plexus
- 33 Th10椎体 Thoracic vertebral body T10
- 34 広背筋 Latissimus dorsi muscle
- 35 下行大動脈 Descending aorta
- 36 椎弓根（関節突起間部）Pedicle of vertebral arch (interarticular portion)
- 37 肝臓 Liver
- 38 黄色靱帯 Ligamentum flavum

424 脊 椎

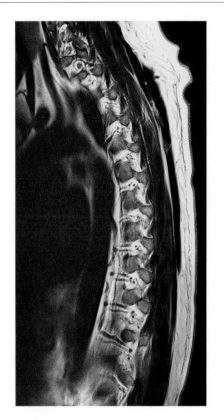

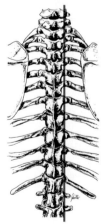

頭側

腹側 □ 背側

尾側

1 **甲状腺** Thyroid gland
2 **頸板状筋** Splenius cervicis muscle
3 **頭長筋** Longus capitis muscle
4 **頸棘筋** Spinalis cervicis muscle,
  多裂筋 Multifidus muscle

胸椎，矢状断 425

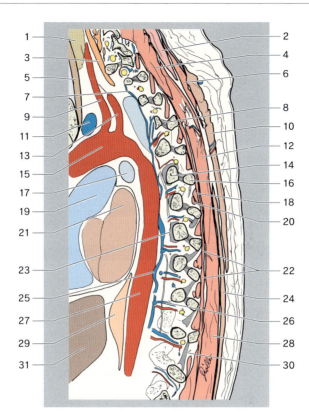

5 胸骨舌骨筋 Sternohyoid muscle
6 大菱形筋 Rhomboid major muscle
7 副半奇静脈 Accessory hemiazygos vein
8 肋横突靱帯 Costotransverse ligament
9 総頸動脈 Common carotid artery
10 僧帽筋 Trapezius muscle
11 左腕頭静脈 Left brachiocephalic vein
12 胸棘筋 Spinalis thoracis muscle
13 鎖骨下動脈 Subclavian artery
14 第6肋骨(頭) Sixth rib (head)
15 大動脈弓 Aortic arch
16 Th6横突起 Transverse process T6
17 左主気管支 Left main bronchus
18 横突間筋 Intertransversarius muscle
19 肺動脈幹 Pulmonary trunk
20 回旋筋 Rotatores muscles
21 左心房 Left atrium
22 多裂筋 Multifidus muscle
23 第8肋骨の放射状肋骨頭靱帯 Radiate ligament of head of rib T8
24 広背筋 Latissimus dorsi muscle
25 半奇静脈 Hemiazygos vein
26 肋間動静脈(背枝) Posterior intercostal artery and vein (dorsal branch)
27 下行大動脈 Descending aorta
28 脊柱起立筋 Erector spinae muscle
29 食道 Esophagus
30 上肋横突靱帯 Superior costotransverse ligament
31 肝臓 Liver

426　脊 椎

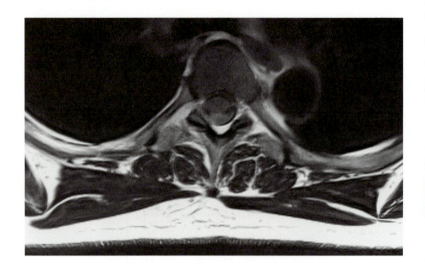

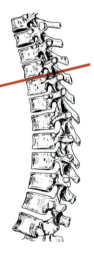

腹側
右 □ 左
背側

胸椎，軸位断 **427**

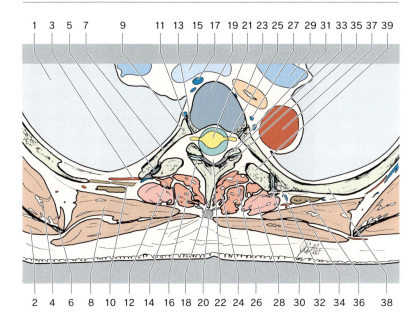

1 右肺 Right lung
2 棘下筋 Infraspinatus muscle
3 肋間動脈 Intercostal artery
4 肩甲下筋 Subscapularis muscle
5 肋横突関節 Costotransverse joint
6 肩甲骨 Scapula
7 肋骨(頸) Rib(neck)
8 大菱形筋 Rhomboid major muscle
9 第5肋骨(頭) Fifth rib(head)
10 肋間筋 Intercostal muscles
11 放射状肋骨頭靱帯 Radiate ligament of head of rib
12 胸回旋筋 Rotatores thoracis muscles
13 肋骨頭関節 Joint of head of rib
14 胸半棘筋 Semispinalis thoracis muscle
15 気管(分岐部) Trachea(bifurcation)
16 Th4/5椎間関節 Zygapophyseal joint T4-5
17 奇静脈 Azygos vein
18 棘突起 Spinous process
19 Th4/5椎間板 Intervertebral disk T4-5
20 棘上靱帯 Supraspinous ligament
21 胸髄 Thoracic spinal cord
22 脊髄後方の脂肪三角(硬膜外脂肪) Retrospinal fatty triangle(epidural fat)
23 食道 Esophagus
24 胸棘筋 Spinalis thoracis muscle
25 脊髄神経節 Spinal ganglion
26 多裂筋 Multifidus muscle
27 副半奇静脈 Accessory hemiazygos vein
28 胸最長筋 Longissimus thoracis muscle
29 左肺動脈 Left pulmonary artery
30 (外側)肋横突靱帯 Costotransverse ligament (lateral)
31 黄色靱帯 Ligamentum flavum
32 第5肋骨(結節) Fifth rib(tubercle)
33 Th5上関節突起 Superior articular process T5
34 僧帽筋 Trapezius muscle
35 Th4下関節突起 Inferior articular process T4
36 胸腸肋筋 Iliocostalis thoracis muscle
37 下行大動脈 Descending aorta
38 第5肋骨(体) Fifth rib(body)
39 Th5横突起 Transverse process T5

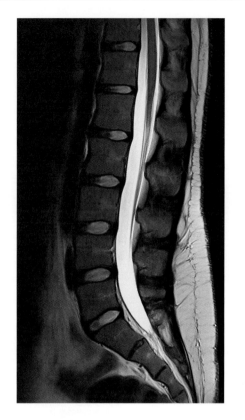

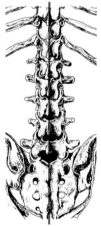

頭側
腹側　　背側
尾側

腰椎，矢状断 **429**

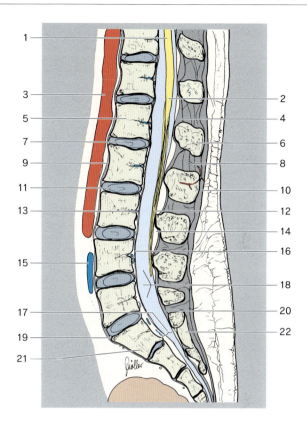

1 脊髄 Spinal cord
2 脊髄円錐 Conus medullaris
3 腹部大動脈 Abdominal aorta
4 黄色靱帯 Ligamentum flavum
5 L1椎体 lumbar vertebral body L1
6 L1棘突起 Spinous process L1
7 L1/2椎間板(髄核) Intervertebral disk L1-2 (nucleus pulposus)
8 棘間靱帯 Interspinous ligament
9 前縦靱帯 Anterior longitudinal ligament
10 棘上靱帯 Supraspinous ligament
11 L2/3椎間板(線維輪) Intervertebral disk L2-3 (annulus fibrosus)
12 馬尾 Cauda equina
13 椎体静脈 Basivertebral vein
14 硬膜外脂肪織 Epidural fatty tissue
15 左総腸骨静脈 Left common iliac vein
16 後縦靱帯 Posterior longitudinal ligament
17 仙骨管 Sacral canal
18 硬膜嚢(腰椎槽) Thecal sac (lumbar cistern)
19 仙骨の岬角 Promontory of sacrum
20 硬膜 Dura mater
21 仙骨(S1) Sacrum (S1)
22 正中仙骨稜 Median sacral crest

430　脊椎

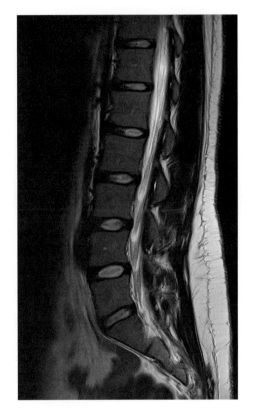

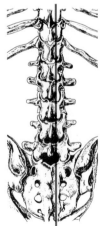

頭側

腹側　　背側

尾側

腰椎，矢状断　　431

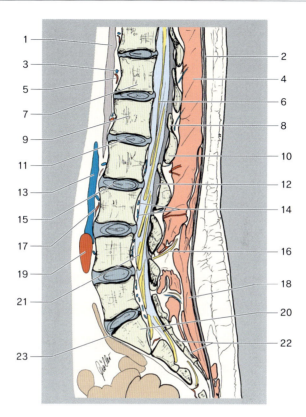

1　横隔膜（腰椎部）Diaphragm (lumbar part)
2　胸腰筋膜　Thoracolumbar fascia
3　前外椎骨静脈叢　Anterior external vertebral venous plexus
4　脊柱起立筋（棘筋）Erector spinae muscle (spinalis muscle)
5　肋間動脈　Posterior intercostal artery
6　神経線維　Nerve filaments
7　Th12椎体　Thoracic vertebral body T12
8　上関節突起　Superior articular process
9　L1椎体　Lumbar vertebral body L1
10　椎弓（椎弓板）Vertebral arch (lamina)
11　L1/2椎間板（髄核）Intervertebral disk L1-2 (nucleus pulposus)
12　黄色靱帯　Ligamentum flavum
13　下大静脈　Inferior vena cava
14　前内椎骨静脈叢　Anterior internal vertebral venous plexus
15　L2/3椎間板（線維輪）Intervertebral disk L2-3 (anulus fibrosus)
16　腰動静脈，神経（背枝の内側皮枝）Lumbar artery and nerve (medial cutaneous branch of dorsal branch)
17　腰動脈　Lumbar artery
18　多裂筋　Multifidus muscle
19　総腸骨動脈　Common iliac artery
20　仙骨（S1）Sacrum (S1)
21　脊髄神経節　Spinal ganglion
22　正中仙骨稜　Median sacral crest
23　仙骨の岬角　Promontory of sacrum

432 脊 椎

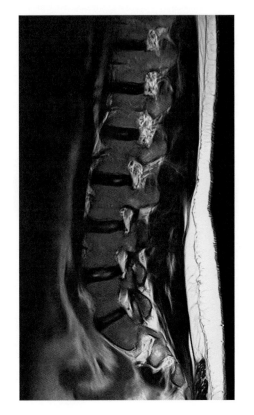

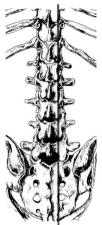

頭側
腹側 　 背側
尾側

腰椎，矢状断　　433

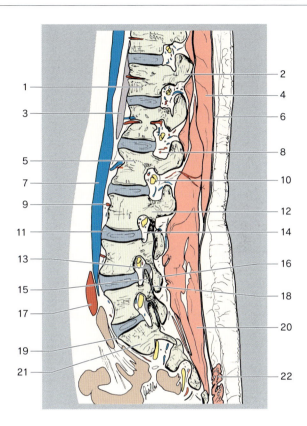

1 Th12椎体 Thoracic vertebral body T12
2 乳頭突起 Mamillary process
3 横隔膜（腰椎部）Diaphragm（lumbar part）
4 脊柱起立筋（棘筋）Erector spinae muscle（spinalis muscle）
5 L2椎体 Lumbar vertebral body L2
6 胸腰筋膜 Thoracolumbar fascia
7 下大静脈 Inferior vena cava
8 腰動脈の脊髄枝（背枝）Spinal branch of lumbar artery（dorsal branch）
9 肋間動脈 Posterior intercostal artery
10 第2腰神経の脊髄神経節 Spinal ganglion L2
11 L3/4椎間板（髄核）Intervertebral disk L3-4（nucleus pulposus）
12 椎弓（椎弓板）Vertebral arch（lamina）
13 黄色靱帯 Ligamentum flavum
14 椎間孔 Intervertebral foramen
15 上関節突起 Superior articular process
16 下関節突起 Inferior articular process
17 総腸骨動脈 Common iliac artery
18 椎間関節 Zygapophyseal joint
19 仙骨の岬角 Promontory of sacrum
20 多裂筋 Multifidus muscle
21 仙骨（S1）Sacrum（S1）
22 大殿筋 Gluteus maximus muscle

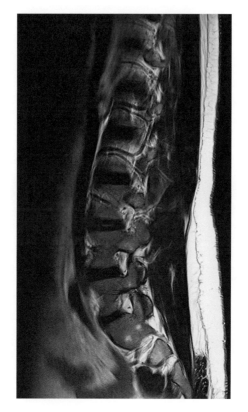

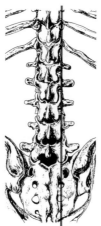

頭側

腹側 　　 背側

尾側

腰椎，矢状断

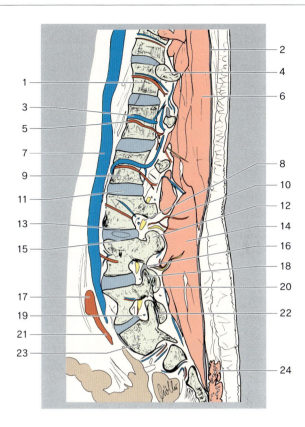

1 **Th12椎体** Thoracic vertebral body T12
2 **胸腰筋膜** Thoracolumbar fascia
3 **腰静脈** Lumbar vein
4 **肋骨(頭)** Rib(head)
5 **腰動脈** Lumbar artery
6 **脊柱起立筋(棘筋)** Erector spinae muscle (spinalis muscle)
7 **下大静脈** Inferior vena cava
8 **第3腰神経** Spinal nerve L3
9 **L2椎体** Lumbar vertebral body L2
10 **腰動脈(背枝)** Lumbar artery (dorsal branch)
11 **椎間板** Intervertebral disk
12 **横突起** Transverse process
13 **椎体下面の終板** Inferior vertebral endplate
14 **多裂筋** Multifidus muscle
15 **椎体上面の終板** Superior vertebral endplate
16 **黄色靱帯** Ligamentum flavum
17 **総腸骨動脈** Common iliac artery
18 **上関節突起** Superior articular process
19 **椎間孔** Intervertebral foramen
20 **下関節突起** Inferior articular process
21 **内腸骨動脈** Internal iliac artery
22 **椎間関節** Zygapophyseal joint
23 **仙骨(S1)** Sacrum(S1)
24 **大殿筋** Gluteus maximus muscle

436　脊椎

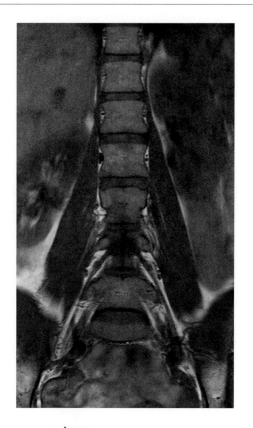

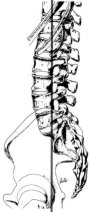

頭側
右 □ 左
尾側

腰椎，冠状断 **437**

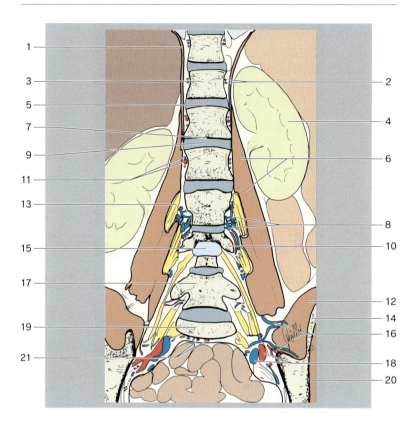

1 横隔膜（腰椎部）Diaphragm（lumbar part）
2 肋間動静脈（背枝）Posterior intercostal artery and vein（dorsal branch）
3 Th12椎体 Thoracic vertebral body T12
4 左腎 Left kidney
5 L1椎体上面の終板 Superior vertebral endplate L1
6 大腰筋 Psoas major muscle
7 L1椎体下面の終板 Inferior vertebral endplate L1
8 前外椎骨静脈叢 Anterior external vertebral venous plexus
9 L1/2椎間板（線維輪）Intervertebral disk L1-L2（anulus fibrosus）
10 L4横突起 Transverse process L4
11 腰動静脈 Lumbar artery and vein
12 腸骨筋 Iliacus muscle
13 腰神経叢 Lumbar plexus
14 腸骨 Ilium
15 硬膜嚢（腰椎槽）Thecal sac（lumbar cistern）
16 腸腰動静脈 Iliolumbar artery and vein
17 L5椎体 Lumbar vertebral body L5
18 内腸骨動静脈 Internal iliac artery and vein
19 仙骨の岬角 Promontory of sacrum
20 中殿筋 Gluteus medius muscle
21 正中仙骨動静脈 Median sacral artery and vein

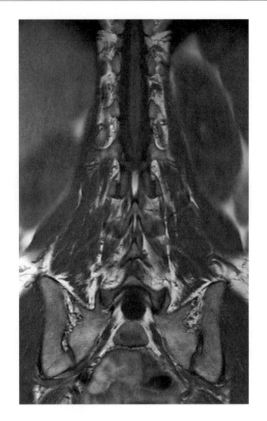

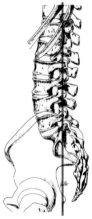

頭側

右 　　 左

尾側

1 **右肺** Right lung
2 **硬膜嚢内の脳脊髄液（腰椎槽）** Cerebrospinal fluid in thecal sac (lumbar cistern)
3 **Th12椎弓根** Pedicle of vertebral arch T12
4 **大腰筋** Psoas major muscle
5 **第12肋骨（頭）** Twelfth rib (head)
6 **脊髄円錐** Conus medullaris

腰椎，冠状断 **439**

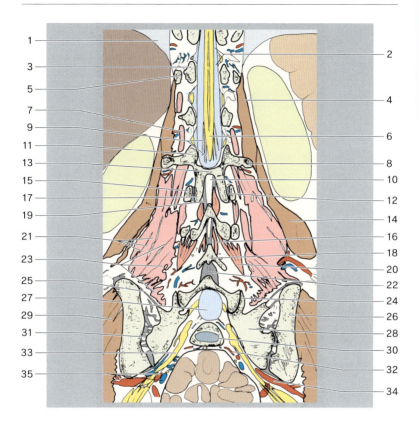

- 7 横突間筋 Intertransversarius muscle
- 8 L2横突起 Transverse process L2
- 9 馬尾 Cauda equina
- 10 後硬膜外脂肪（脊髄後方の脂肪，背側脂肪）Posterior epidural fat (retrospinal fat, dorsal fat)
- 11 L2椎弓（椎弓板）Vertebral arch L2 (lamina)
- 12 椎間関節 Zygapophyseal joint
- 13 第2腰椎の椎弓根 Pedicle of vertebral arch L2
- 14 腰方形筋 Quadratus lumborum muscle
- 15 L3上関節突起 Superior articular process L3
- 16 棘間筋 Interspinales muscles
- 17 L2下関節突起 Inferior articular process L2
- 18 L4棘突起 Spinous process L4
- 19 黄色靱帯 Ligamentum flavum
- 20 多裂筋 Multifidus muscle
- 21 腰腸肋筋 Iliocostalis lumborum muscle
- 22 棘間靱帯 Interspinous ligament
- 23 最長筋 Longissimus muscle
- 24 L5/S1椎間関節 Lumbosacral zygapophyseal joint L5–S1
- 25 仙腸靱帯 Sacroiliac ligaments
- 26 腸骨 Ilium
- 27 硬膜囊（腰椎槽）Thecal sac (lumbar cistern)
- 28 仙骨（外側部）Sacrum (lateral mass)
- 29 中殿筋 Gluteus medius muscle
- 30 S1/2椎間腔 Intervertebral space S1–2
- 31 仙腸関節 Sacroiliac joint
- 32 外側仙骨動静脈 Lateral sacral artery and vein
- 33 仙骨神経叢 Sacral plexus
- 34 上殿動脈 Superior gluteal artery
- 35 内腸骨動静脈 Internal iliac artery and vein

440 脊 椎

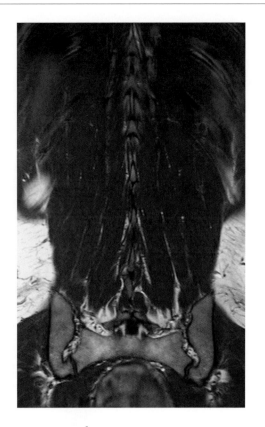

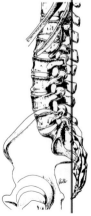

頭側
右 左
尾側

腰椎，冠状断 441

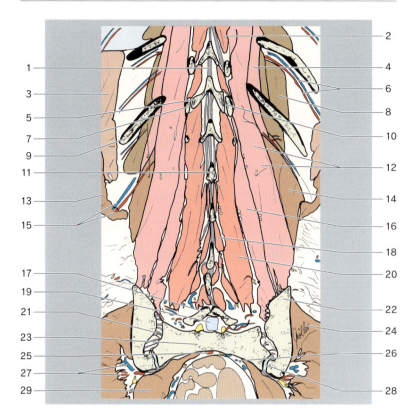

1 棘間靱帯 Interspinous ligament
2 胸棘筋 Spinalis thoracis muscle, 胸回旋筋 Rotatores thoracis muscle
3 前鋸筋 Serratus anterior muscle
4 肋骨挙筋 Levatores costarum muscles
5 Th12下関節突起 Inferior articular process T12
6 肋間動静脈(背枝) Posterior intercostal artery and vein (dorsal branch)
7 L1上関節突起 Superior articular process L1
8 肋間筋 Intercostal muscles
9 第11肋骨 Eleventh rib
10 椎間関節 Zygapophyseal joint
11 L2棘突起 Spinous process L2
12 腰腸肋筋 Iliocostalis lumborum muscle
13 広背筋 Latissimus dorsi muscle
14 腰方形筋 Quadratus lumborum muscle
15 腰動静脈 Lumbar artery and vein
16 最長筋 Longissimus muscle
17 S1椎弓(椎弓板) Vertebral arch S1 (lamina)
18 腰棘間筋 Interspinales lumborum muscles
19 硬膜嚢内の脳脊髄液(腰椎槽) Cerebrospinal fluid in thecal sac (lumbar cistern)
20 多裂筋 Multifidus muscle
21 仙腸靱帯 Sacroiliac ligaments
22 腸骨 Ilium
23 仙骨 Sacrum
24 中殿筋 Gluteus medius muscle
25 正中仙骨動静脈 Median sacral artery and vein
26 外側仙骨動静脈 Lateral sacral artery and vein
27 上殿動静脈 Superior gluteal artery and vein
28 仙腸関節 Sacroiliac joint
29 梨状筋 Piriformis muscle

442　脊椎

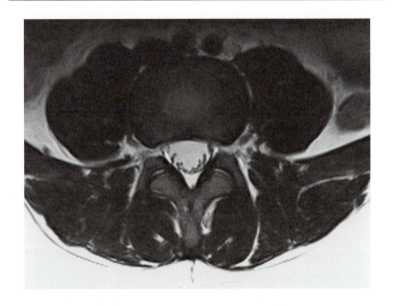

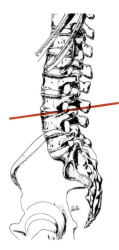

腹側
右 □ 左
背側

腰椎，軸位断 443

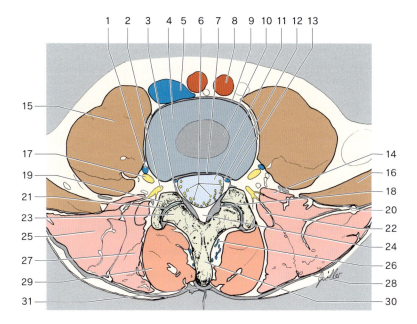

1 腰静脈 Lumbar vein
2 脊髄神経（後枝） Spinal nerve (dorsal branch)
3 神経孔の靱帯 Neuroforaminal ligament
4 L3/4椎間板（線維輪） Intervertebral disk L3-4 (anulus fibrosus)
5 下大静脈（合流部） Inferior vena cava (confluence)
6 馬尾 Cauda equina
7 後縦靱帯 Posterior longitudinal ligament
8 左総腸骨動脈 Left common iliac artery
9 前縦靱帯 Anterior longitudinal ligament
10 L3/4椎間板（髄核） Intervertebral disk L3-4 (nucleus pulposus)
11 硬膜嚢（腰椎槽） Thecal sac (lumbar cistern)
12 脊髄硬膜 Spinal dura mater
13 内椎骨静脈叢 Internal vertebral venous plexus
14 脊柱起立筋（外側筋列） Erector spinae muscle (lateral tract)：
外側横突間筋 Intertransversarii laterales muscle
15 大腰筋 Psoas major muscle
16 腰方形筋 Quadratus lumborum muscle
17 第3腰神経の脊髄神経節 Spinal ganglion L3
18 黄色靱帯 Ligamentum flavum
19 下関節突起 Inferior articular process

20 胸腰筋膜（前葉） Thoracolumbar fascia (anterior layer)
21 椎間関節 Zygapophyseal joint
22 脊柱起立筋（外側筋列） Erector spinae muscle (lateral tract)：
内側横突間筋 Intertransversarii mediales muscle
23 上関節突起 Superior articular process
24 硬膜外脂肪織（脊柱後方・背側脂肪三角） Epidural fatty tissue (retrospinal/dorsal fatty triangle)
25 脊柱起立筋（外側筋列） Erector spinae muscle (lateral tract)：
腰腸肋筋 Iliocostalis lumborum muscle
26 後外椎骨静脈叢 Posterior external vertebral venous plexus
27 脊柱起立筋（外側筋列） Erector spinae muscle (lateral tract)：
最長筋 Longissimus muscle
28 胸腰筋膜（後葉） Thoracolumbar fascia (posterior layer)
29 脊柱起立筋（内側筋列） Erector spinae muscle (medial tract)：
多裂筋 Multifidus muscle
30 棘突起 Spinous process
31 棘上靱帯 Supraspinous ligament

444 脊 椎

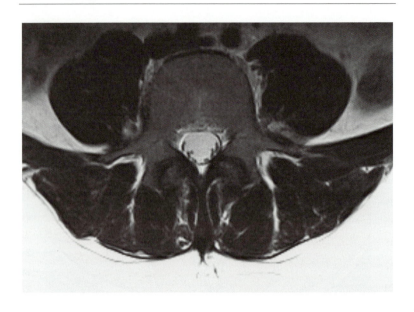

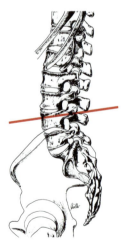

腹側
右 □ 左
背側

腰椎，軸位断

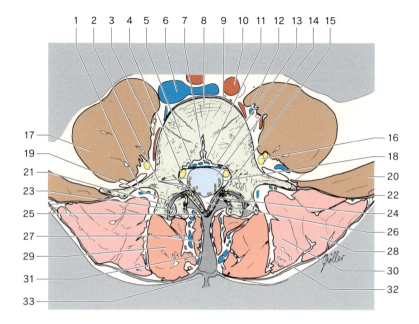

1 肋骨突起 Costal process
2 馬尾 Cauda equina
3 腰動脈 Lumbar artery
4 第4腰神経の脊髄神経節（外側嚢内） Spinal ganglion in lateral recess L4
5 前内椎骨静脈叢 Anterior internal vertebral venous plexus
6 下大静脈（合流部） Inferior vena cava (confluence)
7 栄養孔 Nutrient foramen
8 L4椎体 Lumbar vertebral body L4
9 前縦靱帯 Anterior longitudinal ligament
10 左総腸骨動脈 Left common iliac artery
11 椎体静脈 Basivertebral vein
12 上行腰静脈 Ascending lumbar vein
13 後縦靱帯 Posterior longitudinal ligament
14 硬膜嚢（腰椎槽） Thecal sac (lumbar cistern)
15 L4関節突起間部 Interarticular portion L4
16 第3腰神経の脊髄神経節 Spinal ganglion L3
17 大腰筋 Psoas major muscle
18 脊髄硬膜 Spinal dura mater
19 椎間関節 Zygapophyseal joint
20 腰方形筋 Quadratus lumborum muscle
21 上関節突起 Superior articular process
22 胸腰筋膜（前葉） Thoracolumbar fascia (anterior layer)
23 下関節突起 Inferior articular process
24 黄色靱帯 Ligamentum flavum
25 椎弓（椎弓板） Vertebral arch (lamina)
26 硬膜外脂肪織（脊髄後方・背側脂肪三角） Epidural fatty tissue (retrospinal/dorsal fatty triangle)
27 後外椎骨静脈叢 Posterior external vertebral venous plexus
28 脊柱起立筋（外側筋列） Erector spinae muscle (lateral tract):
   腰腸肋筋 Iliocostalis lumborum muscle
29 脊柱起立筋（内側筋列） Erector spinae muscle (medial tract):
   多裂筋 Multifidus muscle
30 脊柱起立筋（外側筋列） Erector spinae muscle (lateral tract):
   最長筋 Longissimus muscle
31 棘間靱帯 Interspinous ligament
32 胸腰筋膜（後葉） Thoracolumbar fascia (posterior layer)
33 棘上靱帯 Supraspinous ligament

446 脊 椎

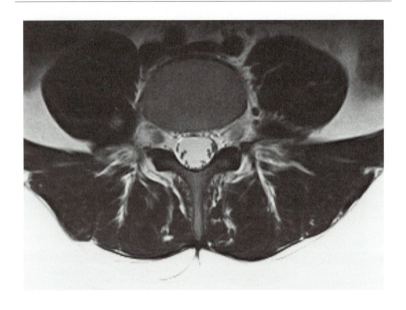

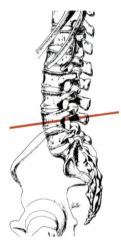

腹側
右 □ 左
背側

腰椎，軸位断　**447**

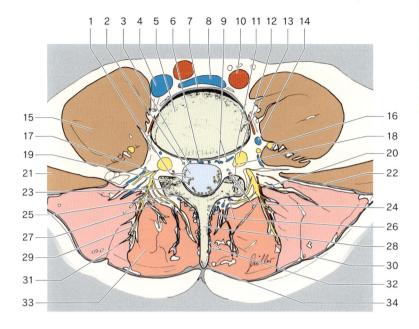

1 馬尾　Cauda equina
2 硬膜嚢(腰椎槽)　Thecal sac (lumbar cistern)
3 脊髄硬膜　Spinal dura mater
4 右総腸骨静脈　Right common iliac vein
5 L4椎体　Lumbar vertebral body L4
6 椎体静脈　Basivertebral vein
7 前縦靱帯　Anterior longitudinal ligament
8 左総腸骨静脈　Left common iliac vein
9 前内椎骨静脈叢　Anterior internal vertebral venous plexus
10 左総腸骨動脈　Left common iliac artery
11 後縦靱帯　Posterior longitudinal ligament
12 第4腰神経の脊髄神経節　Spinal ganglion L4
13 腰動脈　Lumbar artery
14 上行腰静脈　Ascending lumbar vein
15 大腰筋　Psoas major muscle
16 第3腰神経の脊髄神経節　Spinal ganglion L3
17 脊髄神経(後枝)　Spinal nerve (dorsal branch)
18 椎間孔　Intervertebral foramen
19 椎間関節　Zygapophyseal joint
20 腰動脈(背枝の外側皮枝)　Lumbar artery (lateral cutaneous branch of dorsal branch)
21 腰方形筋　Quadratus lumborum muscle
22 胸腰筋膜(前葉)　Thoracolumbar fascia (anterior layer)
23 下関節突起　Inferior articular process
24 根動静脈　Radicular artery and vein
25 椎弓(椎弓板)　Vertebral arch (lamina)
26 後外椎骨静脈叢　Posterior external vertebral venous plexus
27 脊髄神経(内側背側枝)　Spinal nerve (medial dorsal branch)
28 棘突起　Spinous process
29 脊髄神経(外側背側枝)　Spinal nerve (lateral dorsal branch)
30 胸腰筋膜(後葉)　Thoracolumbar fascia (posterior layer)
31 脊柱起立筋(外側筋列)　Erector spinae muscle (lateral tract):
   腰腸肋筋　Iliocostalis lumborum muscle,
   最長筋　Longissimus muscle
32 傍脊椎脂肪織　Paraspinal fatty tissue
33 脊柱起立筋(内側筋列)　Erector spinae muscle (medial tract):
   多裂筋　Multifidus muscle
34 棘上靱帯　Supraspinous ligament

448 脊 椎

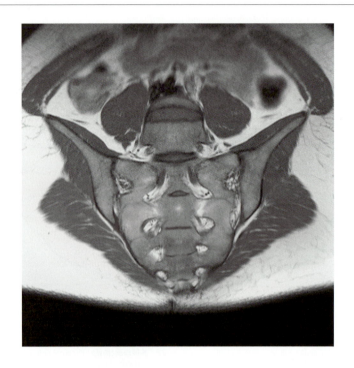

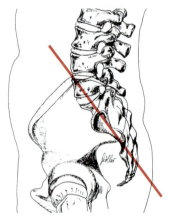

頭側
腹側

右 　　　　　左
外側 □ 外側

尾側
背側

仙骨 449

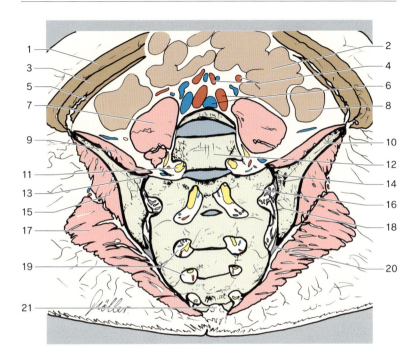

1 外腹斜筋 External oblique muscle
2 回腸 Ileum
3 内腹斜筋 Internal oblique muscle
4 腸骨動脈 Iliac arteries
5 腹横筋 Transversus abdominis muscle
6 (左)総腸骨動静脈 Common iliac artery and vein(left)
7 大腰筋 Psoas major muscle
8 下行結腸 Descending colon
9 腸骨筋 Iliacus muscle
10 腸骨(翼) Ilium(wing)
11 第5腰神経 Fifth lumbar nerve root
12 第5腰椎(椎体) Fifth lumbar vertebra(body)
13 前仙腸靱帯 Anterior sacro-iliac ligaments
14 仙腸関節 Sacro-iliac joint
15 中殿筋 Gluteus medius muscle
16 仙骨(外側部) Sacrum(lateral mass)
17 大殿筋 Gluteus maximus muscle
18 骨間仙腸靱帯 Interosseous sacro-iliac ligaments
19 前仙骨孔 Anterior sacral foramina
20 後仙腸靱帯 Posterior sacro-iliac ligaments
21 仙骨管 Sacral canal

450 脊 椎

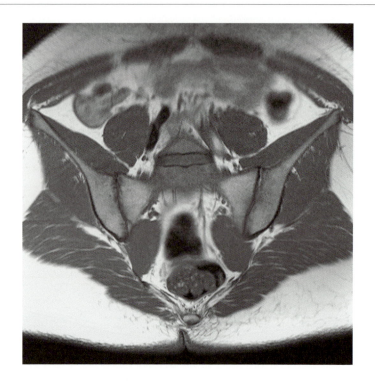

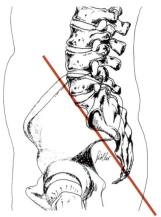

頭側
腹側

右　　　　左
外側　□　外側

尾側
背側

仙骨　451

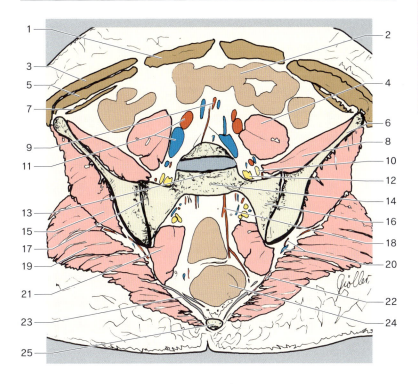

1　腹直筋　Rectus abdominis muscle
2　回腸　Ileum
3　外腹斜筋　External oblique muscle
4　大腰筋　Psoas major muscle
5　内腹斜筋　Internal oblique muscle
6　腸骨（翼）　Ilium (wing)
7　腹横筋　Transversus abdominis muscle
8　腸骨筋　Iliacus muscle
9　腸骨動脈　Iliac arteries
10　大腿神経　Femoral nerve
11　総腸骨動静脈　Common iliac artery and vein
12　仙骨神経叢　Sacral plexus
13　岬角　Promontory
14　仙骨（S1椎体）　Sacrum (body of first sacral vertebra)
15　中殿筋　Gluteus medius muscle
16　仙骨（外側部）　Sacrum (lateral mass)
17　仙腸関節　Sacro-iliac joint
18　正中仙骨動脈　Median sacral artery
19　大殿筋　Gluteus maximus muscle
20　下殿動静脈　Inferior gluteal artery and vein
21　梨状筋　Piriformis muscle
22　尾骨筋　Coccygeus muscle
23　仙棘靱帯　Sacrospinous ligament
24　直腸　Rectum
25　尾骨　Coccyx

参考文献

Braun H, Kenn W, Schneider S, Graf M, Sandstede J, Hahn D. Direkte MR-Arthrographie des Handgelenkes. Rofo 2003;175:1515–1524

Bulling A, Castrop F, Agneskirchner J, et al. Body Explorer 2.0. Heidelberg: Springer Electronic Media; 2001

Burgener FA, Aeyers SP, Tan RK. Differential Diagnosis in MRI. Stuttgart: Thieme; 2002

Cahill DR, Orland MJ, Reading CC. Atlas of Human Cross-Sectional Anatomy. New York, NY: Wiley-Liss; 1995

Chacko AK, Katzberg RW, MacKay A. MRI Atlas of Normal Anatomy. New York, NY: McGraw-Hill; 1991

Clavero JA, Alomar X, Monill JM, et al. MR imaging of ligament and tendon injuries of the fingers. Radiographics 2002; 22:237–256

Clavero JA, Golanó P, Fariñas O, Alomar X, Monill JM, Esplugas M. Extensor mechanism of the fingers: MR imaging–anatomic correlation. Radiographics 2003;23:593–611

Connell DA, Koulouris G, Thorn DA, Potter HG. Contrast-enhanced MR angiography of the hand. Radiographics 2002;22:583–599

Dauber W. Pocket Atlas of Human Anatomy. 5th ed. Stuttgart: Thieme; 2007

Delfaut EM, Demondion X, Bieganski A, Thiron MC, Mestdagh H, Cotton A. Imaging of foot and ankle entrapment syndromes. Radiographics 2003;23:613–623

El-Khoury GY, Bergman RA, Montgomery EJ. Sectional Anatomy by MRI/CT. New York, NY: Churchill-Livingstone; 1990

El-Khoury GY, Bennett D, Stanley MD. Essentials in Musculoskeletal Imaging. New York, NY: Churchill Livingstone; 2003

Garcia-Valtuille R, Abascal F, Cerezal L, et al. Anatomy and MR imaging appearances of synovial plicae of the knee. Radiographics 2002;22:775–784

Grumme T, Kluge W, Kretzmar K, Roesler A. Zerebrale und spinale CT. Berlin: Blackwell; 1998

Harnsberger R. Diagnostic Imaging. Head and Neck. Salt Lake City, UT: Amirsys; 2004

Hosten N, Liebig T. CT of the Head and Spine. Stuttgart: Thieme; 2001

Huk WJ, Gademann G, Friedmann G. MRI of Central Nervous System Diseases. Berlin: Springer; 1990

Kang MS, Resnick D. MRI of the Extremities: An Anatomic Atlas. Philadelphia, PA: Saunders; 2002

Koritke JG, Sick H. Atlas of Sectional Human Anatomy. Baltimore, MD: Urban & Schwarzenberg; 1988

Kretschmann H-J, Weinrich W. Cranial Neuroimaging and Clinical Neuroanatomy. Stuttgart: Thieme; 2003

Leblanc A. Encephalo-peripheral Nervous System. Berlin: Springer; 2001

Lustrin ES, Karakas SP, Ortiz AO, et al. Pediatric cervical spine: normal anatomy, variants, and trauma. Radiographics 2003;23:539–560

Mayerhöfer ME, Breitenseher MJ: MR-Diagnostik der lateralen Sprunggelenksbänder. Rofo 2003;175:670–675

Mengiardi B, Zanetti M, Schöttle PB, et al. Spring ligament complex: MR imaging–anatomic correlation and findings in asymptomatic subjects. Radiology 2005;237:242–249

Meschan I. Synopsis of Radiologic Anatomy. Philadelphia, PA: Saunders; 1978

Mohana-Borges AV, Theumann NH, Pfirrmann CW, Chung CB, Resnick DL, Trudell DJ. Lesser metatarsophalangeal joints. Radiology 2003;227:175–182

Moeller TB, Reif E. MR Atlas of the Musculoskeletal System. Boston, MA: Blackwell Science; 1994

Moeller TB, Reif E. Neuroradiologische Schnittbilddiagnostik. Constance: Schnetztor; 2002

Moeller TB, Reif E. Pocket Atlas of Radiographic Anatomy. 3rd ed. Stuttgart: Thieme; 2010

参考文献 **453**

Morag Y, Jacobson JA, Shields G, et al. MR Arthrography of rotator interval, long head of the biceps brachii, and biceps pulley of the shoulder. Radiology 2005;235:21–30

Munshi M, Pretterklieber ML, Chung CB, et al. Anterior bundle of ulnar collateral ligament: evaluation of anatomic relationship by using MR imaging, MR arthrography, and gross anatomic and histologic analysis. Radiology 2004; 231:797–803

Netter FH. Atlas der Anatomie des Menschen. 3rd ed. Stuttgart: Thieme; 2003

Nowicki BH, Haughton VM. Neural foraminal ligament of the lumbar spine: appearance at CT and MR imaging. Radiology 1992;183:257–264

Oae K, Takao M, Naito K, et al. Injury of the tibiofibular syndesmosis: value of MR imaging for diagnosis. Radiology 2003; 227:155–161

Pech P, Daniels DL, Williams AL, Haughton VM. The cervical neural foramina: correlation of microtomy and CT anatomy. Radiology 1985;155:143–146

Platzer W. Color Atlas and Textbook of Human Anatomy. Vol. 1: Locomotor System. 6th ed. Stuttgart: Thieme; 2009

Richter E, Feyerabend T. Normal lymph node topography. Berlin: Springer; 1991

Robinson P, White LM. Soft-tissue and osseous impingement syndromes of the ankle. Radiographics 2002;22:1457–1471

Rummeny EJ, Reimer P, Heindel W. MR Imaging of the Body. Stuttgart: Thieme; 2008

Schäfer FKW, Order B, Bolte H, Heller M, Brossmann J. Sport injuries of the extensor mechanism of the knee. Radiologe 2002;42(10):799–810

Schmitt R, Lanz U. Diagnostic Imaging of the Hand. 2nd ed. Stuttgart: Thieme; 2007

Schnitzlein HN, Reed Murtagh F. Imaging Atlas of the Head and Spine. Baltimore: Urban & Schwarzenberg; 1990

Schünke M, Schulte E, Schumacher U, Voll M, Wesker K. Prometheus—Lernatlas der Anatomie. 3 vols. Stuttgart: Thieme; 2004–2006

Schünke M, Schulte E, Schumacher U. Thieme Atlas of Anatomy. General Anatomy and Musculoskeletal System. 2nd ed. Stuttgart: Thieme; 2014

Stark DD, Bradley WG. Magnetic Resonance Imaging. St. Louis, MO: Mosby; 1999

Strobel K, Hodler J. MRT des Kniegelenkes. Radiologie up2date. Stuttgart: Thieme; 2003

Stoller DW. MRI, Arthroscopy, and Surgical Anatomy of the Joints. Philadelphia, PA: Lippincott Williams & Wilkins; 1999

Stoller DW, Tirman B. Diagnostic imaging: Orthopaedics. Salt Lake City, UT: Amirsys; 2004

Theumann NH, Pfirrmann CW, Drapé JL, Trudell DJ, Resnick D. MR imaging of the metacarpophalangeal joints of the fingers. Radiology 2002;222:437–445

Theumann NH, Pfirrmann CW, Antonio GE, et al. Extrinsic carpal ligaments: normal MR arthrographic appearance in cadavers. Radiology 2003;226:171–179

Tiedemann K. Anatomy of the Head and Neck. Weinheim: VCH; 1993

Uhlenbrock D. MR Imaging of the Spine and Spinal Cord. Stuttgart: Thieme; 2004

Vahlensieck M, Linneborn G, Schild HH, Schmidt HM. MRT der Bursae des Kniegelenk. Rofo 2001;173:195–199

Vahlensieck M. Anatomie der Schulterregion. Radiologe 2004;44:556–561

Vahlensieck M, Genant HK, Reiser M. MRI of the Musculoskeletal System, Stuttgart: Thieme; 1999

和文索引

あ

アキレス腱　235-247,355-357,387-391
アキレス腱前脂肪体　355,389

い

陰部神経　263

う

右心室　423
烏口肩峰靱帯　71-73,89-91
烏口鎖骨靱帯　3-7,71,93-95,98-102,118,123
烏口上腕靱帯　5-7,71-73,89-91,98
烏口突起　5-7,71,91-93,96-104,120-123
烏口腕筋　9-17,71-75,87-91,97-100,117-123

え

腋窩陥凹　75-77
腋窩神経　13,73-83,89-93
腋窩静脈　9-15,73,93-95,98
腋窩動脈　9-15,73,93-95,98
円回内筋　27-37,97-105,123-129,133-139,143-149,161-163
　尺骨頭　137-139
延髄　406
遠位指節間関節　168,172,176,182
遠位趾節間関節　253

お

黄色靱帯　399-403,421-423,427-435,439,443-445
横隔膜　431-433,437
横膝蓋支帯　215
横上腕靱帯　87-89
横靱帯　→環椎横靱帯,膝横靱帯
横突間筋　425,439
横突起　405,413-415,419,425-427,435-437

か

下顎後静脈　411-415
下顎骨　411-415
　下顎枝　413-415
下関節上腕靱帯　89
下関節突起　401-407,417,423,427,433-435,439-447
下脛腓関節　231,341
下行結腸　449
下行膝動脈　305
下行大動脈　421-427
下前腸骨棘　189
下双子筋　193,263,273-279
下腿骨間膜　219-229
下腿三頭筋　229-233
下大静脈　256,431-435,443-445
　合流部　443-445
下殿静脈　261-265,271,451
下殿神経　263-265,273,277-279
下殿動脈　261-265,271,277,451
下頭斜筋　401-409,413-415
下腓骨筋支帯　247
下腹壁静脈　187-189
下腹壁動脈　187-189
顆間窩　213,307-313,340
顆間結節　340
鵞足　→深鵞足,浅鵞足
鵞足腱　357
鵞足包　337
回外筋　31-35,97-99,109-113,127-131,137-141,145-161
回旋筋　425-427,441
　胸―　427,441
回腸　279,449-451
外果　233-237,341,345,349-351,363-365
外頸動脈　415
外肛門括約筋　288
外耳道　404
外側横突間筋　443
外側下膝静脈　307-311,321-327,339
外側下膝動脈　305-311,319-327,339
外側顆間結節　309-313

和文索引　***455***

外側環軸関節　405
外側関節陥凹　319
外側胸静脈　15
外側胸動脈　15
外側楔状骨　243-249,373-375,383-387
外側広筋　195-209,255-265,269,281-295,303-
　313,319-323
外側膝蓋支帯　209-217,281-283,303,319-321,
　349-352
外側手根側副靱帯　171,181-183
外側上顆
　（上腕骨）27,129-131
　（大腿骨）309
外側上膝静脈　209,293,305-309,321-325,354
外側上膝動脈　209,293,305-311,321-325,354
外側仙骨静脈　439-441
外側仙骨動脈　439-441
外側足根動脈　235
外側足底静脈　243-253,361-375,383-391
外側足底神経　247-251,361-379,383-391
外側足底動脈　243-253,361-375,383-391
外側足背皮神経　367-369
外側側副靱帯
　（手関節）→外側手根側副靱帯
　（肘関節）29,127-129,139-141,157-159
　（膝関節）211-217,311-315,338,342-347
外側大腿回旋静脈　197,259,267,281,287,293-
　301
外側大腿回旋動脈　197,255-259,267-275,281,
　287,293-301
外側頭直筋　405,411
外側半月板　215,305-313,319-325,338-344,
　351-353
　　後角　215,311-313,321-325,351-353
　　前角　215,305,321-323,353
　　体部　215,307-309,319,338-344
外腸骨静脈　187-191
外腸骨動脈　187-191
外腹斜筋　255,258,267,449-451
外閉鎖筋　195,259-261,271-287,298,301
外肋間筋　5-17
蓋膜　398,405
顎動脈　411-413
顎二腹筋　405-407,411-415
肩関節　9,73-79,91
滑車切痕　135-137,143
肝臓　421-425
貫通静脈　199,203-209
貫通動脈　199,203-205,209,269,273,291-299
寛骨臼窩　191-193,275
関節下結節　91

関節窩　5-11,73-79,98-106,116-118
関節窩上腕関節　9,73-79,91
関節上腕靱帯　73,83-87,117
関節唇
　（肩関節）5-11,73-77,116
　（股関節）191-193,257-259,269-275,280
関節突起　419
関節突起間部　423,445
関節包
　（肩関節）11,27,45-53,57,71,79-81,85,91,115-
　　121
　（股関節）271-273
　（膝関節）211-217,291,313-315,319,323-337,
　　351
　（手関節）150,167,170-172,175-178
　（足関節）235,249,361
　（肘関節）29,133,139-141
関節包靱帯　193
環椎（C1）399-415
　　横突起　405,413-415
　　外側塊　400-405,411-413
　　関節突起　415
　　後弓　399-401,407-411
　　前弓　399,411
環椎横靱帯　399,405,411-413
環椎後頭関節　400-405
環椎十字靱帯　399,411
　　横靱帯　→環椎横靱帯
　　縦束　399,411

き

気管　421-422,427
　　分岐部　427
奇静脈　421,427
基節骨
　（足）248-253,383,389-393
　（手）65-69,165-182
弓状膝窩靱帯　315,349
臼蓋　257-261,280-286
距骨　235-243,339-341,353-357,361-369,385-
　393
　　頸　239
　　後突起　241
　　体　239-241
　　頭　239-243
距骨下関節　241,355-357,361-363,385-389
距舟関節　239-241,357,389
距舟靱帯　389-391
距踵関節　→距骨下関節
距腿関節　233-237,339,355-357,361-365,387-
　389

456 和文索引

距腓関節　339-341,363
胸回旋筋　427,441
胸棘筋　425-427,441
胸肩峰動脈　91-95
胸骨　421-423
胸骨舌骨筋　421-422,425
胸鎖乳突筋　405-419
胸最長筋　427
胸神経　401,407-409
胸髄　397,409,421,427
胸腸肋筋　427
胸椎　397-403,407-409,421-427,431-441
胸背静脈　102-105
胸背神経　17,71
胸背動脈　17,102-105
胸半棘筋　423,427
胸腰筋膜　431-435,443-447
棘下筋　5-17,77-95,102-106,109-112,115-118,
　121-123,427
棘間筋　399,421,439-441
　　頸—　421
　　腰—　441
棘間靱帯　265,397-399,409,421,429,439-441,
　445
棘筋　401-403,409,417-419,424-427,441
　　胸—　425-427,441
　　頸—　401-403,409,417-419,424
棘上筋　3-7,71-95,98-123
棘上靱帯　397-399,421,427-429,443-447
棘突起　265,397-399,409,413,417,421,427-429,
　439-443,447
近位指節間関節　168-178
近位趾節間関節　253
筋間中隔
　　（大腿）197-199
　　（足底）373
筋皮神経　17-23,37,91

く

クモ膜下腔　399,413-417
屈筋支帯　47-59,175-181,235-247,363-365

け

茎状突起
　　（尺骨）47,154,169-171
　　（橈骨）183
茎突咽頭筋　415
茎突舌骨筋　411,415
茎乳突孔　404
脛骨　217-231,285-289,293-299,303-315,319-

357,361-365,385-393
　　外側顆　293-295,305-315,319-323,340,347
　　粗面　219,303,323-325,354
　　体　305-309,329,339-344,353-354,357
　　頭　217,285-289,297,325-327,339,342-344,
　　　349-354,357
　　内果　233-235,339-341,363-365,393
　　内側顆　299,305-315,331-337,340,347
　　内側顆間結節　329
脛骨神経　203-243,291,295,315-317,325-329,
　347,353-354,355-359
脛腓関節　311-313,319-321,344,349
脛腓靱帯結合　233,385
脛腓動脈幹　221,353
頸棘間筋　421
頸棘筋　401-403,409,417-419,424
頸最長筋　417-419
頸神経　401-407,415-419
頸神経叢　405
頸髄　399
頸長筋　401-405,415-419
頸椎　397-401,405-421　→環椎（C1）,軸椎
　（C2）,隆椎（C7）も参照
頸半棘筋　401,407-409,417-419
頸板状筋　401,407-409,419,422-424
結節間溝　7,83
楔舟関節　241,389
月状骨　47-51,144-148,158-160,167-177
肩甲下筋　9,13-15,71-75,87-95,100-107,119-
　123,427
肩甲下静脈　71-81,104
肩甲下神経　9,73,81
肩甲下動脈　71-81,104
肩甲回旋動静脈　13,77-79,93-95,123
肩甲挙筋　405-409,417-419
肩甲骨　9-15,71-81,93-95,123,427
　　烏口突起　5-7,71,91-93,96-104,120-123
　　棘　3-7,79-81,95
　　頸　77,121
　　肩峰　3,73-81,87-95,100-106,109-112,115-
　　　120,123
　　体　95
肩甲上静脈　3,7-11,71-79,95,123
肩甲上神経　9-11,71-79
肩甲上動脈　3,7-11,71-79,95,123
肩甲舌骨筋　3
肩鎖関節　3,73-75,91,104-106
肩鎖靱帯　73-75,91,110-112
肩峰　3,73-81,87-95,100-106,109-112,115-120,
　123
肩峰下包　73,77,89

和文索引　457

こ

固有掌側指神経　165-168,182
固有掌側指動脈　165-168,182
固有底側趾静脈　379-381
固有底側趾神経　379-381
固有底側趾動脈　377-381
股関節　257-259,269-273,281-284,301
口蓋咽頭筋　401
広背筋　13-17,71-81,87-95,99-107,117-123,
　423-425,441
甲状腺　417-424
肛門　288
肛門挙筋　191-195,259-265,288
岬角(仙骨)　397,429-433,437,451
後外椎骨静脈叢　417-419,423,443-447
後環椎後頭膜　399
後距腓靱帯　235-237,341-343,361-363,385-389
後鋸筋　11
後脛骨筋　221-247,311-313,319-323,341-347,
　351-357,361-373,389-393
後脛骨神経　347
後脛骨静脈　221-241,343,347,355-361
後脛骨動脈　223-241,315,343,347,355-359,393
後脛骨反回動静脈　347
後脛腓靱帯　231-235
後骨間静脈　35-37,151,155,158-161
後骨間神経　35-37
後骨間動脈　35-37,151,155,158-161
後根　→脊髄神経根
後斜角筋　405-409,417
後十字靱帯　211-217,297,309-313,327-333,340-
　344,354-356
後縦靱帯　399,407-409,421,429,443-447
後上腕回旋動静脈　13,73-93,102,105,109-119
後神経束　100
後仙腸靱帯　449
後前腕皮神経　21-29,33,39,47-49
後大腿皮神経　203
後頭下静脈叢　409
後頭下神経　409
後頭顆　400-404
後頭骨　398-400
後半月大腿靱帯　313,329
　(=Wrisberg靱帯)
後腓骨頭靱帯　315,319
鉤状突起
　(頚椎)405
　(尺骨)111,129-131,135-137,143-145,159-161
鉤突窩　27,129,135
喉頭　419

硬膜　413,429
硬膜外脂肪織　421,427-429,439,443-445
硬膜　397,429,437-439,443-447
項靱帯　397,409-413,417-419
骨間距踵靱帯　239-243,355-357,367,387-389
骨間筋　67-69,167-170,179-180,371-377,387-
　389
骨間楔中足靱帯　244
骨間楔立方靱帯　383-385
骨間手根間靱帯　171
骨間舟状月状靱帯　169
骨間仙腸靱帯　449
骨間中手靱帯　171
骨間静脈　127,137-139,157
　後―　35-37,151,155,158-161
　前―　35-41,141,156,159-160
　総―　131
　反回―　33,155
骨間動脈　127,137-139,157
　後―　35-37,151,155,158-161
　前―　35-41,141,156,159-160
　総―　131
　反回―　31-33,155
骨間膜
　(下腿)219-229
　(前腕)37-39,171
骨性脊柱管　399
根動静脈　447

さ

左心房　421-425
鎖骨　3-7,71-75,91-106,110-123
鎖骨下筋　3-9,97-98,102
鎖骨下静脈　96-98
鎖骨下動脈　98,405,425
坐骨　191-193,263,273-275,288,291,298,301
坐骨棘　191,265
坐骨結節　195,265,277-279
坐骨肛門窩　289
坐骨神経　191-201,263-265,271-277,289-291,
　295,299
坐骨大腿靱帯　193-195,261,275
坐骨直腸窩　195
最長筋　409-419,427,439-447
　胸―　427
　頚―　417-419
　頭―　409-415,419
最内肋間筋　13-17
三角筋　3-17,71-123
　肩甲棘部　3-9,91-95
　肩峰部　3-9,83-93,109-112,115-118,121-123

鎖骨部 3-9,89-95
三角筋下包 87
三角骨 49-53,144-148,154-156,169-175
三角靱帯 233-243,339,361-369,391-393
　脛舟部 233-243,367,393
　脛踵部 239-241,365,393
　後脛距部 237-239,363-365,391-393
　前脛距部 233-237,369,393
三角線維軟骨 47,144-146,173
三角線維軟骨複合体 169

し

子宮 187-191,255-263
子宮静脈叢 191
矢状索 67-69
指屈筋 168,172,175-178,181-182
指伸筋 31-69,97-99,129-131,141,151-163,171-
183
指動脈 182
指背腱膜 65-67
趾屈筋群 253
趾伸筋 383,387-389 →長趾伸筋, 短趾伸筋
示指伸筋 39-61,67,146-150,155-158
耳下腺 404,411-415
軸椎(C2) 397-401,405-415
　後弓 413-415
　歯突起 397-399,405,411-413
　椎弓 407
　椎体 399-401,405,415
膝横靱帯 307,325-333
膝窩 335
膝窩筋 209-219,307-333,338-357
膝窩静脈 209-219,289-291,295,313-317,325-
327,346,353-356
膝窩動脈 209-219,289-291,295,311-317,325-
327,346,353-356
膝蓋下脂肪体 213-217,303,323-333,354-356
(＝Hoffa 脂肪体)
膝蓋下皮下包 325-327
膝蓋骨 209-211,281-283,295-299,323-335,356
膝蓋骨後面軟骨 209-211
膝蓋上脂肪体 303
膝蓋上包 303,323-335
膝蓋靱帯 209-219,297-299,303,323-333,353-
356
膝蓋前皮下包 325-333
膝蓋動静脈網 325-331
膝関節 285-289,293-299,321,335,339-340,350,
353
膝関節動脈網 303-305
脂肪体

アキレス腱前― 355,389
　膝蓋下― 213-217,303,323-333,354-356
　膝蓋上― 303
斜角筋 98-106
斜膝窩靱帯 211-213,217,315,325-327,335
尺側手根屈筋 31-53,105-107,115-123,127,131,
145-147,155-159,165,175
尺側手根伸筋 31-55,99-101,139-141,146,149-
151,155,171-173
尺側側副静脈 117
尺側側副動脈 117-119
尺側皮静脈 19-53,89,101-103,121-125,143,
155-163
尺骨 31-45,99-101,115,129-131,143,144-150,
154-156,169-173
　茎状突起 47,154,169-171
　鉤状突起 111,129-131,135-137,143-145,
159-161
　体 139,143-145,155
尺骨静脈 23-25,33-61,119-121,135,143-147,
156-161
尺骨神経 17-63,73-75,91,103,117-123,131-135,
143,154-159,173-181
尺骨動脈 23-25,33-61,97,119-121,125,135,143-
147,157-161,173-175
尺骨反回動脈 133
手関節 158-160,163,169,177
手根間関節
　舟状有頭 177-179
　有頭有鈎 55
手根中手関節 169-171,175-183
　第1― 167
手掌腱膜 55-61,65,175-180
手掌手根動脈弓 169
種子骨 63,167-169,253,381,391
舟状骨 47-53,144-148,163-171,177-183,239-
245,357,369-371,387-393
終糸 421
小円筋 11-13,77-81,87-95,102,105-106,109-
112,115-118,121-123
小胸筋 7-17,89-97,121-123
小結節 7-11,83
小後頭直筋 399-400,403,411-413
小指外転筋 51-65,154,165-169,173
小指屈筋 165-167,173
小指伸筋 35-67,141,149-156
小指対立筋 57-63,165-167,173
小趾外転筋 249-253,341-343,361-377,379-
389
小趾対立筋 375-377
小腸 187-189,255-256,269-272,275-279
小転子 197,261,269-271,287,296-299

和文索引　*459*

小殿筋　187-195,257-261,267-273,280-286,300
小内転筋　261,271,275-279,285-289
小伏在静脈　215-239,359,379
小菱形筋　419
小菱形骨　53-55,148,169-171,181-183
掌側骨間筋　59-65,173-175,183
掌側指静脈　174,177
掌側指神経　65-69,174
（母指）61,65,69
掌側指動脈　65-69,174-176
掌側尺骨手根靱帯　45-51,154,167,173-175
掌側手根間靱帯　49,53-59,175-179
掌側手根中手靱帯　175-177,183
掌側靱帯　65-67,172-178,182
掌側中手動脈　173,182
掌側橈骨手根靱帯　47-51,165-167,177-181
掌側橈尺靱帯　173
踵骨　241-253,339-347,355-369,383-393
　載距突起　243-245
　踵骨結節　243-245,249-253,355
　踵骨隆起　391
踵骨腱　→アキレス腱　235-247,355-357,387-
　391
踵骨動脈網　391
踵腓靱帯　239-241,341-343,351,363-365,383
踵立方関節　383-387
上咽頭収縮筋　415-419
上関節上腕靱帯　89
上関節突起　401-407,417,423,427,431-435,439-
　445
上行大動脈　421-423
上行腰静脈　445-447
上後鋸筋　422
上尺側側副動静脈　29-31
上尺側側副動脈,神経　27
上双子筋　263,273-279
上殿静脈　187-191,260,265,269,273-279,441
上殿神経　193,265,273-277
上殿動脈　187-193,260,265,269,439-441
上殿皮神経　263
上頭斜筋　407-413
上橈尺関節　31,137
上腓骨筋支帯　237-239
上肋横突靱帯　425
上腕筋　19-33,97-103,109-121,125-163
上腕骨　5-29,71-89,97-119,127-153,157-161
　外側上顆　27,129-131
　滑車　99-101,115,119,127-135,143-147,159-
　　161
　頸　97.110
　小結節　7-11,83
　小頭　29,97-99,109-113,127-129,137-141,

　149-153,157-161
　体　17-25,75-87,99-100,103-105,109-112,
　　129-131,137-139,145-151
　大結節　5-9,73-77,81-83,98,109-112
　大結節稜　83
　頭　5-9,71,81,85-89,97-112,115-118
　内側上顆　27-29,103-107
上腕三頭筋　13-29,77-81,85-93,101-121,129-
　157
　外側頭　13-21,25,77-81,101-113
　長頭　13-21,77-81,89-93,105,109-121
　内側頭　17-21,25,85-87,105-107,113-117
上腕静脈　15-31,71,75,91,97,119-125,133,163
上腕深静脈　19-25,101-109,117
上腕深動脈　19-25,101-109,117,137
上腕動脈　15-31,71,75,91,97,119-125,133,145-
　147,163
上腕二頭筋　7-31,75-73,75-83-91,96-121,125-129,
　133-139,145-153,157,161-163
　腱膜　29-31
　短頭　9-13,19-25,89-91,97
　長頭　7-13,19-25,73-75,83-91,96-121
上腕二頭筋溝　→結節間溝
食道　399,405,417-422,425-427
伸筋支帯　19-63,169,173-183
神経線維　431
深会陰横筋　259-261
深横中手靱帯　65
深下腿筋膜　331-335
深鵞足　309-315,337
深頸静脈　399-403,409-419
深指屈筋　31-69,103-107,111-119,127-137,143-
　145,155-167,173-179
深膝蓋下包　325-333
深掌動脈弓　59-63,169,173-183
深足底動脈弓　373-375,385-389
深腓骨神経　221-235,340,343-344,367,369,373-
　375

せ

正中環軸関節　399,411
正中神経　17-61,71-75,91,97-101,115-127,
　133-135,145,157-158,161-165,177-179,182
正中仙骨静脈　437,441
正中仙骨動脈　437,441,451
正中仙骨稜　429-431
脊髄　407,411-419,429
脊髄円錐　397,421,429,438
脊髄硬膜　407-409,443-447
脊髄神経　443,447
脊髄神経節　401-409,413-417,423,427,431-

433,443-447
　後根　413-419,423
　前根　415-419,423
脊柱管　263,397,407-409
脊柱起立筋　423-425,431-435,443-447
　外側筋列　443-447
　内側筋列　443-447
舌咽神経(第Ⅸ脳神経)　413
舌下神経(第Ⅻ脳神経)　411-415
仙棘靱帯　451
仙結節靱帯　189-195,277-279,291
仙骨　187-189,260-265,291,397,429-441,449-451
　外側部　263-265,439,449-451
　岬角　397,429-433,437,451
仙骨管　429,449
仙骨神経叢　187,259-261,279,439,451
仙腸関節　261-265,439-441,449-451
仙腸靱帯　263,439-441
浅鵞足　307-313,331-337,340
浅指屈筋　31-69,99-105,119,129-137,143-146, 158-163,173-174,177-179
　橈骨頭　139
浅掌動脈弓　175-182
浅腸骨回旋動脈　269
浅腓骨神経　221-231,345,349-351
前外果動脈　383
前外椎骨静脈叢　431,437
前環椎後頭膜　398
前距腓靱帯　235-237,339,385
前鋸筋　3-17,71-75,95-106,441
前脛骨筋　219-245,305-309,319-321,339-342, 349-357,367-368,371-375,391
前脛骨静脈　221-233,340,343-344,349-351
前脛骨動脈　221-233,321-323,340,343-344,349-351,367-374
前脛骨反回静脈　307-309
前脛骨反回動脈　307-309
前脛腓靱帯　231-233,385
前骨間静脈　35-41,141,156,159-160
前骨間神経　35-41
前骨間動脈　35-41,141,156,159-160
前根　→脊髄神経根
前斜角筋　417-419
前十字靱帯　211-215,289,297,307-313,325-327, 339-347,353-354-356
前縦靱帯　399,413,421,429,443-447
前上腸骨棘　187,255-258,267
前上腕回旋静脈　13,71,83-89,98-100
前上腕回旋動脈　13,71,83-89,98-100
前仙骨孔　449
前仙骨靱帯　449

前内果動脈　389
前内椎骨静脈叢　419,431,445-447
前腓骨頭靱帯　307,319
前腕帽膜　45
前腕骨間膜　37-39
前腕正中皮静脈　125

そ

粗線　203
鼠径靱帯　187-189
双子筋　193,263,267-279,286-288,298
　下—　193,263,273-279
　上—　263,273-279
爪体　69
僧帽筋　3,71-81,93-95,98-106,115-120,123,398-403,411-419,423-427
総頸動脈　417-419,425
総骨間静脈　131
総骨間動脈　131
総掌側指神経　63,181-182
総掌側指動脈　179-180
総腸骨動脈　429,447-451
総腸骨動脈　256,431-435,443-447,451
総腓骨神経　203-219,291-295,315-323
足関節　233-237,339,355-357,361-365,387-389
足根中足関節　242,383,387
　第1—　242
足底筋　211-227,293,311-327,338,342,349-355
足底腱膜　253,343,347,359-377,385-393
足底動脈弓　249
足底方形筋　245-251,339-345,359-373,389-391
足背趾皮神経　379
足背静脈　393
足背静脈弓　379
足背動脈　235-247,387
側副靱帯　27,63-69,168-174,182
　遠位指節間関節　178
　中手指節関節　180

た

多裂筋　265,401,409,417-419,423-427,431-435, 439-447
大孔　398,406
大後頭孔　398,406
大門筋　13-17,73-81,87-95,100-107,115-123
大胸筋　7-17,85-97,119-123
大結節　5-9,73-77,81-83,98,109-112
大結節稜　83
大後頭神経　409
大後頭直筋　401-403,409-415

大槽 409
大腿筋膜張筋 187-197,255-257,281-283,293-298
大腿骨 191-215,257-261,267-275,281-315,319-344,351-356
　外側顆 213-215,285-289,293-295,303-315,319-325,338-344,351-353
　外側上顆 309
　顆間部 327
　頸 193,259,267,283-287,297
　小転子 197,261,269-271,287,296-299
　体 259-261,267-269,283-287,295-297,305-309,325-333
　大転子 193,259-263,267,281-286,293-295
　頭 191-193,257-261,269-275,281-286,298,301
　内側顆 211-215,285-291,299-315,329-344
　内側上顆 309
大腿骨頭窩 275
大腿骨頭靱帯 191,283-284
大腿四頭筋腱 281-283,293-295,299,303,323-333,356
大腿膝蓋関節 209-211
大腿神経 187-191,205,255-259,451
大腿深静脈 197-201,259-261,273-275,285-287,297-299
大腿深動脈 197-201,257-261,273-275,285-287,297-301
大腿直筋 191-207,255-257,267-271,281,295-299,329-333
大腿静脈 193-199,201-207,255-259,275-289,295-301
大腿神経 193-199
大腿動脈 193-199,201-207,255-259,275-289,295-301,329
大腿二頭筋 197-217,265,269-277,289-301,313-325,340-344,350-352
　短頭 201-207,293,321-323
　長頭 201-207,265,269-289-301,321-323
大腿方形筋 195-197,263,267-275,289,293-298,301
大転子 193,259-263,267,281-286,293-295
大殿筋 187-199,261-279,288,291-295,296-300,433-435,449-451
大動脈
　─弓 425
　─分岐部 256
　下行─ 421-427
　上行─ 421-423
　腹部─ 429
大内転筋 197-209,261-279,287-291,295-301,309-311,337

大伏在静脈 197-241,255,281-291,301,313,341-347,363-375
大腰筋 257-260,275,279,437-438,443-451
大菱形筋 422,425-427
大菱形骨 53-55,165-169,183
第1指間間関節 169
第1手根中手関節 167
第1足根中足関節 242
短趾屈筋 253,339,343-345,361-381,387-389
短趾伸筋 237-247,367-385
短小指屈筋 55-65,173-175
短小趾屈筋 253,373-377,381-385
短小趾伸筋 375-381
短掌筋 53-61,173
短橈側手根伸筋 31-55,97,109,127,149-153,159-163,181
短内転筋 195-201,257-261,273-289,301
短腓骨筋 221-247,339-351,359-371,383-385
短母指外転筋 53-65,179-183
短母指屈筋 59-65,165-169,179-183
　深頭 59-63,165,179-183
　浅頭 59-63,181-182
短母指伸筋 37-63,149-160,167
短母趾屈筋 247-253,373-379,391-393
　外側頭 249-251,375-379,391
　内側頭 249-251,375,391
短母趾伸筋 367-381

ち

恥骨 191-195,255-261,279-287
　上枝 191-193,281
　下枝 195,261,283-287
恥骨筋 193-197,255-259,271-285,299-301
恥骨結合 255,281-283
恥骨大腿靱帯 195
腔 193-195,259-263,285-287
中間楔状骨 240-245,373-375,387-389
中間広筋 197-207,257-261,267-269,281-287,293-299,321-323
中関節上腕靱帯 5-9,89
中膝関節 211,311
中斜角筋 405-407,417-419
中手骨 57-67,165-183
　第1─ 57-63,165-171
　第2─ 57-65,168-171,181-183
　第3─ 55,65,181
　第4─ 57-65
　第5─ 55-65,167
中手指節関節 167-178
中節骨
　足 253,383,389

手　168-178,182
中足骨　251,379,383
　第1—　242-249,377-381,389-393
　第2—　242-249,375-377,381,387-389
　第3—　247,375-377,381,385
　第4—　249,373-375,381-385
　第5—　371-377,381-383
中足趾節関節　248,383
中側副動脈　25
中殿筋　187-195,255-263,267-272,275,280-286,293-300,437-441,449-451
虫様筋　63-67,166,173-182,253,387
肘筋　27-33,101-109,139-141,145-147,155
肘正中皮静脈　27-35,117-119,125,133,151-153
肘頭　27-29,103-113,117,131-137,143-147,155-161
肘頭窩　103,111-113,131,135-137,161
肘頭滑液包　135-137
肘頭皮下包　27-29
長胸神経　13,97
長趾屈筋　223-253,341-345,353-393
長趾伸筋　219-250,305-309,339-340,349-351,355-357,365-387
長掌筋　29-53,127-129,161
長足底靱帯　245,249-251,365-375,385-387
長橈側手根伸筋　23-55,99,109-113,127-131,139-141,147-153,161-163,171,183
長内転筋　197-201,255-261,277-287,301
長腓骨筋　219-251,305-313,319-321,340-351,361-377,383-389
長母指外転筋　35-55,141,146-159,165
長母指屈筋　35-67,145-149,161-166,179-183
長母指伸筋　35-63,147-150,159,169-171
長母趾屈筋　223-253,343-347,351-381,387-393
長母趾伸筋　223-247,339-343,349-355,367-381,389-393
腸脛靱帯　191-217,257-259,263,283-289,303-311,315-319,338-340,347-349,350-352
腸骨　187-189,255-257,261-300,437-441,449-451
　臼蓋　269-275
　翼　267,279,449-451
腸骨筋　255-260,275,279,286,437,449-451
腸骨大腿靱帯　191-195,257-259,280,296
腸骨動脈　449-451
腸骨稜　260
腸腰筋　187-197,255-259,267-272,277,281-287,299-300
腸腰静脈　437
腸腰動脈　437
跳躍靱帯　245
腸肋筋

胸—　427
腰—　263-265,439-447
直腸　189-195,265,451

つ

椎間関節　401-407,417,423,427,433-435,439-447
椎間孔　401-403,423,433-435,447
椎間静脈　423
椎間板　397-401,407,435
椎弓　265,409,417-419,431-433,439-441,445-447
椎弓板　417-419,431-433,439-441,445-447
椎弓根　419,423,438-439
椎骨静脈　404,417
椎骨動脈　400,403-407,411-419
椎体　397-409,415-423,429-437,445-447,449
　終板　399,423,435-437
椎体静脈　399,417,421,429,445-447

て

底側骨間筋　248,251-253,379-385
底側趾静脈　249
底側趾神経　249
底側趾動脈　249-250
底側踵舟靱帯　245,367-369,387-391
底側中足静脈　249,379
底側中足神経　249
底側中足動脈　249—251,377-379
転子間稜　261-263

と

豆鈎靱帯　53,165-167
豆状骨　49-53,143,154,165-167,173
豆中手靱帯　53-55
頭最長筋　409-415,419
頭長筋　399-403,411-415,424
頭半棘筋　398-400,403,411-417,422
頭板状筋　401-403,406,409-419
橈骨　31-47,97-99,109-113,127-131,137-141,144-163,167-171,175-183
　茎状突起　183
　頸　137
　粗面　129,137,145-147,155-157
　体　113,127-129,137-139,149-151,161-163
　頭　31,97-99,109-111,127-131,137-141,149-159
橈骨手根関節　175,179
橈骨神経　15-39,43-55,71-75,91,101,105-107,

和文索引　　***463***

113,121-127,131,135-139,159,163
橈骨粗面　129,137,145-147,155-157
橈骨静脈　33-57,135,145-147,161-163
橈骨動脈　33-57,125,135,145-147,161-171,
181-183
橈骨輪状靱帯　31,127,131,139-141,155-157,
161
橈尺関節　31,137,147
橈側手根屈筋　29-55,99-101,125-129,133,143,
163,181
橈側正中皮静脈　125
橈側側副動静脈　27-29
橈側反回動脈　159
橈側皮静脈　9-33,37-61,83-97,113-115,121-
125,137-143,146,149,163
　母指　61

な

内果　233-235,339-341,363-365,393
内頸静脈　96,404,411-419
内頸動脈　403,411-415
内後頭隆起　398
内側横突間筋　443
内側下膝静脈　307-313,329-335,339
内側下膝動脈　305-313,329-335,339
内側顆間結節　307-311,327
内側距踵靱帯　241
内側楔状骨　240-247,373-375,389-393
内側広筋　197-207,255,259,267,271-275,281-
289,297-311,325-337
内側膝蓋支帯　209-219,281-283,303,335-337
内側手根側副靱帯　47,146,167-171
内側上顆
（上腕骨）117,129-131,163
（大腿骨）309
内側上膝静脈　209,305-311,329-337
内側上膝動脈　209,305-311,329-337
内側前腕皮神経　33,37-39,43,121
内側足根動脈　367,389,393
内側足底静脈　243-247,251-253,361-375,391
内側足底神経　247-253,361-375,391-393
内側足底動脈　247-253,361-375,391-393
内側側副靱帯
（手関節）→内側手根側副靱帯
（肘関節）129,133
（膝関節）213-217,305-311,338-342
内側大腿回旋静脈　261
内側大腿回旋動脈　259-261,269
内側半月板　215,299,305-313,331-344,356
　後角　215,299,311-313,331-337,356
　前角　215,305,335-337

体部　215,307-309,337-344
内側腓腹皮神経　219-221
内側翼突筋　415
内腸骨静脈　187-189,259,277,437-439
内腸骨動脈　187-189,259,277,435-439
内椎骨静脈叢　443
内腹斜筋　187-191,255-258,267,449-451
内閉鎖筋　189-197,259-273,277-279,283-288,
291,298
内肋間筋　5-17

に

二分靱帯　241-243,369,383-387
乳頭突起　433
乳様突起　404-406,409
尿管　187-193

の

脳神経
　第Ⅸ脳神経　→舌咽神経
　第Ⅹ脳神経　→迷走神経
　第Ⅺ脳神経　→副神経
　第Ⅻ脳神経　→舌下神経

は

ばね靱帯　387,391
歯尖靱帯　398
馬尾　397,421,429,439,443-447
肺　7,11-17,71-73,405-409,427,438
肺動脈　421-427
背側距舟靱帯　235-236,239,387
背側骨間筋　59-65,173,183,244,247-248,251-
253,379-385
背側指静脈　67-69,174,180-182
背側指神経　65-69,170,181
　母指　59-65
背側指動脈　65-69,170,181-182
　母指　59-65
背側趾静脈　251
背側趾神経　251,381
背側趾静脈　251
背側手根間靱帯　51-53,175-179,183
背側手根中手靱帯　173-179,183
背側足根靱帯　238,243-245,371-373,385-387
背側中手静脈　170
背側中手靱帯　57
背側中手動脈　171,183
　（母指）171
背側中足靱帯　383-385

464 和文索引

背側中足静脈　379-381
背側中足動脈　379-381
背側橈骨手根靱帯　47,150,171-179
背側橈骨靱帯　173
薄筋　197-219,257-265,285-291,301,313-317,
　337,342-346
反回骨間静脈　33,155
反回骨間動脈　31-33,155
半奇静脈　423-425
半棘筋　398-400,403,411-417,422-423,427
　胸—　423,427
　頸—　401,407-409,417-419
　頭—　398-400,403,411-417,422
半月板　→外側半月板,内側半月板
半腱様筋　197-219,265,273,279,289-291,295-
　301,311-317,337
半膜様筋　197-217,273,279,289-291,295-301,
　309-317,325-337,346
板状筋
　頸—　401,407-409,419,422-424
　頭—　401-403,406,409-419

ひ

ヒラメ筋　219-231,293-297,315-327,342,345-
　357
皮静脈
　尺側—　19-53,89,101-103,121-125,143,155-
　163
　前腕正中—　125
　肘正中—　27-35,117-119,125,133,151-153
　橈側—　9-33,37-61,83-97,113-115,121-125,
　137-143,146,149,163
　橈側正中—　125
　副橈側—　33,45
腓骨　219-237,309-315,319-321,339-351,361-
　365,383-385
　外果　233-237,341,345,349-351,363-365
　体　345-351
　頭　219,309-315,319-321,344,347-349
腓骨筋支帯　237-247
　下—　247
　上—　237-239
腓骨静脈　223-237,341-347,351,361
腓骨動脈　221-237,341-347,351,361
腓腹筋　209-227,289-297,311-357
　外側頭　209-221,289-297,311-333,338-356
　内側頭　209-221,289-291,311-317,329-346,
　355-357
腓腹神経　223-239,359-365
腓腹静脈　315
腓腹動脈　315

尾骨　397,451
尾骨筋　451

ふ

伏在神経　201-209,231-233,257-259,285-289,
　301,313-317,337
副神経(第XI脳神経)　413-415
副橈側皮静脈　33,45
副半奇静脈　425-427
腹横筋　187-191,255-256,267,449-451
腹直筋　187-195,269-272,275-279,451
腹部大動脈　429

へ

閉鎖静脈　187-193
閉鎖神経　187-195,257-259,279,287
閉鎖動脈　187-193,279

ほ

母指
　掌側指神経　65,69
　掌側指動脈　65,69
　背側指神経　59-65
　背側指動脈　59-65
　背側中手神経　171
　背側中手動脈　171
母指外転筋　161,165
母指主動脈　61
母指伸筋(腱膜)　65-67
母指対立筋　53-63,165-167,181-183
母指内転筋　57-65,165-169,177-182
　横頭　63,165-169,177-182
　斜頭　57-63,167-169,179-182
　深頭　177
母趾外転筋　247-251,339-343,359-381,391-
　393
母趾内転筋　249,253,369-381,387-389
　横頭　253,379-381,387-389
　斜頭　249,253,369-379,387-389
方形回内筋　41-43,146,156-163,167-169,173-
　181
放射状肋骨頭靱帯　425-427
放射性手根靱帯　167
縫工筋　189-219,255-257,267-291,298,301,311-
　313,331-337,342-346
膀胱　187-193,255-261,281-282

和文索引　　**465**

ま

末節骨
　（足）250-253,383,389-393
　（手）69,166-168,172,176,182

め

迷走神経（第Ⅹ脳神経）　411-415

ゆ

有鈎骨　53-57,144-148,156,165-171,175,181
有鈎骨鈎　55-57,165-167,181
有頭骨　49-55,144-148,158-160,169-171,177-
　179

よ

腰棘間筋　441
腰筋　→大腰筋
腰静脈　431,435-437,441-447
　上行―　445-447
腰神経　431-435,443-449
腰神経叢　260,437
腰仙骨神経叢　189
腰腸肋筋　263-265,439-447
腰椎　258,397,429-449
腰動脈　431-435,445-447
腰椎槽　429,437-447
腰方形筋　439-447
翼状靱帯　405,411
翼突筋静脈叢　411

ら

卵管　189
卵巣　189,259

り

梨状筋　187-191,263-265,271-279,286-288,298,
　441,451
立方骨　245-251,369-373,383-387
隆椎（C7）　397-401,405-409,421
菱形筋　401,419,422,425-427
　大―　422,425-427

小―　419
輪状軟骨　417
輪帯　261

ろ

肋横突関節　427
肋横突靱帯　425-427
肋間筋　5-17,71-75,97-104,107,409,427,441
　外―　5-17
　最内―　13-17
　内―　5-17
肋間静脈　9-11,17,97-107,401-403
肋間神経　9-11,17,97-107
肋間動脈　9-11,17,97-107,401-403,421-425,
　427,431-433,437,441
肋骨　3-17,71-75,95-107,407-409,425-427,438-
　441
　頸　407,427
　結節　409,427
　体　407,427
　頭　407,425-427,435,438
肋骨挙筋　441
肋骨頭関節　427
肋骨突起　445

わ

腕尺関節　27-29,101,109-115,129,133,143-147,
　157-161
腕神経叢　7-13,93-95,100
腕頭静脈　421-425
腕頭動脈　421-423
腕橈関節　99,109-111,129,137-139,149-153,
　157-159
腕橈骨筋　21-43,97-103,109-121,125-131,135-
　141,145-153,163-165,169-171

欧文

DIP関節　→遠位指節間関節,遠位指趾節間
　関節
Hoffa脂肪体　→膝蓋下脂肪体
PIP関節　→近位指節間関節,近位趾節間関節
S状結腸　187,261-263
S状静脈洞　406-409
Wrisberg靱帯　→後半月大腿靱帯

欧文索引

A

abdominal aorta 429
abductor digiti minimi muscle
(foot) 249-253,341-343,361-369
(hand) 51-65,154,165-169,173
abductor hallucis muscle 247-251,339-343,
359-381,391-393
abductor pollicis brevis muscle 53-65,179-
183
abductor pollicis longus muscle 35-55,141,
146-159,165
abductor pollicis muscle 161,165
accessory cephalic vein 33,45
accessory hemiazygos vein 425-427
accessory nerve(XI) 413-415
acetabular fossa 191-193,275
acetabular labrum 191-193,257-259,269-275,
280
acetabulum 257-261,280-286
Achilles tendon 235-247,355-357,387-391
acromioclavicular joint 3,73-75,91,104-106
acromioclavicular ligament 73-75,91,110-112
acromion 3,73-81,87-95,100-123
adductor brevis muscle 195-201,257-261,
273-289,301
adductor hallucis muscle 249,253,369-381,
387-389
oblique head 249,253,369-379,387-389
transverse head 253,379-381,387-389
adductor longus muscle 197-201,255-261,
277-287,301
adductor magnus muscle 197-209,261-279,
287-291,295-301,309-311,337
adductor minimus muscle 261,271,275-279,
285-289
adductor pollicis muscle 57-65,165-169,177-
182
deep head 177
oblique head 57-63,167-169,179-182
transverse head 63,165-169,177-182

alar ligament 405,411
anconeus muscle 27-33,101-109,139-141,145-
147,155
ankle joint 233-237,339,355-357,361-365,387-
389
anserine bursa 337
antebrachial fascia 45
anterior atlanto-occipital membrane 398
anterior circumflex humeral artery 13,71,
83-89,98-100
anterior circumflex humeral vein 13,71,83-
89,98-100
anterior cruciate ligament 211-215,289,297,
307-313,325-327,339-347,354-356
anterior external vertebral venous plexus
431,437
anterior internal vertebral venous plexus
419,431,445-447
anterior interosseous artery 35-41,141,156,
159-160
anterior interosseous nerve 35-41
anterior interosseous vein 35-41,141,156,
159-160
anterior lateral malleolar artery 383
anterior longitudinal ligament 399,413,421,
429,443-447
anterior medial malleolar artery 389
anterior sacral foramina 449
anterior sacro-iliac ligaments 449
anterior superior iliac spine 187,255-258,
267
anterior talofibular ligament 235-237,339,
385
anterior tibial artery 221-233,321-323,340,
343-344,349-351,367-374
anterior tibial recurrent artery 307-309
anterior tibial recurrent vein 307-309
anterior tibial vein 221-233,340-344,349-351
anterior tibiofibular ligament 231-233,385
anular ligament(radius) 31,127,131,139-141,
155-157,161
anus 288

欧文索引　**467**

aorta　256,421-429
　　abdominal— 429
　　ascending— 421-423
　　bifurcation　256
　　descending— 421-427
aortic arch　425
arcuate popliteal ligament　315,349
articular process　419
ascending aorta　421-423
ascending lumbar vein　445-447
atlanto-occipital joint　400-405
atlas（C1）　399-415
　　anterior arch　399,411
　　articular process　415
　　lateral mass　400-405,411-413
　　posterior arch　399-401,407-411
　　transverse process　405,413-415
axillary artery　9-15,73,93-95,98
axillary nerve　13,73-83,89-93
axillary recess　75-77
axillary vein　9-15,73,93-95,98
axis（C2）　399-401,405-407,413-415
　　body　401,415
　　dens　397-399,405,411-413
　　posterior arch　413-415
　　vertebral arch　407
　　vertebral body　399,405
azygos vein　421,427

B

basilic vein　19-53,89,101-103,121-125,143,
　　155-163
basivertebral vein　399,417,421,429,445-447
biceps brachii muscle　7-31,73-75,83-91,96-
　　121,125-129,133-139,145-153,157,161-163
　　long head　7-13,19-25,73-75,83-91,96-121
　　short head,9-13,19-25,89-91,97
biceps femoris muscle　197-217,265,269-277,
　　289-301,313-325,340-344,350-352
　　long head　201-207,265,269,289-301,321-
　　323
　　short head　201-207,293,321-323
bicipital aponeurosis　29-31
bicipital groove　7,83
bifurcate ligament　241-243,369,383-387
brachial artery　91,145-147
brachial artery and vein　15-31,71,75,97,119-
　　125,133,163
brachial plexus　7-13,93-95,100

brachial vein　91
brachialis muscle　19-31,97-103,109-121,125-
　　163
brachiocephalic trunk　421-423
brachiocephalic vein　421-425
brachioradialis muscle　21-43,97-103,109-121,
　　125-131,135-141,145-153,163-165,169-171

C

calcaneal anastomosis　391
calcaneal tuberosity　243,355
calcaneocuboid joint　383-387
calcaneofibular ligament　239-241,341-343,
　　351,363-365,383
calcaneus　241-253,339-347,355-369,383-393
　　talar shelf　243-245
　　tuber　391
　　tuberosity　245,249-253
calcaneal tendon　235-247,355-357,387-391
calcaneal tuberosity　245,249-253
capitate　49-55,144-148,158-160,169-171,177-
　　179
capitatohamate intercarpal joint　55
capsular ligament　193
carpometacarpal joint　167-171,175-183
cauda equina　397,421,429,439,443-447
cephalic vein　9-33,37-61,83-97,113-115,121-
　　125,137-143,146-149,163
cervical plexus　405
cervical spinal cord　399
cervical vertebra　397,401,405,417-419
　　→atlas（C1）,axis（C2）,vertebra prominens
　　（C7）も参照
circumflex scapular artery　13,77-79,93-95,
　　123
circumflex scapular vein　13,77-79,93-95,123
cisterna magna　409
clavicle　37,71-75,91-106,110-115,120-123
coccygeus muscle　451
coccyx　397,451
collateral ligament　27,63-69,168-174,178-182
　　distal interphalangeal joint　178
　　metacarpophalangeal joint　180
　　palmar— 172-174,182
　　→lateral collateral ligament,
　　　medial collateral ligament も参照
collateral ulnar artery　117-119
collateral ulnar vein　117
common carotid artery　417-419,425

common fibular nerve 203-219,291-295,315-323

common iliac artery 256,431-435,443-451

common iliac vein 429,447-451

common interosseous artery 131

common interosseous vein 131

common palmar digital artery 179-180

common palmar digital nerve 63,181-182

conus medullaris 397,421,429,438

coracoacromial ligament 71-73,89-91

coracobrachialis muscle 9-17,71-75,87-91, 97-100,117-123

coracoclavicular ligament 3-7,71,93-95,98-102,118,123

coracohumeral ligament 5-7,71-73,89-91,98

coracoid process 5-7,71,91-93,96-104,120-123

coronoid fossa 27,129,135

coronoid process 111,135-137,143-145,159-161

costal process 445

costotransverse joint 427

costotransverse ligament 425-427

cranial nerve

IX →glossopharyngeal nerve

X →vagus nerve

XI →accessory nerve

XII →hypoglossal nerve

cricoid cartilage 417

cruciate ligament(atlas) 411

cuboid 245-251,369-373,383-387

cuneocuboid interosseous ligament 383-385

cuneometatarsal interosseous ligament 244

cuneonavicular joint 241,389

D

deep artery of thigh(=deep femoral artery) 197-201,257-261,273-275,285-287,297-301

deep brachial artery 19-25,101-109,117,137

deep brachial vein 19-25,101-109,117

deep cervical vein 399-403,409-419

deep fascia of leg 331-335

deep femoral artery 285-287,299

deep fibular nerve 221-235,340-344,367-369, 373-375

deep infrapatellar bursa 325-333

deep palmar arch 59-63,169,173-183

deep pes anserinus 309-315,337

deep plantar arch 373-375,385-389

deep transverse metacarpal ligament 65

deep transverse perineal muscle 259-261

deep vein of thigh(=deep femoral vein) 197-201,259-261,273-275,285-287,297-299

deltoid ligament 233-243,339,361-369,391-393

anterior tibiotalar part 233-237,369,393

posterior tibiotalar part 237-239,363-365, 391-393

tibiocalcaneal part 239-241,365,393

tibionavicular part 233-243,367,393

deltoid muscle 3-17,71-123

acromial part 3-9,83-93,109-123

clavicular part 3-9,89-95

spinal part 3-9,91-95

dens(axis) 397-399,405,411-413

descending aorta 421-427

descending colon 449

descending genicular vein 305

diaphragm 431-433,437

digastric muscle 405-407,411-415

digital artery 182

digital fibrous sheath 67-69

distal interphalangeal joint(DIP) 168,172, 176,182,383

(foot) 253,383

(hand) 168,172,176,182

distal phalanx

(foot) 250-253,383,389-393

(hand) 69,166-168,172,176,182

dorsal aponeurosis 67

dorsal capsule 361

dorsal carpometacarpal ligament 173-179, 183

dorsal digital artery 65-69,170,181-182

thumb 59-65

dorsal digital cutaneous nerve of foot 379

dorsal digital nerve 65-69,170,181

thumb 59-65

dorsal digital nerves of foot 381

dorsal digital vein 67-69,174,180-182

dorsal intercarpal ligament 51-53,175-179, 183

dorsal interosseous muscle

(foot) 244-253,379-385

(hand) 59-65,173,183

dorsal lateral cutaneous nerve 241

dorsal metacarpal artery 171,183

dorsal metacarpal ligament 57

dorsal metacarpal nerve 171

欧文索引 **469**

dorsal metacarpal vein 170
dorsal metatarsal artery 379-381
dorsal metatarsal ligaments 383-385
dorsal metatarsal vein 379-381
dorsal radiocarpal ligament 47,150,171-179
dorsal radioulnar ligament 173
dorsal root 413-419
dorsal talonavicular ligament 235-239,387
dorsal tarsal ligaments 238,243-245,371-373,
385-387
dorsal venous arch（foot） 379
dorsalis pedis artery 235-247,387
dorsalis pedis vein 393
dura mater 413,429

E

epidural fatty tissue 421,429,443-445
erector spinae muscle 423-425,431-435,443-
447
lateral tract 443-447
medial tract 443-447
spinalis muscle 431-435
esophagus 399,405,417-427
extensor carpi radialis brevis muscle 31-
55,97,109,127,149-153,159-163,181
extensor carpi radialis longus muscle
23-55,99,109-113,127-131,139-141,147-153,
161-163,171,183
extensor carpi ulnaris muscle 31-55,99-101,
139-141,146-151,155,171-173
extensor digiti minimi brevis muscle 375-
381
extensor digiti minimi longus muscle 381
extensor digiti minimi muscle 35-67,141,
149-156
extensor digitorum brevis muscle 237-247,
367-385
extensor digitorum longus muscle 219-250,
305-309,339-340,349-351,355-357,365-387
extensor digitorum muscle
（foot） 383,387-389
（arm/hand） 31-69,97-99,129-131,141,151-
163,171-183
extensor hallucis brevis muscle 367-381
extensor hallucis longus muscle 223-247,
339-343,349-355,367-381,389-393
extensor indicis muscle 39-61,67,146-150,
155-158
extensor pollicis brevis muscle 37-63,149-

160,167
extensor pollicis longus muscle 35-63,147-
150,159,169-171
extensor pollicis muscle 65-67
extensor retinaculum
（foot） 235
（hand） 41,45-49
external anal sphincter muscle 288
external auditory canal 404
external carotid artery 415
external iliac artery 187-191
external iliac vein 187-191
external intercostal muscle 5-17
external oblique muscle 255,258,267,449-451

F

fat body →fat pad も参照
infrapatellar— 213-217
pre-Achilles— 355,389
（elbow）anterior— 135
posterior— 131,135
fat pad →fat body も参照
Hoffa— →infrapatellar fat pad
infrapatellar— 303,323-333,354-356
suprapatellar— 303
femoral artery 193-207,255-259,275-289,295-
301,329
femoral nerve 187-199,205,255-259,451
femoral vein 193-207,255-259,275-289,295-
301
femoropatellar joint 209-211
femur 191-215,257-263,267-275,281-315,319-
344,351-356
greater trochanter 193,259-263,267,281-
286,293-295
head 191-193,257-261,269-275,281-286,298-
301
intercondylar part 327
lateral condyle 213-215,285-289,293-295,
303-315,319-325,338-344,351-353
lateral epicondyle 309
lesser trochanter 197,261,269-271,287,296-
299
medial condyle 211-215,285-291,299-315,
329-344
medial epicondyle 309
neck 193,259,267,283-287,297
shaft 259-261,267-269,283-287,295-297,
305-309,325-333

fibula 219-237,309-315,319-321,339-351,361-365,383-385
  head 219,309-315,319-321,344-349
  lateral malleolus 233-237,341,345,349-351, 363-365
  shaft 345-351
fibular artery 223-237,341-347,351,361
fibular collateral ligament 311-315,338,344, 347
fibular vein 223-237,341-347,351,361
fibularis brevis muscle 221-247,339-351,359-371,383-385
fibularis longus muscle 219-251,305-313,319-321,340-351,361-377,383-389
filum terminale 421
flexor carpi radialis muscle 29-39,41-55,99-101,125-129,133,143,163,181
flexor carpi ulnaris muscle 31-53,105-107, 115-123,127,131,145-147,155-159,165,175
flexor digiti minimi brevis muscle
  (foot) 253,373-377,381-385
  (hand) 55-65,173-175
flexor digiti minimi longus muscle 381
flexor digiti minimi muscle 165-167,173
flexor digitorum brevis muscle 253,339,343-345,361-381,387-389
flexor digitorum longus muscle 233-253, 341-345,353-393
flexor digitorum muscle 168,172-175,178-182,253
flexor digitorum profundus muscle 31-69, 103-107,111-119,127-137,143-145,155-167, 173-179
flexor digitorum superficialis muscle 31-69, 99-105,119,129-139,143-146,158-163,173-179
  radial head 139
flexor hallucis brevis muscle 247-253,373-379,391-393
  lateral head 249-251,375-379,391
  medial head 249-251,375,391
flexor hallucis longus muscle 223-253,343-347,351-381,387-393
flexor pollicis brevis muscle 59-65,165-169, 179-183
  deep head 59-63,165,179-183
  superficial head 59-63,181-182
flexor pollicis longus muscle 35-67,145-149, 161-166,179-183
flexor retinaculum 47-59,175-181,235-247, 363-365

foramen magnum 398,406
fovea 275

G

gastrocnemius muscle 209-227,289-297,311-357
  lateral head 209-221,289-297,311-333,338-356
  medial head 209-221,289-291,311-317,329-346,355-357
gemellus muscle 193,263,267-279,286-288, 298
  inferior 193,263,273-279
  superior 263,275-279
genicular anastomosis 303-305
glenohumeral joint 9,73-79,91
glenohumeral ligament 73,83-87,117
glenoid 5-11,73-79,98-106,116-118
glenoid labrum 9-11,73-77,116
glossopharyngeal nerve(Ⅸ) 413
gluteus maximus muscle 187-199,261-279, 288-300,433-435,449-451
gluteus medius muscle 187-195,255-263, 267-275,280-286,293-300,437-441,449-451
gluteus minimus muscle 187-195,257-261, 267-273,280-286,300
gracilis muscle 197-219,257-265,285-291, 301,313-317,337,342-346
great saphenous vein 197-241,255,281-291, 301,313,341-347,363-375
greater trochanter 193,259-263,267,281-286, 293-295
greater tubercle 5-9,73-77,81-83,98,109-112

H

hamate 53-57,144-148,156,165-171,175,181
  hook 55-57,165-167,175,181
hemiazygos vein 423-425
hip joint 257-259,269-273,281-284,301
Hoffa fat pad→infrapatellar fat pad
humeroradial joint 99,109-111,129,137-139, 149-153,157-159
humeroulnar joint 27-29,101,109-115,129, 133,143-147,157-161
humerus 5-29,59,73-89,97-118,127-131,135-141,145-153,157-163,309
  capitulum 29,97-101,109-119,127-153,157-161

欧文索引　**471**

greater tubercle　5-9,73-77,81-83,98,109-112

head　59,71-81,85-89,97-98,104-118

lateral epicondyle　27,129-131

lesser tubercle　7-11

medial epicondyle　27-29,103-107,117,129-131,163

neck　97,110

shaft　17-25,75-87,99-105,109-112,129-131,137-139,145-151

trochlea　99-101,115,119,127-135,143-147,159-161

hypoglossal nerve（Ⅻ）　411-415

I

ileum　449-451

iliac artery　449-451

iliac crest　260

iliacus muscle　255-260,275,279,286,437,449-451

iliocostalis lumborum muscle　263-265,439-447

iliocostalis thoracis muscle　427

iliofemoral ligament　191-195,257-259,280,296

iliolumbar artery　437

iliolumbar vein　437

iliopsoas muscle　187-197,255-259,267-272,277,281-287,299-300

iliotibial tract　191-217,257-259,263,283-289,303-311,315-319,338-340,347-352

ilium　187-189,255-279,300,437-441,449-451

iliac spine　187-189,255-258,267

anterior superior—　187,255-258,267

inferior anterior—　189

joint socket　277

roof of acetabulum　269-275

wing　267,279,449-451

inferior anterior iliac spine　189

inferior articular process　401-407,417,423,427,433-435,439-447

inferior epigastric artery　187-189

inferior epigastric vein　187-189

inferior fibular retinaculum　247

inferior glenohumeral ligament　89

inferior gluteal artery　261-265,271,277,451

inferior gluteal nerve　263-265,273,277-279

inferior gluteal vein　261-265,271,451

inferior lateral genicular artery　305-311,

inferior lateral genicular vein　307-311,321-327,339

inferior medial genicular artery　305-313,329-335,339

inferior medial genicular vein　307-313,329-335,339

inferior tibiofibular joint　231,341

inferior vena cava　256,431-435,443-445

confluence　443-445

infraglenoid tubercle　91

infrapatellar fat pad（fat body）　213-217,303,323-333,354-356

infraspinatus muscle　5-17,77-95,102-123,427

inguinal ligament　187-189

innermost intercostal muscle　13-17

intercarpal joint

capitatohamate　55

scaphocapitate　177-179

intercondylar fossa　213,307-313,340

intercondylar tubercle　340

intercostal artery　9-11,17,97-107,427

intercostal muscle　5-17,71-75,97,104-107,409,427,441

external—　5-17

innermost—　13-17

internal—　5-17

intercostal nerve　9-11,17,97-107

intercostal vein　9-11,17,97-107

intermediate cuneiform　240-245,373-375,387-389

internal carotid artery　403,411-415

internal iliac artery　187-189,259,277,435-439

internal iliac vein　187-189,259,277,437-439

internal intercostal muscle　5-17

internal jugular vein　96,404,411-419

internal oblique muscle　187-191,255-258,267,449-451

internal occipital protuberance　398

internal vertebral venous plexus　443

interosseous artery　127,137-139,157

interosseous intercarpal ligament　171

interosseous ligament

cuneocuboid　383-385

cuneometatarsal　244

scapholunate　169

talocalcaneal　239,243,355-357,367,387-389

interosseous membrane　37-39,171,219-229

（forearm）　37-39,171

（leg）　219-229

472 欧文索引

interosseous metacarpal ligament 171

interosseous muscle 67-69,167-170,179-180, 371-377,387-389

interosseous sacro-iliac ligaments 449

interosseous talocalcaneal ligament 241-243

interosseous vein 127,137-139,157

interphalangeal joint I 169

interspinales cervicis muscles 421

interspinales lumborum muscles 441

interspinales muscles 399,439

interspinous ligament 265,397-399,409,421, 429,439-441,445

intertransversarii laterales muscle 443

intertransversarii mediales muscle 443

intertransversarius muscle 425,439

intertrochanteric crest 261-263

intertubercular sulcus 7,83

intervertebral disk 397-401,405-407,421-423, 427-437,443

   anulus fibrosus 421,429-433,437

   nucleus pulposus 421,429-431,443

intervertebral foramen 401-403,423,433-435, 447

intervertebral space C5/C6 417,439

intervertebral vein 423

ischial spine 191,265

ischial tuberosity 195,265,277-279

ischioanal fossa 289

ischiofemoral ligament 193-195,261,275

ischiorectal fossa 195

ischium 191-193,263,273-275,288-291,298-301

J

joint capsule 11,27,45-53,57,71,79-81,85,91, 115-121,133,139-141,150,167,170-178,211-217,235,249,271-273,291,313-315,319,323-337,351,361

   ankle 235,249,361

   elbow 133,139-141

   hip 271－273,

   knee 211-217,291,313-315,319,323-337,351

   shoulder 11,27,45-53,57,71,79-81,85,91,115-121,

   wrist 150,167,170-178

joint of head of rib 427

K

knee joint 285-289,293-299,321,335,339-340, 350-353

L

larynx 419

lateral atlantoaxial joint 405

lateral circumflex femoral artery 197,255-259,267-275,281,287,293-301

lateral circumflex femoral vein 197,259,267, 281,287,293-301

lateral collateral ligament

   (elbow) 29

   (knee) 211-217,342

lateral condyle

   (femur) 213-215,285-289,293-295,303-315, 319-325,338-344,351-353

   (tibia) 293-295,305-315,319-323,340,347

lateral cuneiform 243-249,373-375,383-387

lateral cutaneous nerve of forearm 37,43, 125

lateral dorsal cutaneous nerve 367-369

lateral epicondyle

   (femur) 309

   (humerus) 27,129-131

lateral femoral condyle→lateral condyle (femur)

lateral femoral intermuscular septum 197-199

lateral intercondylar tubercle 309-313

lateral joint recess 319

lateral malleolus 233-237,341,345,349-351, 363-365

lateral meniscus 215,293-295,305-313,319-325,338-344,351-353

   anterior horn 215,305,321-323,353

   body 215,307-309,319,338-344

   posterior horn 215,295,311-313,321-325, 351-353

lateral patellar retinaculum 209-217,281-283, 303,319-321,349-352

lateral plantar artery 243-253,361-375,383-391

lateral plantar nerve 247-251,361-379,383-391

lateral plantar vein 243-253,361-375,383-391

lateral sacral artery 439-441

欧文索引　**473**

lateral sacral vein　439-441
lateral tarsal artery　235
lateral thoracic artery　15
lateral thoracic vein　15
lateral tibial condyle　293-295,305-315,319-323,340,347
latissimus dorsi muscle　13-17,71-81,87-95,99-107,117-123,423-425,441
left atrium　421-425
lesser trochanter　197,261,269-271,287,296-299
lesser tubercle　83
levator ani muscle　191-195,259-265,288
levator scapulae muscle　405-409,417-419
levatores costarum muscles　441
ligament of head of femur　191,283-284
ligamentum flavum　399-403,421-423,427-435,439,443-445
linea aspera　203
liver　421-425
long plantar ligament　245,249-251,365-375,385-387
long thoracic nerve　13,97
longissimus capitis muscle　409-415,419
longissimus cervicis muscle　417-419
longissimus muscle　439-447
longissimus thoracis muscle　427
longitudinal fasciculi　65,399
longus capitis muscle　399-403,411-415,424
longus colli muscle　401-405,415-419
lumbar artery　431-437,441,445-447
lumbar cistern　429,437-447
lumbar nerve　431
lumbar plexus　260,437
lumbar vein　435-437,441-443,
lumbar vertebra　258,397,429-437,445-449
　body　397,449
lumbosacral plexus　189
lumbosacral zygapophyseal joint L5-S1　439
lumbrical muscle　63-67,166,173-182,253,387
lunate　47-51,144-148,158-160,167-177
lung　7,11-17,71-73,405-409,427,438

M

major occipital nerve　409
mamillary process　433
mandible　411-415
　ramus　413-415
mastoid process　404-406,409

maxillary artery　411-413
medial circumflex femoral artery　259-261,269
medial circumflex femoral vein　261
medial collateral artery　25
medial collateral ligament
　（elbow）　129
　（foot）　338-342
　（knee）　213-217,305-311,338-342
medial cuneiform　240-247,373-375,389-393
medial cutaneous nerve of forearm　33,37-39,43,121
medial dorsal cutaneous nerve I　381
medial epicondyle
　（femur）　309
　（humerus）　27-29,103-107,117,129-131,163,309
medial femoral condyle　211-215,285-291,299-315,329-344
medial genicular artery　311
medial intercondylar tubercle　307-311,327-329
medial malleolus（tibia）　233-235,339-341,363-365,393
medial meniscus　215,299,305-313,331-344,356
　anterior horn　215,305,335-337
　body　215,307-309,337-344
　posterior horn　215,299,311-313,331-337,356
medial patellar retinaculum　209-219,281-283,303,335-337
medial plantar artery　243-253,361-375,391-393
medial plantar nerve　247-253,361-375,391-393
medial plantar septum　373
medial plantar vein　243-247,251-253,361-375,391
medial pterygoid muscle　415
medial talocalcaneal ligament　241
medial tarsal artery　367,389,393
medial tibial condyle　299,305-315,331-337,340,347
median atlanto-axial joint　399,411
median cephalic vein　125
median cubital vein　27-35,117-119,125,133,151-153
median nerve　17-61,71-75,91,97-101,115-127,133-135,145,157-163,177-179,182

median sacral artery 437,441,451
median sacral crest 429-431
median sacral vein 437,441
median vein of forearm 125
medulla oblongata 406
metacarpal 57-67,165-183
   I 57-63,165-171
   II 57-65,168-171,181-183
   III 57-65,181
   IV 57-65
   V 55-65,167
metacarpophalangeal joint 167-178
metatarsal 242-253,371-393
   I 242-249,377-381,389-393
   II 242-249,375-377,381,387-389
   III 247,375-377,381-385
   IV 249,373-375,381-385
   V 371-377,381-383
metatarsophalangeal joint 248,383
metatarsophalangeal joint IV 383
middle genicular artery 211
middle glenohumeral ligament 59,89
middle phalanx
  （foot）253,383,389
  （hand）168,172-178,182,
multifidus muscle 265,401-403,409,417-419,
423-427,431-435,439-447
musculocutaneous nerve 17-23,91

N

navicular 239-245,357,369-371,387-393
nerve filaments 431
neuroforaminal ligament 443
nuchal ligament 397,409-413,417-419
nutrient foramen 445

O

oblique popliteal ligament 211-213,217,315,
325-327,335
obliquus capitis inferior muscle 401-409,413-
415
obliquus capitis superior muscle 407-413
obturator artery and nerve 279
obturator artery,vein,and nerve 187-193
obturator externus muscle 195,259-261,271-
287,298-301
obturator internus muscle 189-197,259-273,
277-279,283-291,298

obturator nerve 195,257-259,287
occipital bone 398-400
  internal occipital protuberance 398
occipital condyle 400-404
olecranon 27-29,103-113,117,131-137,143-147,
155-161
olecranon bursa 135-137
olecranon fossa 103,111-113,131,135-137,161
omohyoid muscle 3
opponens digiti minimi muscle 57-63,165-
167,173,375-377
opponens pollicis muscle 53-63,165-167,181-
183
ovary 189,259

P

palatopharyngeus muscle 401
palmar aponeurosis 55-61,65,177-180
palmar aponourosis 175
palmar carpal arch 169
palmar carpometacarpal ligament 175-177,
183
palmar collateral ligament 172-174,182
palmar digital artery 65-69,174-176
  thumb 65,69
palmar digital nerve 65-69,174
  thumb 61,65,69
palmar digital vein 174-177
palmar intercarpal ligament 49,53-59,175-
179
palmar interosseous muscle 59-65,173-175,
183
palmar ligament 65-67,176-178
palmar metacarpal artery 173,182
palmar radiocarpal ligament 47-51,165-167,
177-181
palmar radioulnar ligament 173
palmar ulnocarpal ligament 45-51,154,167,
173-175
palmaris brevis muscle 53-61,173
palmaris longus muscle 29-39,41-53,127-
129,161
parotid gland 404,411-415
patella 209-211,281-283,295-299,323-356
patellar anastomosis 325-331
patellar ligament 209-219,297-299,303,323-
333,353-356
pectineus muscle 193-197,255-259,271-285,
299-301

欧文索引 *475*

pectoralis major muscle 7-17,85-97,119-123
pectoralis minor muscle 7-17,89-97,121-123
pedicle(vertebral arch) 419,423,438-439
perforating artery 199,203-205,209,269,273,
291-299
perforating vein 199,203-209
peroneal retinaculum 241-245
peroneus brevis muscle 221-247,339-351,
359-371,383-385
peroneus longus muscle 219-251,305-313,
319-321,340-351,361-377,383-389
pes anserinus 307-315,331-337,340
deep 309-315,337
superficial 307-313,331-337,340
pes anserinus tendon 357
piriformis muscle 187-191,263-265,271-279,
286-288,298,441,451
pisiform 49-53,143,154,165-167,173
pisohamate ligament 53,165-167
pisometacarpal ligament 53-55
plantar aponeurosis 253,343,347,359-377,385-
393
plantar arch 249
plantar calcaneonavicular ligament 245,367-
369,387-391
plantar digital artery 249-251
plantar digital artery proper 381
plantar digital nerve 249-251
plantar digital vein 249-251
plantar digital vein proper 381
plantar interosseous muscle 248-253,379-
385
plantar metatarsal artery 249-251,377-379
plantar metatarsal nerve 249
plantar metatarsal vein 379
plantaris muscle 211-227,293,311-327,338,
342,349-355
popliteal artery 209-219,289-291,295,311-317,
325-327,346,353-356
popliteal fossa 335
popliteal vein 209-219,289-291,295,313-317,
325-327,346,353-356
popliteus muscle 209-219,307-333,338-357
posterior atlanto-occipital membrane 399
posterior circumflex humeral artery 13,73-
93,102-105,109-119
posterior circumflex humeral vein 13,73-93,
102-105,109-119
posterior cruciate ligament 211-217,297,309-
313,327-333,340-344,354-356

posterior cutaneous nerve of forearm 21-
29,33,39,47-49
posterior(dorsal) funiculus 100
posterior external vertebral venous plexus
417-419,423,443-447
posterior femoral cutaneous nerve 203
posterior intercostal artery 401-403,423-427,
437,441
posterior intercostal vein 401-403,425-427,
437,441
posterior interosseous artery 35-37,151,155,
158-161
posterior interosseous nerve 35-37
posterior interosseous vein 35-37,151,155,
158-161
posterior longitudinal ligament 313,329,399,
407-409,421,429,443-447
posterior meniscofemoral ligament 329
posterior sacro-iliac ligaments 449
posterior talofibular ligament 235-237,341-
343,361-363,385-389
posterior tibial artery 223-241,315,343,347,
355-361,393
posterior tibial nerve 347
posterior tibial recurrent artery 347
posterior tibial recurrent vein 347
posterior tibial vein 223-241,343,347,355-361
posterior tibiofibular ligament 231-235
pre-Achilles fat body 355,389
princeps pollicis artery 61
promontory(sacrum) 397,429-433,437,451
pronator quadratus muscle 41-43,146,156-
163,167-169,173-181
pronator teres muscle 27-37,97-105,123-129,
133-139,143-149,161-163
ulnar head 137-139
proper palmar digital artery 165-168,182,
377-379
proper palmar digital nerve 165-168,182,
379-381
proper palmar digital vein 379
proximal interphalangeal joint 253,383
(foot) 253,383
(hand) 168-178
proximal phalanx
foot 248-253,383,389-393
hand 65-69,165-182
proximal radioulnar joint 31,137
psoas(major)muscle 257-260,275,279,437-
438,443-451

476　欧文索引

pterygoid venous plexus　411
pubic symphysis　255,281-283
pubis　191-195,255-261,279-287
　inferior ramus　195,261,283-287
　superior ramus　191-193,281
pubofemoral ligament　195
pudendal nerve　263
pulmonary artery　421-427

Q

quadratus femoris muscle　195-197,263,267-
　275,289,293-301
quadratus lumborum muscle　439-447
quadratus plantae muscle　245-251,339-345,
　359-373,389-391
quadriceps femoris muscle　281-283,293-295,
　299,303,323-333,356
quadriceps tendon　281-283,293-295,299,303,
　323-333,356

R

radial artery　33-57,97,125,135,145-147,161-
　171,181-183
radial collateral artery　27-29
radial collateral ligament
　（elbow）　29,127-129,139-141,157-159
　（wrist）　171,181-183
radial collateral vein　27-29
radial nerve　15-39,43-55,71-75,91,101,105-
　107,113,121-127,131,135-139,159,163
radial recurrent artery　159
radial tuberosity　129,137,145-147,155-157
radial vein　33-57,135,145-147,161-163
radiate carpal ligament　167
radiate ligament of head of rib　425-427
radicular artery　447
radicular vein　447
radiocarpal joint　175,179
radioulnar joint　31,137,147
radius　31-47,97-99,109-113,127-131,137-141,
　144-151,158-163,167-171,175-183
　head　31,97-99,109-111,127-131,137-141,149-
　　159
　neck　137
　shaft　113,127-129,137-139,149-151,161-163
　styloid process　183
rectum　189-195,265,451
rectus abdominis muscle　187-195,269-279,

451
rectus capitis lateralis muscle　405,411
rectus capitis posterior major muscle
　401-403,409-415
rectus capitis posterior minor muscle　399-
　403,411-413
rectus femoris muscle　191-207,255-257,267-
　271,281,295-299,329-333
recurrent interosseous artery　31-33,155
recurrent interosseous vein　33,155
retromandibular vein　411-415
retropatellar cartilage　209-211
rhomboid major muscle　422-427
rhomboid minor muscle　419
rhomboid muscle　401,419,422-427
　major　422-427
　minor　419
rib　3-17,71-75,95-97,107,407-409,425-427,
　435,438-441
　body　407,427
　head　407,425-427,435,438
　neck　407-409,427
　tubercle　409,427
right atrium　423
rotatores muscles　425-427,441
rotatores thoracis muscle　427,441

S

sacral canal　429,449
sacral plexus　187,259-261,279,439,451
sacroiliac joint　261-265,439-441,449-451
sacroiliac ligament　263,439-441
sacrospinous ligament　451
sacrotuberous ligament　189-195,277-279,291
sacrum　187-189,260-265,291,397,429-441,449-
　451
　lateral mass　263-265,439,449-451
　promontory　397,429-433,437
sagittal ligament　67-69
saphenous nerve　201-209,231-233,257-259,
　285-289,301,313-317,337
sartorius muscle　189-219,255-257,267-291,
　298-301,311-337,342-346
scalenus anterior muscle　417-419
scalenus medius muscle　405-407,417-419
scalenus muscle　98-106
　anterior　417-419
　medius　405-407,417-419
　posterior　405-409,417

欧文索引 **477**

scalenus posterior muscle 405-409,417
scaphocapitate intercarpal joint 177-179
scaphoid 47-53,144-148,163-171,177-183
scapholunate interosseous ligament 169
scapula 9-15,71-81,93-95,121-123,427
  body 95
  neck 77,121
  spine 79-81,95
sciatic nerve 191-201,263-265,271-277,289-291,295,299
semimembranosus bursa 291
semimembranosus muscle 197-217,273,279, 289-291,295-301,309-317,325-337,346
semispinalis capitis muscle 398-403,411-417, 422
semispinalis cervicis muscle 401,407-409,417-419
semispinalis thoracis muscle 423,427
semitendinosus muscle 197-219,265,273,279, 289-291,295-301,311-317,337
serratus anterior muscle 3-17,71-75,95-106, 441
serratus posterior muscle 11
serratus posterior superior muscle 422
sesamoid bone 63,167-169,253,381,391
sigmoid colon 187,261-263
sigmoid sinus 406,409
small intestine 187-189,255-256,269-279
small saphenous vein 215-239,359,379
soleus muscle 219-231,293-297,315-327,342-357
spinal canal 263,407
spinal cord 407,411-419,429
spinal dura mater 407-409,443-447
spinal ganglion 401-409,415-417,423,427,431-433,443-447
spinal nerve 401-407,417-419,435,443,447
  dorsal branch 443,447
spinalis cervicis muscle 401-403,409,417-419, 424
spinalis thoracis muscle 425-427,441
spinous process 265,397-399,409,413,417,421, 427-429,439-443,447
splenius capitis muscle 401-403,406-419
splenius cervicis muscle 401,407-409,419, 422-424
spring ligament →plantar calcaneonavicular ligament
sternocleidomastoid muscle 405-419
sternohyoid muscle 421-425

sternum 421-423
styloglossus muscle 415
stylohyoid muscle 411
styloid process (ulna) 47,154,169-171
stylomastoid foramen 404
stylopharyngeus muscle 415
subacromial bursa 73,77,89
subarachnoid space 399,413-417
subclavian artery 98,405,425
subclavian vein 96-98
subclavius muscle 39,97-98,102
subcutaneous infrapatellar bursa 325-327
subcutaneous olecranon bursa 27-29
subcutaneous prepatellar bursa 325-333
subdeltoid bursa 87
suboccipital fatty tissue 399-403
suboccipital nerve 409
suboccipital venous plexus 409
subscapular artery 71-81,104
subscapular nerve 9,73,81
subscapular vein 71-81,104
subscapularis muscle 9,13-15,71-75,85-95, 100-107,119-123,427
subtalar joint 241,355-357,361-363,385-389
superficial circumflex iliac artery 269
superficial femoral artery →femoral artery
superficial femoral vein →femoral vein
superficial fibular nerve 221-231,345,349-351
superficial palmar arch 175-182
superficial pes anserinus 307-313,331-337, 340
superior articular process 401-407,417,423, 427,431-435,439-445
superior clunial nerves 263
superior collateral ulnar artery 27-29
superior collateral ulnar nerve 27
superior collateral ulnar vein 29
superior constrictor muscle of pharynx 415-419
superior costotransverse ligament 425
superior fibular retinaculum 239
superior gemellus muscle 273
superior glenohumeral ligament 89
superior gluteal artery 187-193,260,265,269, 273-279,439-441
superior gluteal nerve 193,265,273-277
superior gluteal vein 187-191,260,265,269, 273-279,441
superior lateral genicular artery 209,293,

305-311,321-325,354

superior lateral genicular vein 209,293,305-309,321-325,354

superior medial genicular artery 209,305-311,329-337

superior medial genicular vein 209,305-311,329-337

superior peroneal retinaculum 237

superior ulnar collateral artery 31

superior ulnar collateral vein 31

supinator muscle 31-35,97-99,109-113,127-131,137-141,145-161

suprapatellar bursa 303,323-335

suprapatellar fat pad 303

suprascapular artery 3,7-11,71-79,95,123

suprascapular nerve 9-11,71-79

suprascapular vein 3,7-11,71-79,95,123

supraspinatus muscle 3-5,57,71-95,98-123

supraspinous ligament 397-399,421,427-429,443-447

sural arteries and veins 315

sural nerve 223-239,359-365

T

talocalcaneal interosseous ligament 239,355-357,367,387-389

talocalcaneal joint→subtalar joint

talocrural joint 233-237,339,355-357,361-365,387-389

talofibular joint 339-341,363

talonavicular joint 239-241,357,389

talonavicular ligament 389-391

talus 235-243,339-341,353-357,361-369,385-393

　body 239-241

　head 239-243

　neck 239

　posterior process 241

tarsometatarsal joint 242,383,387

tectorial membrane 398,405

tensor fasciae latae muscle 187-197,255-257,281-283,293-298

teres major muscle 13-17,73-81,87-95,100-107,115-123

teres minor muscle 11-13,77-81,87-95,102-123

thecal sac 397,429,437-447

thoracic spinal cord 397,409,421,427

thoracic vertebra 397-403,407-409,421-423,431-437

　body 397,403,409

thoracoacromial artery 91-95

thoracodorsal artery 17,102-105

thoracodorsal nerve 17,71

thoracodorsal vein 102-105

thoracolumbar fascia 431-435,443-447

thyroid gland 417-424

tibia 217-235,285-289,297-299,305-315,325-357,361-365,385-393

　head 217-285-289,297,325-327,339,342-344,349-357

　medial condyle 299,305-315,331-337,340,347

　medial malleolus 233-235,339-341,363-365,393

　shaft 305-309,329,339-344,353-357

tibial nerve 203-243,291,295,315-317,325-329,347,353-359

tibial tuberosity 219,303,323-325,354

tibialis anterior muscle 219-245,305-309,319-321,339-342,349-357,367-375,391

tibialis posterior muscle 221-247,311-313,319-323,341-347,351-357,361-373,389-393

tibiofibular joint 311-313,319-321,344,349

　proximal 313,321

　superior 349

tibiofibular syndesmosis 233,385

tibiofibular trunk 221,353

trachea 421-422,427

　bifurcation 427

transverse humeral ligament 87-89

transverse ligament 307,325-333,399,411-413

　(atlas) 399,411-413

　(knee) 307,325-333

transverse patellar retinaculum 215

transverse process 405,419,425-427,435-439

transversus abdominis muscle 187-191,255-256,267,449-451

trapezium 53-55,165,169,183

　tubercle 183

trapezius muscle 3,71-81,93-95,98-106,115-123,398-403,411-419,423-427

　descending part 398-403

　transverse part 401-403

trapezoid 53-55,148,169-171,181-183

欧文索引 **479**

triangular fibrocartilage 47,144-146
triangular fibrocartilage complex(TFC) 169,
173
triceps brachii muscle 13-29,77-81,85-93,
101-121,129-157
　lateral head 13-21,25,77-81,101-113
　long head 13-21,77-81,89-93,105,109-121
　medial head 17-21,25,85-87,105-107,113-
　117
triquetrum 49-53,144-148,154-156,169-175
trochlear notch 135-137,143

U

ulna 31-45,99-101,115,129-131,139,143-150,
154-156,169-173
　coronoid process 129-131
　shaft 139,143-145,155
　styloid process 47,154,169-171
ulnar artery 23-25,33-61,97,119-121,125,135,
143-147,157-161,173,175
ulnar articular disk 171
ulnar collateral ligament(wrist joint) 47,146,
167-171
ulnar nerve 17-63,73-75,91,103,117-123,131-
135,143,154-159,165,173-181
ulnar recurrent artery 133
ulnar styloid process 47,154,169
ulnar vein 23-25,33-61,119-121,135,143-147,
156-161
uncinate process 405
ureter 187-193
urinary bladder 187-193,255-261,281-282
uterine tube 189
uterine venous plexus 191
uterus 187-191,255-263

V

vagina 193-195,259-263,285-287
vagus nerve(X) 411-415
vastus intermedius muscle 197-207,257-261,
267-269,281-287,293-299,321-323
vastus lateralis muscle 195-209,255-265,269,
281-295,303-313,319-323
vastus medialis muscle 197-207,255,259,267,
271-275,281-289,297-311,325-337
ventral root 413-419
vertebra prominens(C7) 397-401,405-409,
421
vertebral arch 265,409,417-419,431-433,439-
441,445-447
　pedicle 419,423,438-439
vertebral artery 400-407,411,419
vertebral body 397-409,415-423,429-437,
445-447,449
vertebral canal 397,409
vertebral endplate 399,421-423,435-437
vertebral vein 404,417

W

Wrisberg ligament →posterior meniscofemoral ligament
wrist joint 158-163,169,177

Z

zona orbicularis 261
zygapophyseal joint 401-407,417,423,427,
433-435,439-447

CT・MRI 画像解剖ポケットアトラス

③ 脊椎/四肢/関節　　　第4版　定価：本体 4,800 円＋税

2008 年 3 月 31 日発行　第 3 版第 1 刷
2018 年 3 月 30 日発行　第 4 版第 1 刷©
2022 年 3 月 30 日発行　第 4 版第 2 刷

著　者　トルステン B. メーラー
　　　　エミール レイフ

監訳者　町田　徹
　　　　まちだ　とおる

発行者　株式会社 メディカル・サイエンス・インターナショナル
　　　　代表取締役　金子　浩平
　　　　東京都文京区本郷 1-28-36
　　　　郵便番号 113-0033　電話 (03) 5804-6050

印刷：三報社印刷/表紙装丁：岩崎邦好デザイン事務所

ISBN 978-4-8157-0120-8　C 3047

本書の複製権・翻訳権・上映権・譲渡権・貸与権・公衆送信権(送信可能化権を含む)は(株)メディカル・サイエンス・インターナショナルが保有します．本書を無断で複製する行為(複写，スキャン，デジタルデータ化など)は，「私的使用のための複製」など著作権法上の限られた例外を除き禁じられています．大学，病院，診療所，企業などにおいて，業務上使用する目的(診療，研究活動を含む)で上記の行為を行うことは，その使用範囲が内部的であっても，私的使用には該当せず，違法です．また私的使用に該当する場合であっても，代行業者等の第三者に依頼して上記の行為を行うことは違法となります．

[JCOPY] 〈出版者著作権管理機構　委託出版物〉
本書の無断複製は著作権法上での例外を除き禁じられています．複製される場合は，そのつど事前に，出版者著作権管理機構（電話 03-5244-5088，FAX 03-5244-5089，info@jcopy.or.jp）の許諾を得てください．